Pharmacology

For Churchill Livingstone

Publisher: Timothy Horne
Project Editor: Barbara Simmons
Copy Editor: Jane Ward
Production Controllers: Debra Barrie, Nancy Arnott
Design Direction: Erik Bigland, Charles Simpson
Indexer: Laurence Errington

Churchill's Mastery of Medicine

Pharmacology

Peter Winstanley

MD MRCP DTM&H

Senior Lecturer in Clinical Pharmacology
University of Liverpool;
Honorary Consultant Physician
Royal Liverpool University Hospital

Tom Walley

MD FRCP(London) FRCPI

Professor of Clinical Pharmacology
University of Liverpool;
Honorary Consultant Physician
Royal Liverpool University Hospital

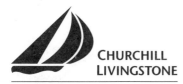

CHURCHILL
LIVINGSTONE

CHURCHILL LIVINGSTONE
NEW YORK EDINBURGH LONDON MADRID MELBOURNE
SAN FRANCISCO AND TOKYO 1996

CHURCHILL LIVINGSTONE
Medical Division of Pearson Professional Limited

Distributed in the United States of America by Churchill
Livingstone Inc., 650 Avenue of the Americas, New York,
N.Y. 10011, and by associated companies, branches and
representatives throughout the world.

First published 1996

ISBN 0 443 049483

British Library of Cataloguing in Publication Data
A catalogue record for this book is available from the British
Library.

Library of Congress Cataloging in Publication Data
A catalog record for this book is available from the Library of
Congress.

Medical knowledge is constantly changing. As information
becomes available, changes in treatment, procedures, equipment
and the use of drugs become necessary. The authors and
publisher have, as far as it is possible, taken care to ensure that
the information given in the text is accurate and up to date.
However, readers are strongly advised to ensure that the
information, especially with regard to drug usage, complies with
current legislation and standards of practice.

The
publisher's
policy is to use
**paper manufactured
from sustainable forests**

Produced by Longman Singapore Publishers (Pte) Ltd.
Printed in Singapore

Contents

Using this book

Philosophy of the book

What drugs are used for hypertension? How do they work? What adverse effects do they have, and who should *not* receive them? This book will help you with these, and similar, questions with the general aims of passing the examination *and* retaining an understanding of pharmacology for your future career.

Drugs have always been, and remain, one of the main ways of treating and preventing disease. Broadly, the discipline of *pharmacology* is concerned with how drugs work and how they reach their site of action, while *therapeutics* is concerned with their clinical use. Most doctors have expertise in therapeutics — they use it every day of practice. However, detailed expertise in pharmacology is not needed by all doctors, but most retain a degree of 'background knowledge', which renders their therapeutic use of drugs more rational.

Your aim should be to develop an understanding of the principles which govern the clinical use of drugs.

Layout of the book

This book is organised along clinical, rather than strictly pharmacological, lines to render it more accessible to medical students. Consequently the chapters focus on anatomical systems (e.g. the cardiovascular system) or the therapy of specific diseases (e.g. cancer chemotherapy) rather than on mechanisms of drug action. In each chapter we have tried to set out mechanisms and principles, rather than lists, and have tried to link together sections of the book where the same topic is dealt with from different angles.

The chapters are subdivided into sections, each dealing with a therapeutic area (e.g. the cardiovascular chapter includes sections on hypertension, angina and arrhythmias) and we have tried to construct these in a reasonably uniform way. Each section starts with a brief description of the clinical context: there would be little point learning about antiepileptic drugs, for example, if you did not understand the nature of epilepsy. Many diverse drugs may be relevant to the therapy used to treat the same condition: we have grouped similar drugs under the same class heading (e.g. the benzodiazepines). For each drug class we describe:

- mode of action: at the molecular, cellular, organ and whole-body levels where relevant
- examples and clinical pharmacokinetics: there are usually several drugs of each class in common use, we describe the commoner examples and contrast their pharmacokinetic properties
- therapeutic uses: a drug class can be used for several indications (e.g. although beta-blockers are described in the ischaemic heart disease section of Chapter 3, they are also used for hypertension, anxiety and migraine)

- adverse effects: are described in detail under subheadings and, because some subgroups of the population are at particular risk from certain drugs (e.g. beta-blockers precipitate asthma), these *contraindications* are listed
- interactions: patients often take more than one drug at a time: potential adverse interactions, and their clinical consequences, are described.

The final section of each chapter allows self-assessment; we have tried to set questions that require thought rather than recollection of facts. The questions are in the form of patient management problems (which require short answers), multiple choice and essays. The answer is given along with a detailed explanation in each case. Some aspects of a topic may be covered for the first time in this section of the book.

Approach to examinations

There is no correct way to revise for an exam and, by this stage in your career, you have already passed many, so your own system cannot be too bad. However, your performance may be improved by reading the brief notes below.

Before starting to prepare for the exam, you need to know:

- the scope of the syllabus in your medical school (these vary quite widely): consult the list of lectures/tutorials given, or the study guides presented at the start of the course
- the format of the examination (consult past papers if you can)
- how many examinations you will be sitting at once (your revision plan will need to divide time between subjects).

The *notes* you made during lectures, tutorials or group sessions are probably the ideal revision material; the subject was described by, or your reading was guided by, those who set the exam, and reading your notes should stimulate your memory. Large *textbooks of Clinical Pharmacology* are useful as a reference source during revision, as they were during the course, but you should not try to read them from cover to cover. Furthermore, it is probably unwise to buy more than one reference text; different books may cover the same topic in differing ways, causing confusion. Condensed 'crammers' which rely heavily on lists are probably best avoided: they encourage retention of facts rather than understanding and, on the whole, Pharmacology does not lend itself to lists. The present book covers most, but not all, of the topics likely to crop up in undergraduate examinations, and may be used to complement your own notes.

Tips on methods of examination

Multiple choice questions (MCQs)

For the most part, these test your recall of facts. Read the stem of the question with care, paying attention to words such as *only, rarely, usually, never* and *always*.

The most common forms of MCQs involve *either* choosing the most appropriate answer from a list (usually one out of five) *or* answering true/false to each part of the question.

Remember to check the marking system — many MCQ exams employ negative marking.

Short notes

The examiners will have decided on a marking system for each important fact. You should set out your knowledge in a concise manner — no marks will be gained for superfluous information.

Essays

There is a need to plan the structure of the essay which allows you to develop an argument or theme.

Subheadings often make an answer more easily accessible to the examiner.

Patient management problems

This type of question may be designed to test both recall of factual knowledge and its application to a clinical therapeutic problem. Formats vary, but a common form is an evolving case history, with information being presented sequentially and responses to specific questions (e.g. on choice of drug or anticipated adverse effects). As with *short notes* you should aim to be concise.

Viva

In many centres vivas are offered to candidates who have either distinguished themselves or who are in danger of failing. Interviews for the two types of candidate vary considerably.

In the 'distinction' setting, the examiner may try to discover what the candidate does *not* know and may also be looking for evidence of knowledge of the current literature. A small number of topics will usually be considered in depth.

In the pass/fail setting, the examiner will try to cover many topics, often quite superficially. She/he will try to establish whether the candidate did badly in the written exam because of ignorance in just a couple of areas, or whether ignorance is wide ranging.

Remember that you may be asked to choose the initial topic of conversation in either distinction or pass/fail vivas ('what would you like to talk about?') so be prepared.

Remember that the examiners will have your written paper in front of them: if you have done particularly badly in one topic, they may well take this up in the viva. This is not an attempt to be unpleasant, but a chance for you to redeem yourself somewhat, so be prepared for this.

Basic principles

1.1 Drugs

There is no succinct definition of a drug, but it can be taken to mean any molecule used to alter body functions thereby preventing or treating disease. Drugs vary widely in size, shape and physicochemical properties. However, most drugs dissolve readily in water and are lipid-soluble when unionised (see below). These common features allow drugs to cross membranes, an essential characteristic because they are usually delivered into a site distant from their 'target' tissue (e.g. they may be given into the gut, but act in the brain) and must be transported across several membranes to reach it.

Though a drug generally produces the same *type* of effect in different people (e.g. anticoagulation), there can be wide variation in the *degree* of that effect: for example, a 10 mg daily maintenance dose of warfarin may be needed for the adequate anticoagulation of a minority of patients, though it would cause life-threatening haemorrhage in the majority. Such *interindividual* variation in drug response has obvious clinical importance and is the main theme of this chapter; it may result from the processes by which a drug travels from its point of delivery to its site of action – pharmacokinetics – or from those processes by which drugs alter body function – pharmacodynamics.

1.2 Pharmacokinetics

Clinical response to a drug can sometimes be directly measured with accuracy, like the effect of insulin on blood sugar or warfarin on clotting, and this measurement alone can be enough to predict how *much* drug is needed and how *often*. More usually, such direct measurements are impossible or impractical and an indirect approach becomes necessary. In in vitro systems, it is easy to demonstrate that the magnitude of drug response is proportional to concentration, and the same relationship can often be assumed to apply in clinical practice. Therefore, measurement of drug concentration, and its rates of change, can be used to predict the magnitude and duration of action of a drug.

When a systemically acting drug is given by any route (other than intravenous [i.v.]), three processes govern its concentration:

- absorption
- distribution to the tissues, including to specialised sites like the central nervous system (CNS)
- elimination, irreversible removal from the body.

Absorption

Most drugs act systemically and need to be absorbed, but topical applications do not require absorption for activity, though adverse effects may result from any which is absorbed. Topical drugs include skin and eye preparations, inhaled drugs, vaginal pessaries, some rectal preparations and local anaesthetics. Systemic drugs may be administered into the gut, mouth, rectum, skin or muscle and must, therefore, cross at least one cell: most do so by passive diffusion (i.e. movement from areas of high concentration to those of lower concentration) but a minority require carrier-mediated transport (e.g. levodopa and fluorouracil).

Factors affecting rate and degree of absorption

Certain factors affect absorption in all sites; their relative importance will vary from site to site (e.g. absorption from the gut or from intramuscular injection):

- lipid solubility
- surface area
- time
- blood flow.

Lipid solubility
The degree of lipid solubility of a drug is largely determined by physicochemical factors such as molecular weight and structure, but that of an individual drug will vary with its degree of ionisation: only *unionised* drug is lipid soluble. Most drugs are weak acids or bases, and their degree of ionisation is determined by the surrounding pH and their pK_a (the pK_a is the pH at which the drug is 50% ionised). The Henderson–Hasselbach equation allows the unionised fraction to be calculated:

for acids: $pH = pK_a + \log$ (ionised conc./unionised conc.)

for bases: $pH = pK_a + \log$ (unionised conc./ionised conc.).

So for aspirin, which is an acid with a pK_a of 3.5, if the pH is 2.5 then the ratio of ionised:unionised is 0.1 (antilog of −1) i.e. 90% of the drug is unionised and it crosses membranes readily. If the pH were 5.5 then the same ratio is 100 (antilog of 2) i.e. 1% of the drug is unionised and it crosses membranes poorly.

Surface area
The greater the surface area available, the faster absorption takes place. In the case of the gut, the surface area of the small bowel exceeds that of the stomach to such a degree that even acidic drugs will usually be more extensively absorbed from this site. So if given orally, the rate of drug absorption will be influenced by the rate of gastric emptying. Small bowel surface area can be reduced by diseases such a gluten-sensitive enteropathy and inflammatory bowel disease.

Time
The drug must spend an adequate time at the absorp-

tion site. Short transit time (e.g. during gastroenteritis) may reduce the degree of absorption.

Blood flow

Gastrointestinal blood flow is usually high, though it may be compromised in some disease states. By comparison, muscle blood flow is very variable: in severe hypotension, flow rate may be low and intramuscular (i.m.) drugs may be absorbed slowly.

Bioavailability

Bioavailability refers to the fraction of the dose which proceeds *unaltered* from the site of administration to the systemic circulation. When given i.v., 100% of the dose enters the systemic circulation, and bioavailability is 1.0. While incomplete absorption often accounts for low bioavailability, there are other possible explanations (Fig. 1):

- it may be broken down by acid conditions, e.g. benzylpenicillin
- it may be metabolised by enzymes in the gut wall or liver before reaching the systemic venous blood (e.g. glyceryl trinitrate). This is termed *first pass* effect.

Distribution

Plasma protein binding

Most drugs travel in the plasma partly in solution in the plasma water and partly bound to plasma proteins – the ratio of one to the other varies between drugs. Binding is reversible and, because the rates of association with and dissociation from the proteins are so fast, the bound and unbound drug fractions are always in a state of dynamic equilibrium. Only the *unbound* drug fraction is available to cross membranes and produce an effect.

Generally, acidic drugs bind to albumin, the most abundant plasma protein, while bases bind more

avidly to α_1-acid glycoprotein. Plasma protein binding becomes clinically important when, because of a disease state (see Ch. 20), plasma protein concentrations fall (e.g. albumin concentrations in liver cirrhosis) or rise (e.g. α_1-acid glycoprotein, which is an acute phase reactant, in acute infection): total drug concentration in the plasma may be unchanged from that recorded in healthy subjects, but the drug is more/less potent because a greater/lower fraction is unbound (Fig. 2). Thus, in Figure 2, the total drug concentration in parts A and B of the diagram are the same, but changes in plasma protein concentration influence the unbound fraction of the drug.

Examples of drugs extensively bound to proteins (90% or more)

- warfarin
- phenylbutazone
- diazepam.

Examples of drugs with less extensive protein binding

- digoxin
- gentamicin
- theophylline.

Tissue distribution

After absorption, most drugs are distributed in the blood to the body tissues where they have their effects,

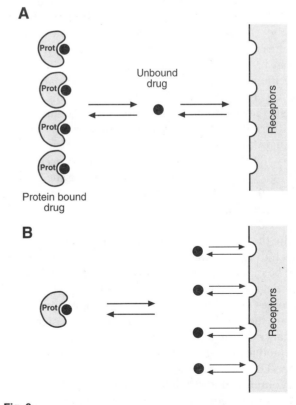

A

Unbound drug

Protein bound drug

Receptors

B

Prot

Receptors

Fig. 2
Variation in plasma protein concentration. **A.** High levels of plasma proteins; **B.** reduced levels of plasma proteins.

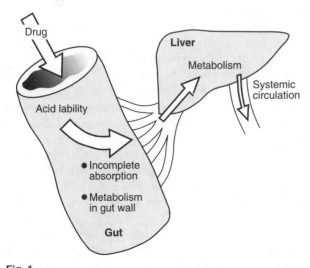

Drug

Liver

Metabolism

Systemic circulation

Acid lability

- Incomplete absorption
- Metabolism in gut wall

Gut

Fig. 1
Causes of incomplete bioavailability.

both therapeutic and toxic. The degree to which a given drug is likely to accumulate in a tissue can be predicted (without accuracy) from knowledge of its lipophilicity and the blood flow of the tissue.

A highly lipophilic drug, largely unionised at pH 7.4, crosses membranes readily even in the presence of tight junctions between endothelial cells, as occurs in the CNS. The principal determinant of tissue distribution of such a drug will, therefore, be organ blood flow. For example, the anaesthetic induction agent thiopentone is highly lipophilic, and after injecting it accumulates to a greater degree in brain than in muscle because of the much higher blood flow to the former (and also its greater lipid content).

In contrast, a hydrophilic drug, largely ionised at physiological pH, crosses membranes poorly. The principal determinant of tissue distribution will, therefore, be the degree of 'leakiness' of the capillary endothelium. For example, the antibiotic gentamicin is a polar compound that crosses membranes poorly, and after injection it accumulates to a greater degree in muscle than in brain because of the leaky nature of muscle capillaries.

Apparent volume of distribution

Once in the tissue, the drug may bind to macromolecules: some of which mediate the drug's effects (including receptors, enzymes and structural proteins – see below) and others to which the drug binds without producing pharmacological effects – so-called 'non-specific' binding. Some drugs, like aspirin, mainly stay in the circulation and undergo little tissue binding whereas others, like the tricyclic antidepressants, are so extensively bound in the tissues (mostly in a non-specific manner) that plasma concentrations are small. Figure 3 shows the effect of tissue binding on the plasma levels of the drug and on its apparent volume of distribution. The apparent volume of distribution (VD) is calculated from the amount of drug in the body, [Drug]$_{body}$ divided by the plasma concentration [Drug]$_{plasma}$. Where drugs have minimal tissue binding (Fig. 3a) the VD is close to the plasma volume. Where tissue binding is high, the apparent VD is high, 100 l in Figure 3b.

In the real world, we never know precisely how much drug is in the tissues of a living subject – it cannot be measured – but VD gives an *indirect* measure of the degree of tissue distribution. Knowing this value becomes clinically useful in the setting of drug overdose: the likely success of measures designed to enhance drug elimination from the plasma (e.g. haemodialysis) are likely to be useful with drugs with low VDs but much less useful if these are high.

Volumes of distribution values range from about 0.1 l/kg (e.g. for salicylate or warfarin), through 1–10 l/kg (e.g. lignocaine, digoxin or propranolol) to 20–200 l/kg (e.g. tricyclics and chloroquine).

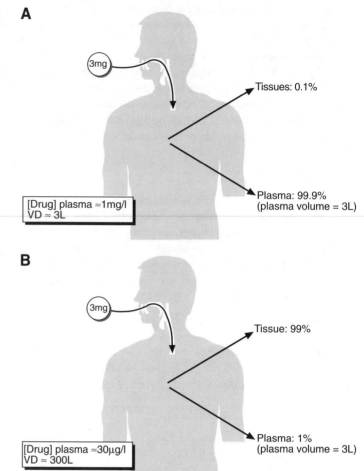

A

3mg

Tissues: 0.1%

Plasma: 99.9%
(plasma volume = 3L)

[Drug] plasma ≈1mg/l
VD ≈ 3L

B

3mg

Tissue: 99%

Plasma: 1%
(plasma volume = 3L)

[Drug] plasma ≈30µg/l
VD ≈ 300L

Fig. 3
Apparent volume of distribution. **A.** A drug that is minimally tissue bound would have 0.1% in the tissues, 99.9% left in the plasma, for example. A 3 mg dose would leave 2.997 mg in the plasma. In a 70 kg adult with a plasma volume of 3 litres, the plasma concentration would be 0.999 mg/l. VD = [Drug] body ÷ [Drug] plasma = 3 ÷ 0.999 = 3.0031. This is roughly equal to the plasma volume. **B.** An extremely tissue-bound drug might have 99% in the tissues and a 3 mg dose will give a plasma concentration of 30 µg/l and VD of 100 litres.

Biotransformation

Living systems take up many non-nutrient molecules, like drugs, from their environment and have needed to evolve mechanisms to eliminate them. Foremost among these is biotransformation or drug metabolism. Broadly, this process involves the transformation of the drug into a polar, water-soluble compound that can more easily be eliminated in the urine or bile. Metabolites usually lack pharmacological or toxic activity (but there are important exceptions, dealt with below). Of the various pharmacokinetic processes, biotransformation is probably most prone to interindividual variation.

Most biotransformation takes place in the liver, though many compounds are metabolised in other tissues, for example oral contraceptive steroids in the gut wall and succinylcholine in the plasma. There are a number of factors that affect biotransformation efficiency. The importance of each varies from drug to drug and for each drug it will also vary with the state of the patient, e.g. other diseases or drugs.

Genetic factors (genetic polymorphism). Genetically determined differences in the levels of certain enzymes have profound effects on the levels of certain drugs in the body. For example, several drugs are eliminated by acetylation, e.g. the anti-TB drug isoniazid (Ch. 13), the antiarrhythmic procainamide (Ch. 3) and the antihypertensive hydralazine (Ch. 3). Genetically slow acetylators comprise a group at risk of toxicity from these drugs. Other genetically determined variations include poor metabolisers of the muscle-relaxant succinylcholine (Ch. 8) and poor oxidisers of tricyclics or neuroleptics (Ch. 6).

Disease-induced factors. Diseases affecting the liver are particularly important, for example metabolism of opioids is slower in patients with liver disease (see Ch. 20).

Drug-induced factors. Certain drugs may act as enzyme inhibitors or inducers (see later in this chapter) affecting their own metabolism or that of other drugs.

Phases of biotransformation

Most drug-metabolising enzymes are located in the membranes of the endoplasmic reticulum, in the cytosol or in mitochondria. The chemical processes involved are numerous and are broadly classified into *phase I* and *phase II* reactions, which (confusingly) does not mean that phase I necessarily precedes or is followed by phase II.

Some drugs are excreted unchanged (e.g. gentamicin), some can undergo phase I followed by phase II (e.g. diazepam), others undergo phase I only (e.g. theophylline) or phase II only (e.g. morphine), while some undergo a phase II reaction followed by phase I (e.g. isoniazid).

Phase I

Phase I processes include oxidation, reduction and hydrolysis. Of these, oxidation reactions are most commonly encountered and are often catalysed by one of the family of cytochrome P450 enzymes. Phase I usually results in the introduction or exposure of a polar group in the molecule, an increase in water solubility and abolition of pharmacological activity. However, this is not invariable: the phase I products of some drugs have pharmacological activity while the parent compound does not (the so-called *prodrugs*, e.g. enalapril, see Ch. 31) while in other cases the phase I products are highly toxic, for example in paracetamol poisoning (see Ch. 7).

Phase II

Phase II processes (often termed conjugation) involve the attachment to the drug of an endogenous substance, such as glucuronate, sulphate or acetyl groups. The resulting conjugate is almost invariably polar, water soluble and without pharmacological activity. One exception to this is the glucuronide metabolite of morphine, which retains analgesic effects.

Induction and inhibition of cytochrome P450s

Some drugs can increase the rate of synthesis of cytochrome P450s and the resulting enzyme induction can enhance the clearance of other drugs. Usually such induction requires exposure to the inducing agent for some time before effects are seen. Examples of inducing agents are:

- rifampicin
- carbamazepine
- phenobarbitone
- phenytoin.

Other drugs can inhibit cytochrome P450s by a variety of processes; these effects are usually seen rapidly after drug exposure. Examples of enzyme-inhibiting agents are:

- cimetidine
- erythromycin
- ciprofloxacin
- isoniazid.

Concentration-dependent biotransformation

Most drugs are metabolised by concentration-independent mechanisms: in other words the enzyme is not saturated by the drug within the therapeutic range. Under these circumstances, the proportion of drug metabolised in a set time (and, therefore, its half-life, see below) is constant. However, some drugs can saturate a rate-limiting enzyme within the therapeutic range. Under these circumstances (sometimes called zero order processes) the proportion of drug metabolised in a set time diminishes as its concentration rises. A good clinical example of this is the antiepileptic drug phenytoin (Ch. 6) where small increases in the dose result in a disproportionate rise in drug concentration, giving serious adverse effects.

Excretion

Some drugs (e.g. aminoglycosides, atenolol, chlorpropamide and digoxin) are mainly excreted by the kidney without prior metabolism. Most drug metabolites are inactive and their rate of renal excretion is usually without clinical importance; however, if metabolites retain pharmacological activity (like the principal metabolite of acebutolol), drug action my be terminated by excretion not biotransformation. This is of most importance in the setting of renal disease, dealt with in Chapter 20.

Mechanisms of renal excretion

Glomerular filtration. Renal blood flow is about 1.5 l/min, and about 10% of this, by volume, appears as glomerular filtrate. Only unbound drug may be filtered since protein molecules are too large.

Tubular secretion. Cells of the proximal convoluted tubule can actively secrete some compounds, mostly relatively strong acids and bases, into the lumen of the nephron (e.g. penicillin and urate). Under these circumstances and assuming that no reabsorption occurs, the rate of excretion of a drug exceeds its rate of filtration.

Tubular reabsorption. Active reabsorption has evolved to help conserve nutrients including glucose, amino acids and vitamins. Certain drugs too may be extensively reabsorbed: such compounds tend to be lipid soluble and unionised at urine pH (see the Henderson–Hasselbach equation, above). This of most importance in the setting of drug poisoning, when methods are employed to increase renal clearance, for example by increasing urine pH in salicylate or phenobarbitone poisoning.

Other routes of excretion

Biliary. Parent drugs and metabolites with molecular weights greater than 350 may be actively excreted into the bile; examples include: oestradiol, ampicillin and rifampicin. This process may be followed by loss of the drug in the faeces. However, drug conjugates may be hydrolysed by gut bacteria, releasing the parent drug which may be reabsorbed. The resulting *enterohepatic circulation* may have important clinical consequences, as it does for oral contraceptive steroids (see Ch. 12).

Minor routes. Drugs may be excreted in saliva, sweat, tears and expired air, but none of these is a major route. Lactating mothers excrete some drugs in breast milk, with potentially important consequences for the breast-fed infant.

Pharmacokinetic parameters

Drug concentrations change after dosing under the influence of the processes described in Figure 4. Pharmacokinetics allows a number of predictions to be made that have clear clinical implications on dosage regimens:

- magnitude and duration of drug effects
- effect of disease states on drug effects
- degree of interindividual variation in drug disposition
- effect of one drug upon the disposition of another.

To make useful predictions, drug disposition must be 'reduced' to numerical parameters, such as half-life, clearance and VD.

Half-life

Of the various parameters that can be calculated, the half-life is the easiest to envisage and means 'the time

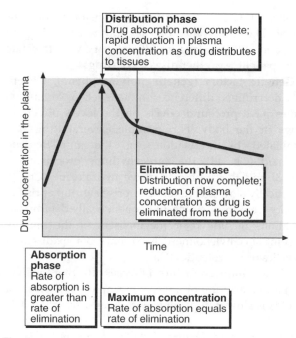

Fig. 4
Drug concentrations after an oral dose.

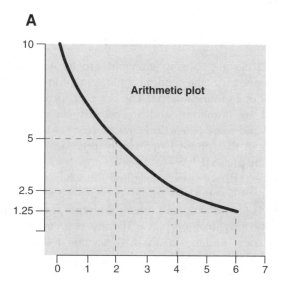

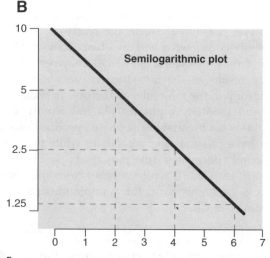

Fig. 5
The half-life of a drug. **A.** Arithmetic plot. **B.** Semilogarithmic plot.

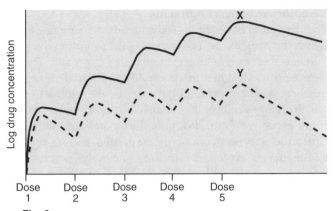

Fig. 6
Two drugs given at the same interval. The half-life of drug X is half that of drug Y, and drug X therefore accumulates to a greater degree.

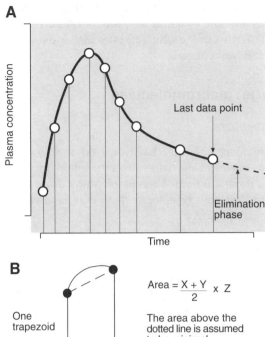

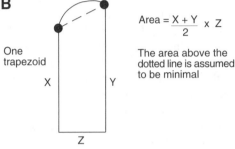

Fig. 7
Calculation of AUC from summation of trapezoids. **A.** Data from multiple oral doses. **B.** One trapezoid.

taken for concentration to fall to half its original value'; the unit of measurement is hours. Drug concentration data are usually plotted against time, as illustrated in Figure 5 for an i.v. bolus injection. When concentration data are plotted arithmetically against time (Fig. 5a) an exponential curve results; the data are often easier to handle if the vertical scale is logarithmic (Fig. 5b). Half-time varies enormously between drugs, and if the drug is to be given over a long term, the half-life is the main influence on dose frequency. In Figure 6, two drugs are being given at the same interval even though half-time of drug X is half that of drug Y. Because some drug always remains in the body from the previous dose, accumulation occurs until the amount lost equals the dose given: this is called *steady state*; in Figure 6 you can see that, because drug X is more slowly eliminated than drug Y, drug X accumulates to a greater degree. A drug achieves 50% of its steady-state concentration after one half-life, 75% after two half-lives, 88% after three, 94% after four and 97% after five half-lives.

Area under the curve (AUC)

AUC is used in the calculation of VD, clearance and bioavailability. In Figure 7, which represents data obtained after an oral dose, AUC can be calculated from the time of dosing to the last data point by summation of trapezoids. Extrapolation of the elimination phase (the dotted line in Fig. 6a) allows calculation of the AUC to infinity; the unit of measurement is in the form mg/h per l.

Clearance (C)

For the majority of drugs the rate of elimination E is directly proportional to the drug concentration c. In other words: $E = kc$, where k is a constant. This constant is termed clearance, and can be envisaged as the *volume* of plasma which is cleared completely of the drug per

unit time; the unit of measurement is, therefore, of the form l/h. Most drugs are partly eliminated by hepatic metabolism and partly by renal excretion of unchanged drug. Separate hepatic and renal clearance values can be measured in experimental settings; their sum is equal to total clearance, unless there is another route of elimination (e.g. biliary excretion or loss in breast milk).

Volume of distribution (VD)

The basic concept of VD has been dealt with above. The units of measurement are those of volume, ml or l.

1.3 Pharmacodynamics

Most drugs exert their effects on the body by interacting with macromolecule 'targets' which are usually on the surface of or within cells.

There are important exceptions to this:

- some drugs act by exerting physical effects, for example the osmotic diuretic mannitol
- some drugs interact directly with ions or other drugs, for example protamine interacts with and is

used to reverse the effects of the anticoagulant heparin and chelating agents (Ch. 17), such as desferrioxamine which chelates iron, are used to bind heavy metals.

Target macromolecules

Receptors

Regulatory molecules have evolved to allow endogenous chemical signals to affect the internal function of cells; these are termed receptors. Many drugs work by interacting with receptors, which may be divided into four groups (Fig. 8).

Intracellular receptors

Some receptors are situated in the cytoplasm, for example those for glucocorticoids, while others are in the nucleus (e.g. those for thyroid hormone). Clearly, in these cases, the ligand must be lipid soluble in order to cross the cell membrane. Once in the cell, the drug can then interact with an intracellular receptor. Where the ligand–receptor complex influences DNA transcription, the resultant mRNA encodes for the synthesis of a new polypeptide which alters cell function. Not surprisingly, such complicated processes entail a delay of up to several hours before drug effects are seen.

Transmembrane enzymes

Here, the receptor is a protein that crosses the cell membrane and has a binding site at the extracellular end and an enzyme moiety at the intracellular end (which is usually a part of the same protein). When the specific hormone binds to the receptor, the enzyme assumes its 'active' configuration and catalyses a reaction. The best characterised reaction is the phosphorylation of protein tyrosine residues by the enzyme tyrosine kinase which is activated by insulin.

Receptors acting via G-proteins

The receptor is again a transmembrane protein to which the drug binds. This activates the receptor which interacts with a signalling protein called G-protein. The G-protein itself, which may amplify the initial signal, interacts with an intracellular enzyme, the product of which changes cell function. Such *second messengers* include cyclic AMP, inositol polyphosphates, and cyclic GMP; the enzymes commonly associated with G-protein-mediated reactions include adenylyl cyclase, guanylyl cyclase and phospholipase C. Endogenous compounds that work in this way include some sympathomimetics and opioids.

Ion channels

The lipid bilayer that envelopes cells is bridged by protein and glycoprotein molecules which, under certain circumstances, allow the passive diffusion of specific ions (e.g. sodium, potassium and calcium). Such channels act as receptors for neurotransmitters such as acetyl choline and gamma-aminobutyric acid. Diffusion of the ion along a concentration gradient changes the transmembrane potential which elicits further intracellular responses. This mechanism of drug action allows for very rapid responses.

Other target molecules

Enzymes

Lipid-soluble drugs often alter cell function by impairing enzyme activity. The drug may resemble the enzyme's natural substrate, with which it may compete for binding. Alternately the drug may bind irreversibly to the active site of the enzyme. Examples of enzymes which may be inhibited by drugs are numerous and include dihydrofolate reductase (methotrexate), xanthine oxidase (allopurinol) and monoamine oxidase (selegiline).

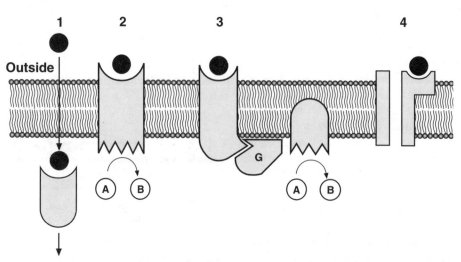

Fig. 8
Drug receptors. **1.** Membrane solubility allows lipid-soluble drugs to cross the cell membrane and bind to intracellular receptors. **2.** Transmembrane proteins bind the drug at the extracellular side of the cell membrane and binding activates an intracellular enzyme site. **3.** The transmembrane protein is linked to an enzyme via a G-protein. **4.** The receptor is a transmembrane ion channel.

Structural proteins

The best example of a drug targeting structural proteins is the binding of colchicine to tubulin (Ch. 9). Drug binding inhibits tubulin polymerisation and, therefore, interferes with the migration and mitosis of cells of the immune system.

Transport mechanisms

Living cells maintain internal concentrations of ions like Na^+, K^+, Cl^- and Ca^{2+} that differ from external concentrations. Therefore, the passive entry of ions via specific channels must be opposed by active 'pumping' in the reverse direction to maintain gradients. Such pumps are usually enzyme systems that consume energy in the form of ATP. Examples include NA^+/K^+-ATPase (which is inhibited by digoxin) and H^+/K^+-ATPase (which is inhibited by omeprazole).

Relationship between dose and response

Agonists

Agonists are compounds that bind to receptors and produce a response. In in vitro systems, the relationship between concentration and response resembles those in Figure 9. The maximum drug effect is often termed E_{max} and the concentration of drug required for half the maximum effect is termed EC_{50}.

Agonists can be subdivided into *full* agonists (Fig. 10, compound A) which induce a maximal response when all receptors are occupied, and *partial* agonists, which produce a sub-maximal response even when all receptors are occupied (Fig. 9, compound B). Compound A in Figure 9 has greater *efficacy* than compound B.

The term *potency* refers to the relative concentration (or dose) of a drug needed to produce a given response. In Figure 9, drugs A and B are equipotent even though A is more efficacious; drug C has greater potency than either A or B.

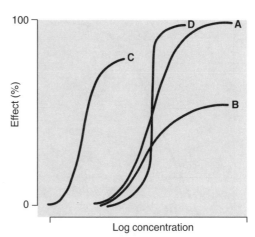

Fig. 10
Full and partial agonists and the concepts of efficacy and potency. Drug A is a full agonist while drug B is a partial agonist. Drugs A and B are equipotent even though drug A is more efficacious, while drug C has greater potency than either A or B. Drug D has similar potency to drug A and is equally efficacious, but has a steeper dose-response curve.

The *shape* of the curve also has clinical significance: drugs A and D have similar E_{max} and EC_{50} values, but drug D has a much steeper curve; this may have clinically important consequences if undesirable effects (like coma) are seen at the higher concentrations.

Antagonists

Antagonists bind to receptors *without* producing a response and by occupying the receptors they prevent access by agonists.

Competitive antagonists. A competitive antagonist (for example, beta-blockers; Ch. 3) form bonds with receptor molecules that are rapidly reversible, just like those of the agonist. As the antagonist concentration rises, progressively more receptors become occupied; however, the effects of a competitive antagonist may be abolished by increasing the agonist concentration (Fig. 11).

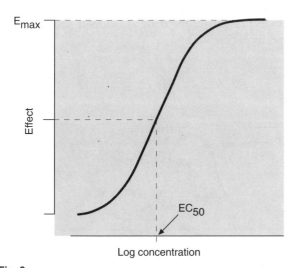

Fig. 9
Dose-response curves.

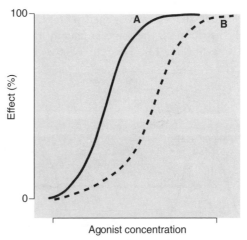

Fig. 11
Competitive antagonist. Curve A is the agonist effect in the absence of antagonist. Curve B is its effect in the presence of a fixed concentration of antagonist. The antagonist effect is abolished at high concentrations of agonist.

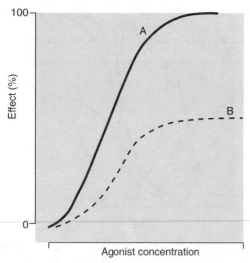

Fig. 12
Non-competitive antagonist. Curve A is the agonist effect in the absence of agonist. Curve B is its effect in the presence of a fixed concentration of antagonist. The antagonist effect cannot be overcome entirely, in contrast to the competitive antagonist (Fig. 11).

Non-competitive antagonists. Antagonists that are non-competitive (e.g. omeprazole) form bonds with the receptor, usually at sites other than the 'natural' agonist-binding site, which are near-irreversible; in some cases, they may be covalent (Fig. 12). When covalent bonding occurs, the inhibition of effect cannot be overcome entirely no matter how high the agonist concentration is raised (Fig. 12). The duration of action of such antagonists is determined by the rate of receptor turnover.

Therapeutic window

Clinicians use drugs to achieve a particular result, which is termed 'therapeutic'. If the dose of any drug is increased sufficiently, unwanted or toxic effects invariably develop. In a given population, the dose of drug required to produce a desired effect varies, usually yielding a bell-shaped curve when plotted, a so-called 'normal' distribution; the same is usually true for undesired effects (Fig. 13). The 'gap' between the dose needed to produce the desired effect in 50% of the population and that needed for the undesired effect is termed the therapeutic window. Drugs with broad therapeutic windows (like penicillins, β_2-agonists and thiazide diuretics) are generally safe and easy to use. Those with narrow therapeutic windows (like digoxin, theophyllines, lithium and phenytoin) can be difficult to use unless plasma concentrations are measured frequently: this is called *therapeutic drug monitoring.*

Inter-individual variation in drug response

There are two main pharmacodynamic reasons for the variation between individuals in their response to drugs.

Variation in concentration of endogenous ligands

The concentration of endogenous regulatory mediators, like catecholamines, can vary between individuals and within the same person. Predictably therefore, specific antagonists or agonists administered against this varying background produce variable responses.

Variation in receptor numbers

Continued stimulation/inhibition of living systems tends to induce compensatory processes, and the area of receptor/ligand interactions is no exception. Thus individuals continually exposed to an agonist/antagonist predictably require larger doses to achieve a given effect than would a naive subject. For example, people continually exposed to gamma-aminobutyric acid agonists (like benzodiazepine sedatives) need bigger doses to achieve an effect. This *tolerance* is thought to result from a decrease in receptor numbers, or *down-regulation*. The opposite may also occur: in patients on long-term beta-blocker therapy, it is thought that catecholamine receptor numbers are increased, *up-regulation*; this explains the tendency to a marked rise in blood pressure if the drug is stopped suddenly (rebound hypertension).

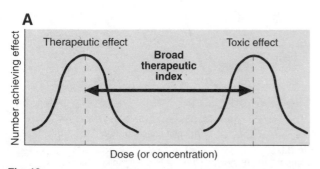
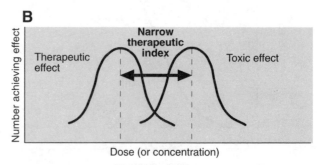

Fig. 13
Therapeutic window. **A.** A broad therapeutic index, where there is a wide gap between the desired effect and toxic effects. **B.** Narrow therapeutic index.

Self-assessment: questions

Multiple choice questions

1. Regarding drug receptors:
   a. A drug usually binds to only one receptor type
   b. Cellular responses to receptors that are ion channels are usually fast
   c. Cellular responses to receptors that work by modifying transcription of the genome are usually slow
   d. G-proteins amplify the effect of receptor stimulation
   e. Receptors are continually being synthesised and destroyed by the cell

2. Antagonists:
   a. Do not themselves bind to receptors, but interfere with the binding of agonists
   b. Bind to receptors but do not stimulate them
   c. May bind covalently to receptors
   d. Usually bind to receptors for very short periods (fractions of a second)
   e. If competitive, can be overcome by increasing the agonist concentration

3. The following statements can be made regarding pharmacodynamic concepts:
   a. All drugs act by binding to cell macromolecules
   b. Drug A is said to be more potent than drug B if drug A's maximal effect is greater than that of drug B
   c. A partial agonist is a drug which binds to a receptor without stimulating it
   d. The expression 'therapeutic index' refers to the difference between the concentration of a drug required to produce its effects and that required to produce toxicity
   e. Drug A is said to be more efficacious than drug B if drug A produces its maximum effect at a lower concentration than drug B

4. The following statements that can be made regarding pharmacokinetic concepts are correct:
   a. Only the unbound (free) drug fraction has pharmacological effects
   b. All drug metabolism takes place in the liver
   c. All drugs must first be metabolised before they can be excreted
   d. Only the unionised drug fraction may cross intact cell membranes
   e. Drug metabolites invariably lack pharmacological effects

Short note questions

1. A new drug is being developed and its manufacturers want to know its oral bioavailability.
   a. What clinical reasons are there for determining this pharmacokinetic parameter?
   b. Should bioavailability be tested with only fasted subjects? If your answer is no, explain why.
   c. How would you go about measuring bioavailability in a group of 12 healthy subjects?

2. An antihypertensive drug is given to 12 volunteers; the concentration of the drug is measured in the plasma, and its effects on blood pressure are recorded. As seen in Figure 14 the drug had a very short half-life (about 30 minutes) and was detectable for only 2 hours. However, as can also be seen in Figure 14 the effect on diastolic blood pressure was maximal 30 minutes after dosing, and returned to predose values after 12 hours.
   Give two possible explanations for these findings.

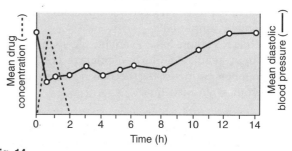

Fig. 14
Plasma concentration of the antihypertensive drug and changes in blood pressure.

3. Consider the following model of drug disposition: water is flowing into a washbasin at a rate of X ml/min, there is a plug, but it has a 5 mm diameter hole in it.
   a. Just after the tap is switched on, is the rate of flow through the hole equal to, greater than or less than that from the tap?
   b. If the tap is left running at X ml/min, what will eventually happen to the level of water in the basin?
   c. If the tap is left running at X ml/min but the diameter of the hole is halved, what will happen to the level of water in the basin?
   d. If the rate of flow is now gradually reduced, what will happen to the level of water?
   e. In this model, is clearance best represented by the rate of flow through the drain, or the diameter of the hole?

4. A new drug is found to be eliminated entirely by renal excretion, with no prior metabolism. Its renal clearance (found from plasma and urine concentration data) in an experiment on six healthy subjects is found to be about 200 ml/min; the mean glomerular filtration rate of the six volunteers is about 125 ml/min. What do these data tell you about the mode of excretion of the drug?

Self-assessment: answers

Multiple choice answers

1. a. **False.** We often classify a drug by the type of receptor relevant to its pharmacological effect, but drugs probably bind to far more cell macro-molecules than documented: some of these interactions produce adverse effects, but many produce no obvious effect.
   b. **True.** The influx of ions induced by receptor activation rapidly changes conditions within the cell.
   c. **True.** Such a mechanism explains the slow response to corticosteroids.
   d. **True.** Once activated, many G-proteins remain active for longer than the receptor is occupied by the drug; the second message is dependent upon active G-protein, not occupied receptors, so the signal is amplified.
   e. **True.** Receptors have a variable life-span; the cell can up-regulate or down-regulate receptor numbers by increasing/decreasing their rate of synthesis/destruction.

2. a. **False.** Antagonists bind to receptors without stimulating them; they, therefore, occupy receptors which would otherwise be occupied by agonist. This has the effect of reducing the effect of the agonist.
   b. **True.**
   c. **True.** Non-competitive (irreversible) antagonists may do this; there are few clinically used examples, the alpha-antagonist phenoxybenzamine is one.
   d. **True.** Competitive antagonists (the group in most common clinical use) usually bind for milli-seconds.
   e. **True.** As agonist concentrations rise, receptor occupancy by agonist molecules becomes more likely at any given moment. Eventually the effect of the antagonist may be nearly completely overcome.

3. a. **False.** Some drugs act via physical effects, for example osmotic diuretics.
   b. **False.** This is the definition of efficacy.
   c. **False.** A partial agonist binds to a receptor and stimulates it; however, the maximal achievable response is lower than that seen with a full agonist.
   d. **True.**
   e. **False.** This is the definition of potency.

4. a. **True.** Only the unbound fraction is available to diffuse across membranes to reach its site of action.
   b. **False.** Other sites include lung, gut wall, plasma and kidney.
   c. **False.** Some polar compounds, like gentamicin and digoxin, are excreted unchanged.
   d. **True.** The unionised fraction is lipid soluble and therefore can pass through the membrane.
   e. **False.** Many drugs act entirely via the effects of their metabolites, for example enalapril and zidovudine.

Short note answers

1. a. The new drug must have been shown to have desired pharmacological effects in vitro and also probably in an animal model to get this far. However, unless the drug gets into the human body, it cannot produce its effects. Bioavailability can vary markedly between species, and even between individuals: this is of obvious impor-tance in deciding dose size.
   b. Food can affect bioavailability, and this needs to be examined since the drug will in due course be in general use. In many cases, food reduces biovailability, for example penicillins, cephalo-

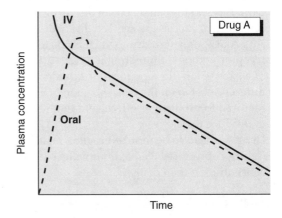

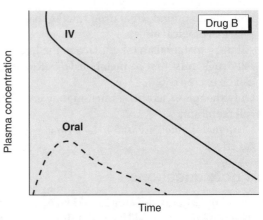

Fig. 15
Measuring bioavailability. Values for two days, A and B, given as an oral dose (---) or as in an i.v. dose (—).

sporins, rifampicin, isoniazid and captopril, but in some cases it is increased (e.g. propranolol, metoprolol, griseofulvin and hydralazine).

c. This is usually determined from the AUC of the drug after oral dosing divided by that (in the same subject, but on a different occasion) after i.v. dosing. So in Figure 15, the two AUC values for drug A are about the same: this drug has a bioavailability of about 1.0. Drug B, however, has a much smaller AUC when it is given orally.

2. a. This could be a prodrug, which produces its effects through an unidentified metabolite; as shown in Figure 16, the metabolite may have a much longer half-life than the parent compound.

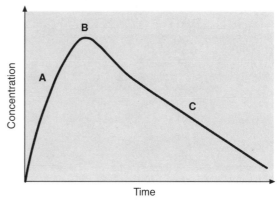

Fig. 17

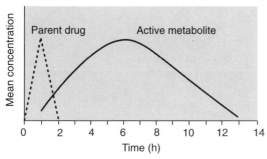

Fig. 16
Plasma concentration for parent drug (---) and active metabolite (—).

b. The drug could be a non-competitive antagonist which binds irreversibly to its receptor. Drug effects would be terminated by receptor turnover, rather than drug elimination from the plasma.

3. This may seem a poor model for drug disposition, but the two have much in common. Soon after the tap is switched on, the rate of drainage from the basin is much less than the rate of entry, and water accumulates in the basin until the two are equal. Analogous with this is the period immediately after drug dosing (phase A in Fig. 17): the rate of drug absorption

exceeds that of elimination, and the plasma concentration rises. Because the rate of elimination is proportional to drug concentration, a time will come when the two are equal (point B in Fig. 17). In the model, narrowing the hole in the plug will reduce the rate of drainage, causing further accumulation of water in the basin until a new equilibrium is reached. The diameter of the hole represents the constant termed *clearance*. Finally, if the tap is gradually turned off over the next half hour or so, the level of water in the basin will fall. The same happens to a finite drug dose: as the proportion of the dose unabsorbed falls, the rate of absorption also falls, so that this is gradually exceeded by the rate of elimination (phase C in Fig. 17).

4. About 25% of the cardiac output (therefore about 1.2 l/min) goes to the kidneys, and of this about 10% is filtered by the glomerulus (the glomerular filtration rate; GFR). The maximum clearance of a drug by this route is, therefore, equal to the GFR; in fact most drugs have much lower filtration rates since only unbound drug can be filtered. The renal clearance of this new drug *exceeds* the GFR; the likeliest explanation is that it is extensively *secreted* by the renal tubules.

The autonomic nervous system

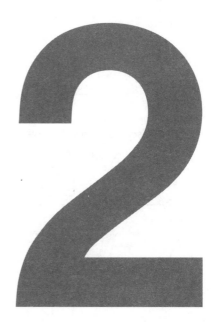

2.1 Organisation

The autonomic nervous system regulates visceral functions, such as cardiac output, gut motility and blood vessel tone, and is not under conscious control. It is separated on anatomical and physiological grounds into *sympathetic* and *parasympathetic* divisions. While a simplification, it is useful to think of stimulation by the sympathetic division inducing conditions for *flight* or *fight*, such as increased heart rate and stroke volume, dilation of the pupils, increased blood sugar, cutaneous vasoconstriction and contraction of sphincters, while stimulation by the parasympathetic system usually, but not always, has the opposite actions.

Many drugs produce their effects by working on the autonomic system, for example anti-hypertensives and bronchodilators, and the same mechanisms explain the adverse effects of many others, for example some neuroleptics and the antiarrhythmics. The main examples will be dealt with in subsequent chapters: this chapter will describe the anatomy and physiology of the autonomic nervous system and will classify the drugs that affect it, some of which will not be dealt with elsewhere.

Anatomy

Both sympathetic and parasympathetic divisions are subject to control by centres in the hypothalamus and brainstem.

The sympathetic system

Nerve fibres that can be identified as sympathetic leave the spinal cord with the nerve roots, between T1 and L2, and pass into the sympathetic trunk where they may or may not synapse: neurones which do not synapse here do so in sympathetic ganglia elsewhere (e.g. the coeliac ganglion). The first-order neurones are referred to as *preganglionic. Postganglionic* fibres then pursue a lengthy course (Fig. 18) finally reaching such structures as the heart, blood vessels, bronchi, pupillary muscle and gut. One exception to this general pattern is innervation of the adrenal medulla, where first-order neurones travel directly to the organ and synapse with modified neurones in the medulla, which secrete catecholamines (including adrenaline) into the circulation.

The parasympathetic system

In the parasympathetic system, preganglionic fibres leave the CNS with the cranial nerves and sacral nerve roots. Unlike sympathetic ganglia, those of the parasympathetic system are very close to their destination, and postganglionic fibres are short (Fig. 18).

Neurotransmitters

The term neurotransmitter is given to any molecule released by neurones that causes depolarisation of the membrane of another cell (another neurone, a muscle fibre or a gland).

Preganglionic neurotransmitters

Preganglionic fibres of both parasympathetic and sympathetic systems release acetyl choline, as do somatic nerve fibres.

Postganglionic neurotransmitters

Postganglionic fibres of the parasympathetic system also release acetyl choline. In contrast, postganglionic fibres of the sympathetic system release noradrenaline. There are two exceptions to this: (a) the transmitter at sweat glands is acetyl choline, and (b) certain postganglionic fibres release dopamine, for example those to the renal vasculature.

Removal of neurotransmitters

The action of acetyl choline in synaptic clefts is terminated very rapidly by the enzyme *acetylcholinesterase*, which cleaves it into acetate and choline molecules: the latter are then reabsorbed by the presynaptic cell and used in the synthesis of more acetyl choline (Fig. 19).

The action of noradrenaline in synaptic clefts is terminated partly by diffusion away from the cleft but mainly by cellular absorption. Absorption into the presynaptic cell (*uptake I*) leads to metabolism of noradrenaline by mitochondrial monoamine oxidase (MAO); absorption into the postsynaptic cell (*uptake II*) leads to metabolism by catechol-O-methyl transferase (COMT) (Fig. 19).

Receptors

Receptors respond to different neurotransmitters and can be divided into groups based on the neurotransmit-

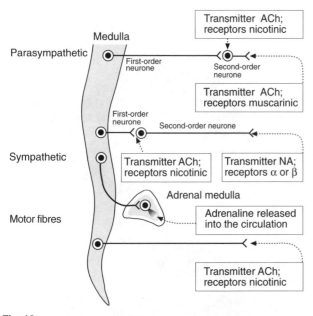

Fig. 18
Anatomy of the autonomic nervous system. ACh, acetyl choline; NA, noradrenaline.

A

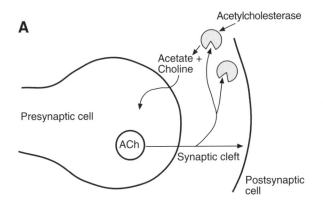

B

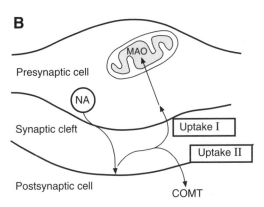

Fig. 19
Metabolism of neurotransmitters. **A.** Removal of acetyl choline (ACh) from the cholinergic synaptic cleft, which terminates its activity. **B.** In adrenergic synaptic clefts, noradrenaline (NA) is absorbed in to the cells where it is metabolised by monoamine oxidase (MAO) or by catechol-O-methyl transferase (COMT).

ter involved and the response to added agonists. These main groups can be subdivided further and this can be used to define the action of drugs more exactly.

Cholinergic receptors

Cholinergic receptors on postganglionic fibres and effector cells differ in their structure, and this explains the selectivity of many of the drugs dealt with below.

Nicotinic receptors. In both sympathetic and parasympathetic divisions, receptors on the postganglionic cell membranes (like those of the motor end plate of skeletal muscle), as well as responding to acetyl choline, can be stimulated by the agonist nicotine and are, therefore, termed nicotinic. After stimulation, the nicotinic receptor, which bridges the cell membrane, 'opens' allowing Na^+ and K^+ to diffuse down their concentration gradients causing depolarisation of the postganglionic fibre.

Muscarinic receptors. Acetyl choline receptors on the membranes of parasympathetic division effector cells, such as smooth muscle or glands, cannot be stimulated by nicotine but are stimulated by muscarine; they are, therefore, termed muscarinic. The cellular events which occur after stimulation of muscarinic receptors are complex: intracellular cyclic GMP levels rise, inositol phospholipid turnover accelerates

and adenyl cyclase is inhibited, but the role of each is not established.

Adrenergic receptors

Adrenergic receptors for sympathetic division catecholamines (adrenoceptors) are classified as follows:

The α_1-receptors. These are mainly postsynaptic and are found especially on smooth muscle. At a cellular level, stimulation causes release of inositol triphosphate and an increase in intracellular Ca^{2+}. At an organ level, stimulation causes contraction of smooth muscle.

The α_2-receptors. These are mainly presynaptic, occurring at 'peripheral' adrenergic nerve terminals. At a cellular level, stimulation causes inhibition of adenyl cyclase and reduction of intracellular cyclic AMP; this leads to inhibition of release of further noradrenaline from the terminal. Stimulation of α_2-receptors, therefore, acts as 'feedback' control of noradrenaline release. In addition α_2-receptors are the predominant adrenoceptors of the CNS.

The β_1-receptors. These are mainly located in the heart. At a cellular level, stimulation causes activation of adenyl cyclase and an increase in intracellular cyclic AMP. At an organ level, stimulation produces an increase in heart rate and contractility.

The β_2-receptors. These are widely distributed, but sites of particular importance include the smooth muscle of blood vessels, bronchi and uterus. The cellular mechanisms are the same as for β_1-receptors. At an organ level, stimulation of β_2-receptors produces smooth muscle relaxation.

Dopamine (D) receptors. These are most numerous within the CNS, but they are also important in control of renal blood flow. Stimulation produces renal vasodilatation.

2.2 Drug actions

Cholinergic agonists

Drugs acting as agonists at cholinergic receptors can do so directly by interacting with the receptor or indirectly by prolonging the life of the neurotransmitter acetyl choline.

Direct agonists

This group includes muscarine and nicotine, used originally to define the subgroup of receptors. Neither is used therapeutically.

Pilocarpine. A direct muscarinic agonist that is applied topically to cause pupillary constriction (miosis) in the treatment of glaucoma (Fig. 20).

Bethanechol. This is another direct muscarinic agonist. It is (infrequently) used to increase smooth muscle tone in the bladder in patients with urinary retention and in the colon in the management of megacolon. It is

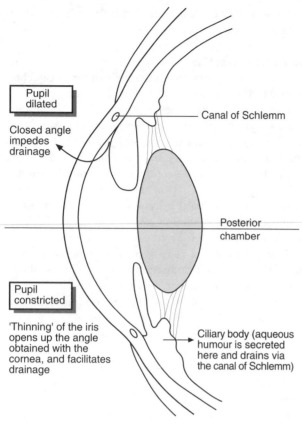

Fig. 20
Use of miotics in closed-angle glaucoma.

incompletely absorbed from the gut. Bethanechol is predictably contraindicated in patients with asthma, bradycardia and urinary/gut outflow obstruction.

Indirect agonists

These act by inhibiting acetylcholinesterase, thereby prolonging the duration of acetyl choline action. They are often termed anticholinesterases and are described in Chapter 8.

Cholinergic antagonists (anticholinergics)

These can be classified as antimuscarinic and antinicotinic drugs, depending on their receptor affinities.

Antimuscarinic drugs

The classical example of this group is atropine, a naturally occurring alkaloid that is a non-selective re-versible muscarinic antagonist. All the other examples described below have structural similarities with atropine. The effects of atropine on various organs is as follows:

- **Eye:** causes pupillary dilatation (mydriasis)
- **CNS:** in standard doses antimuscarinics cause mild sedation; in high doses they produce agitation, seizures, hallucinations and coma; acting in the basal ganglia, they have anti-Parkinsonian effects (see Ch. 6)

- **Gut:** reduces salivation, gastric secretion and gastrointestinal motility (causing constipation)
- **Heart:** causes tachycardia because the effects of the vagus are opposed
- **Bronchi:** causes bronchodilatation
- **Bladder:** causes relaxation of the walls, which may lead to urinary retention (especially in men with prostatic hypertrophy)
- **Sweat glands:** reduces secretion.

Muscarinic receptors in these sites vary slightly in their drug affinities and this has led to a system of classification as subgroups. Detailed knowledge of this classification is of limited value, but the point to remember is that some drugs bind better at some muscarinic receptors than others, and this explains their selectivity.

Examples and clinical pharmacokinetics

- **Atropine** is well absorbed from most sites, and crosses the blood–brain barrier. It has a half-life of about 2 hours. Atropine is an unselective antagonist
- **Pirenzipine** is well absorbed and relatively specific for gastric muscarinic receptors
- **Benztropine.** Like atropine it is well absorbed and readily crosses the blood–brain barrier
- **Ipratropium.** Unlike the other examples, this molecule is polar and poorly absorbed from most sites.

Therapeutic uses

- **Eye:** atropine and derivatives (like tropicamide) are used in iritis as mydriatic agents, thereby preventing the formation of adhesions between the iris and the cornea
- **CNS:** benztropine and others are used in Parkinsonism (Ch. 6); antimuscarinics are also used against motion sickness (Ch. 8)
- **Gut:** pirenzipine is a second-line drug for the healing of peptic ulcer (Ch. 11)
- **Heart:** atropine is given intravenously to increase heart rate in patients with symptomatic bradycardias and during asystolic cardiac arrest
- **Bronchi:** ipratropium is given for asthma, and, because it is not absorbed, it has few systemic adverse effects (Ch. 10)
- **Bladder:** antimuscarinic drugs may be used to relax the bladder wall and increase sphincter tone in a minority of cases of urinary incontinence.

Adverse effects

These are dose related and include: dryness of the mouth, urinary retention, constipation, raised intra-ocular pressure, tachycardia and confusion. In severe poisoning, there may be tachyarrhythmias, coma and seizures (Ch. 17)

Some drugs used for other indications have anti-muscarinic side effects, notably tricyclic antidepressants (Ch. 6), neuroleptics (Ch. 6), and disopyramide and quinidine (Ch. 3).

Contraindications

- Glaucoma: antimuscarinic agents induce mydriasis which narrows the angle between the iris and the cornea, thereby reducing drainage of aqueous humour into the canal of Schlemm
- Prostatic hypertrophy: urinary retention is worsened.

Antinicotinic drugs

Antagonists at skeletal muscle nicotinic receptors (which are not part of the autonomic system) are widely used in anaesthesia as muscle relaxants (Ch. 8). Autonomic antinicotinic drugs (the 'ganglion blockers') were used in the past for hypertension but are now obsolete.

Adrenergic agonists (sympathomimetics)

Endogenous sympathomimetics include noradrenaline, the principal postganglionic neurotransmitter of the sympathetic system, dopamine and adrenaline, secreted by the adrenal medulla. Synthetic sympathomimetics with therapeutic uses include isoprenaline, dobutamine and salbutamol. Each has different receptor affinities, from which its effects can be predicted.

Noradrenaline binds to α_1-, α_2- and β_1-receptors. Injected i.v. noradrenaline tends to cause marked *vasoconstriction* and an increase in myocardial contractility: blood pressure, therefore, rises. Although a positive chronotropic effect would be expected this is usually overcome by vagal homeostatic mechanisms, and there may be a *bradycardia*. Noradrenaline is not used therapeutically.

Adrenaline binds to α_1-, α_2-, β_1- and β_2-receptors. The net effect of an i.v. injection is usually unchanged vascular resistance (vascular resistance increases markedly in some vascular beds, while decreasing in others; this reflects local distribution of α- and β_2-receptors), increased myocardial contractility, increased heart rate, increased systolic blood pressure and little or no change in diastolic pressure.

Isoprenaline binds to β_1- and β_2-receptors. The net effect of an i.v. injection is increased heart rate, increased myocardial contractility and decreased vascular resistance; blood pressure usually falls.

Dopamine. At low concentrations, this binds principally to specific dopamine receptors and causes renal vasodilatation. At progressively higher concentrations dopamine activates β_1-receptors (positive chronotropic and inotropic effects) and subsequently α_1-receptors (vasoconstriction).

Dobutamine. Selective for β_1-receptors, it causes increased heart rate and contractility. Blood pressure rises. Like dopamine, dobutamine activates α_1-receptors at high concentration, causing unwanted vasoconstriction.

Salbutamol. Selective for β_2-receptors, it causes relaxation of vascular and bronchial smooth muscle. At higher concentrations, salbutamol becomes less selective, binding to β_1-receptors, which causes tachycardia.

Ephedrine. A non-selective sympathomimetic with a similar spectrum to adrenaline.

Therapeutic uses

- **Anaphylaxis.** This syndrome of shock (secondary to vasodilatation) and bronchospasm in response to an allergen (Ch. 10) is treated with subcutaneous adrenaline, which induces bronchodilatation and raises blood pressure.
- **Asthma.** Inhaled, oral or parenteral β_2-agonists such as salbutamol are drugs of first choice (Ch. 10).
- **Cardiogenic shock.** Where shock is caused by loss of blood or plasma, or in severe dehydration, treatment comprises replacement of the appropriate fluid. Where there is an acute reduction in myocardial contractility, as in a massive myocardial infarction, plasma expanders will often worsen the situation. Dobutamine, by its β_1-effects, increases stroke volume and heart rate and improves the perfusion of vital structures; however, if the concentration rises too high, dobutamine causes vasoconstriction through α-agonist activity. Dopamine causes useful renal vasodilatation which increases naturesis and reduces the risk of tubular necrosis; at higher concentration dopamine is positively inotropic but causes vasoconstriction at supratherapeutic levels. Dopamine and dobutamine are given as constant-rate i.v. infusions.
- **Asystole.** Adrenaline may be given i.v. during resuscitation from asystole.
- **Reduction of local blood flow.** The local anaesthetic lignocaine is formulated in combination with adrenaline for certain procedures. Local vasoconstriction reduces the rate of removal of the anaesthetic from the site and prolongs its effect, while at the same time reducing blood loss. This drug combination must not be used when anaesthetising extremities because of the risk of avascular necrosis.
- **Nasal decongestants.** Ephedrine is given orally to reduce nasal congestion; it is often present in proprietary cough mixtures.

Drug interactions

Monoamine oxidase (type A) inhibitors. Monoamine oxidase occurs in two forms, type A (MAO-A) and type B (MAO-B). MAO-A is one of the principal enzymes responsible for the breakdown of catecholamines and is inhibited by several antidepressant drugs (see Ch. 6). Ingestion of sympathomimetics (usually in cough mixtures) may cause severe hypertension.

Adrenergic antagonists

These drugs are also known as alpha-blockers and beta-blockers and are considered in Chapter 3.

Self-assessment: questions

Multiple choice questions

1. The following statements are true:
   a. Salbutamol given i.v. causes tachycardia
   b. Dobutamine i.v. is indicated for shock secondary to gastrointestinal haemorrhage
   c. Isoprenaline i.v. causes bronchodilatation
   d. Noradrenaline i.v. causes bronchodilatation
   e. Dobutamine i.v. dilates renal arterioles

2. The action of noradrenaline:
   a. Is terminated by its uptake from the synapse
   b. Is potentiated by inhibitors of monoamine oxidase B
   c. Is potentiated by tricyclic antidepressants
   d. Includes vasodilatation in some arteriolar beds
   e. Is potentiated by cocaine

Case histories

Case history 1

> A 6-year-old girl is brought to casualty because of collapse at home. She had been playing unsupervised in a local wood and had been well previously. She is semi-conscious and confused, her pupils are dilated, her skin is dry and her pulse rate is 200 per minute.

1. What may be the cause of her problem?
2. What should be done?
3. How is the autonomic nervous system involved?

Case history 2

> A farmer is brought as an emergency after an accident with crop-spraying equipment, during which he was copiously sprayed with insecticide. He is salivating profusely and has difficulty breathing; his pulse rate is 40 per minute.

1. What is the mechanism of the poisoning?
2. What should be done?

Case history 3

> A 70-year-old man takes disopyramide (see Ch. 3) as prophylaxis against cardiac arrhythmias. He also has Parkinsonism for which his doctor has put him on benztropine (see Ch. 6). He becomes constipated and, within 2 days of starting the latter drug, he is admitted in acute retention of urine.

What has happened?

Essay question

What is the relevance of the autonomic nervous system to clinical pharmacology and therapeutics?

Self-assessment: answers

Multiple choice answers

1. a. **True.** Salbutamol has higher affinity for β_2- than for β_1-receptors; however, binding to the latter does occur, causing tachycardia.
   b. **False.** Dobutamine dilates splanchnic vessels, including those to the stomach/duodenum and could worsen bleeding.
   c. **True.** Isoprenaline binds to both β_1- and β_2-receptors.
   d. **False.** Noradrenaline has little activity at β_2-receptors.
   e. **False.** Dobutamine is a specific β_1-agonist and has little effect on splanchnic vessels.

2. a. **True.** Noradrenaline is taken up presynaptically (uptake I) and postsynaptically (uptake II).
   b. **False.** Monoamine oxidase A metabolises noradrenaline and 5-HT, while monoamine oxidase B metabolises dopamine.
   c. **True.** Tricyclic antidepressants inhibit uptake I.
   d. **False.** Noradrenaline binds to α_1-, α_2- and β_1-receptors.
   e. **True.** Cocaine interferes with uptake of noradrenaline from the synapse; unlike lignocaine, cocaine need not be formulated with adrenaline for this reason.

Case history answers

History 1

1. This patient has features of anticholinergic poisoning; she may have eaten Deadly Nightshade berries or fungi. She is confused because the alkaloid has crossed her blood–brain barrier.
2. Her airway should be protected and her stomach emptied (even if poisoning was some time ago as anticholinergics delay gastric emptying). Supportive care with attention paid to maintenance of breathing and the circulation, and termination of seizures (usually with diazepam) is indicated. The nearest National Poisons Centre should be phoned. Anticholinesterases (Ch. 8) may be useful to potentiate acetyl choline: physostigmine is then the drug of first choice since it crosses the blood–brain barrier.
3. Secretomotor fibres to her salivary and sweat glands have been blocked, as have parasympathetic fibres of the vagus.

History 2

1. Organophosphorus insecticides are potent and long-acting anticholinesterases: over-activity at parasympathetic receptors is responsible for the clinical features, and his breathlessness may be caused by bronchospasm.
2. Contaminated clothes should be removed, and he should be washed in copious water — the compound can cross the skin. Bronchospasm should be treated according to asthma guidelines (Ch. 10), and he should be given frequent doses of i.v. atropine for its antimuscarinic effects. Pralidoxime is a specific antidote capable of regenerating active cholinesterase by releasing it from covalent binding to the insecticide.

History 3

Benztropine is an antimuscarinic, and disopyramide has antimuscarinic side effects. Both tend to increase the tone of the bladder sphincter, decrease the tone of the bladder wall and cause constipation. Hard faecal masses pressing on an already large prostate has finally caused painful urinary retention. In addition, disopyramide can occasionally *cause* tachyarrhythmias through its antimuscarinic activity (though this complication has not happened here).

Essay answer

1. a. Many drugs produce their effects by working on the autonomic system, and the same mechanisms explain the adverse effects of many others. Dealing with such drugs (which include antihypertensives, antiarrhythmics, bronchodilators, neuroleptics) as agonists and antagonists at autonomic receptors allows better understanding of their therapeutic use, and adverse effects.
   b. Define what you mean by agonists and antagonists.
   c. Deal with cholinergic receptors.
   Nicotinic agonists. None in regular clinical use (mention 'indirect' agonists, i.e. the cholinesterase inhibitors, which are used for their effects on the motor system, rather than on the autonomic system).
   Nicotinic antagonists. None in regular clinical use (ganglion blockers are obsolete).
   Muscarinic agonists. For example, pilocarpine which causes pupillary constriction and is used in glaucoma or bethanechol which causes increased muscle tone in the bladder.
   Muscarinic antagonists. For example, atropine (also list several other antimuscarinics and their uses). Give the adverse effects of antimuscarinic drugs. Mention drugs that either achieve their effect through antagonism of muscarinic receptors (e.g. pirenzipine, benztropine and ipratropium) or that produce adverse effects by the

same mechanism (e.g. quinidine, disopyramide, tricyclics).

d. Deal with adrenergic receptors. Cover the effects of stimulation of α_1-, α_2-, β_1- and β_2-receptors and describe their anatomical locations. Describe the clinical use of the agonists: salbutamol, adrenaline, noradrenaline, isoprenaline, dobutamine and dopamine. Describe the clinical use of the antagonists: propranolol, atenolol, prazosin and phenoxybenzamine.

Drugs used in cardiovascular disease

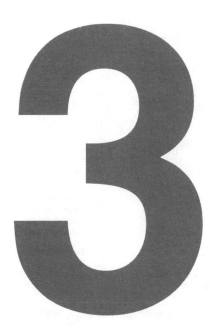

3.1 Ischaemic heart disease

Ischaemic heart disease is usually caused by athero-sclerosis, narrowing the coronary arteries. Risk factors include smoking, hyperlipidaemia, hypertension, heredity and diabetes. The most frequent manifestations of ischaemic heart disease are sudden death, angina pectoris or myocardial infarction.

Angina pectoris

Angina pectoris occurs when there is an imbalance between the oxygen supply (reduced because of the narrowed vessels or in some patients because of spasm of a coronary artery) and oxygen demand (typically during exercise) and presents most commonly as an intermittent chest pain of short duration (Fig. 21).

The **management of angina** involves:

1. Treating the acute attack:
   a. rest
   b. glyceryl trinitrate (GTN) tablets or spray
   c. patients whose attacks do not respond within minutes to a first or second GTN tablet should seek medical attention (they may be in the early stages of a myocardial infarction)
2. Prophylactic therapy. This should be taken regularly. Three types of drugs are used:
   - beta-blockers
   - calcium-channel blockers
   - oral nitrates.

   Each acts in a different way and they can usefully be combined in the same patient. Aspirin is also used, provided there are no contraindications, to reduce the risk of serious thrombotic complications. In patients who have had a previous myocardial infarction, aspirin may reduce the risks of further infarcts.

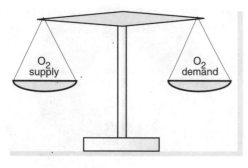

Decreased by:
Coronary artery
disease
Anaemia

Increased by:
Exercise
Tachycardia
Hypertension

Increased by:
Nitrates
Calcium-channel blockers
Beta-blockers

Decreased by:
Nitrates
Calcium-channel blockers
Beta-blockers

Fig. 21
The balance of oxygen demand and supply in the heart.

3. Correct risk factors where possible.
4. Many patients may benefit from interventions to relieve blockages in coronary vessels. Selection of patients for this depends on investigation, including treadmill exercise testing and angiography.

Myocardial infarction

Myocardial infarction occurs when thrombosis occurs on a ruptured atherosclerotic plaque, occluding a coronary artery, so that part of the myocardium dies. The patient usually suffers severe chest pain. Apart from loss of myocardium, the patient is also at risk from potentially fatal arrhythmias. Prompt action may reduce the loss of myocardium and improve survival.

Management of a myocardial infarction involves:

1. sublingual GTN (it may be a severe attack of angina, and not a myocardial infarction)
2. aspirin (if there is no contraindication) orally (improves survival)
3. pain relief, i.v. opiates (perhaps with an antiemetic)
4. thrombolytic drugs (if there is no contraindication)
5. other treatments can also decrease mortality but are less widely used, including intravenous atenolol, or nitrates.

Drugs to treat ischaemic heart disease

Nitrates

Mode of action

Cellular: nitrates are converted in the body to nitric oxide (NO), which combines with sulphydryl (–SH) groups to form nitrosothiols. These activate the enzyme guanylyl cyclase to produce the second messenger cyclic GMP. Cyclic GMP causes smooth muscle relaxation and vasodilatation (Fig. 22).

In the body: nitrates dilate blood vessels in three areas: the venous circulation, which decreases venous return and the preload on the heart; the arterioles, reducing peripheral resistance and the afterload (both of these reduce the stress on the myocardial wall and lower oxygen demand); and the coronary arteries, especially if there is coronary spasm (this improves oxygen supply).

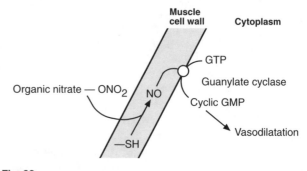

Fig. 22
The actions of nitrates.

Nitrate tolerance

Many patients become tolerant to the antianginal effects of nitrates if they receive them for prolonged periods (>24 hours), as a result of depletion of the essential –SH groups. When prescribing, a nitrate-free period should be built into the regimen. For example, isosorbide dinitrate to be taken at 8 a.m. and 2 p.m. leaves the patient free of nitrates overnight and prevents tolerance. The best regimen must be individualised for each patient.

Examples and clinical pharmacokinetics

Glyceryl trinitrate (GTN) is well absorbed when given sublingually; if taken orally, it is broken down by first-pass metabolism in the liver. GTN is volatile, and the tablets should be kept in a sealed dark container; tablets from an opened container will lose their effect after about 4 weeks. It can also be given i.v., or in the form of GTN ointment or GTN transdermal patches as it can be absorbed through the skin. It acts very rapidly after sublingual use, within 1–2 minutes and the effects last for 30–60 minutes.

Isosorbide dinitrate is taken sublingually, orally or i.v. It is absorbed more slowly but has a longer action. It is partly metabolised by the liver to isosorbide mononitrate, and both the dinitrate and mononitrate contribute to its effects. Its half-life is 2–4 hours. **Isosorbide mononitrate** can also be given orally. It is not metabolised by the liver, and so more reliable plasma nitrate levels are obtained after mononitrate than dinitrate — this is usually of little practical importance.

Therapeutic uses

- Angina pectoris — acute treatment and prophylaxis
- Congestive cardiac failure
- Myocardial infarction.

Adverse effects

These result from vasodilatation and include:

1. Headache (from vasodilatation of cerebral blood vessels) and facial flushing — very common
2. Hypotension and tachycardia — less common.

Beta-blockers

Mode of action

These drugs competitively block the β-adrenoceptors in the heart and reduce the production of cyclic AMP. The β-adrenoceptors in the heart were thought to be all β_1-receptors but β_2-receptors are also present. Beta-blockers can be non-selective and block both types of β-receptor, or relatively selective for β_1-receptors. They slow the heart and reduce its force of contraction and so decrease oxygen demand. They may also increase oxygen supply because diastole, during which most blood flow in the coronary arteries occurs, is lengthened.

They also block β-receptors elsewhere and must be avoided in asthmatics (even the relatively β_1-selective drugs). They may cause peripheral vasoconstriction by blocking β_2-receptors in the peripheral circulation. Some have partial agonist activity (intrinsic sympathomimetic activity) at the β-receptor in addition to beta-blocking properties and partially stimulate β-receptors as well as blocking them. These may cause less bradycardia and peripheral vasoconstriction than other beta-blockers. When blocked by prolonged use of a beta-blocker, the β-adrenoceptor may undergo 'up-regulation', i.e. the number and sensitivity of the receptors increase. This may make sudden withdrawal of beta-blockers unwise, as the patient may suffer a rebound worsening of his angina.

Examples and clinical pharmacokinetics

Beta-blockers may be lipophilic (penetrate lipids and cell membranes well and are metabolised by the liver) or hydrophilic (do not penetrate lipids and membranes so well and are excreted unchanged by the kidney rather than metabolised). The three beta-blockers most widely used are:

Propranolol: a lipophilic non-selective beta-blocker
Atenolol: a hydrophilic β_1-selective blocker
Metoprolol: a lipophilic β_1-selective blocker.

Therapeutic uses

- Angina pectoris
- Hypertension
- After myocardial infarction (reduces risk of recurrence)
- Antiarrhythmic
- Anxiety (reduces manifestations of anxiety such as tremor).

Adverse effects

- Bradycardia, including heart block
- Bronchospasm
- Congestive cardiac failure
- Peripheral vasoconstriction: cold hands and feet
- Fatigue, depression, vivid dreams (especially the lipophilic drugs).

Contraindications

- Asthma or any obstructive airway disease
- Congestive cardiac failure
- Raynaud's phenomenon or peripheral vascular disease
- Heart block of any degree
- Insulin-dependent diabetes mellitus — may decrease awareness of hypoglycaemia by masking somatic effects.

Calcium-channel blockers

Mode of action

In cardiac muscle or vascular smooth muscle, a change

in membrane potential causes Ca^{2+} to enter the cell through voltage-dependent calcium channels. Calcium is essential in the interaction between actin and myosin filaments causing muscle contraction. Calcium-channel blockers inhibit the voltage-dependent calcium channels, and reduce Ca^{2+} entry. They reduce the force of contraction of the heart, slow the heart rate in vitro and reduce smooth muscle contraction. They have no effect on skeletal muscle which is less dependent on exogenous Ca^{2+}. They are effective in hypertension and in angina, especially caused by coronary artery spasm.

Examples and clinical pharmacokinetics
There are three types of calcium channel blocker, which bind to different but related receptor sites on the Ca^{2+} channel and whose effects vary in different tissues.

Dihydropyridines (e.g. **nifedipine**) mainly cause intense arterial vasodilatation and lower the blood pressure and the afterload (i.e. the load against which the heart must eject blood) on the heart. Because of the vasodilatation, a sympathetic reflex occurs, which increases the heart rate and force of contraction (in isolated hearts without sympathetic reflexes, nifedipine behaves like other calcium-channel blockers and tends to slow the heart and decrease the force of contraction). Nifedipine is well absorbed orally and is metabolised by the liver.

Verapamil, unlike nifedipine, tends to have less effect on the peripheral circulation and more effect on the heart, slowing the heart and reducing force of contraction. It also slows conduction through the AV node (where the action potential is largely dependent on Ca^{2+}) and has a special role in treating supraventricular tachycardia. Verapamil can be given orally or intravenously. It is metabolised by the liver, and there is extensive first-pass metabolism.

Diltiazem has more effect on the heart than nifedipine, and more effect on the peripheral circulation than verapamil. Diltiazem is metabolised by the liver.

Therapeutic uses
All are used for angina and hypertension. Nifedipine is also used for Raynaud's phenomenon; verapamil is also used for supraventricular tachycardia.

Adverse effects
These mainly result from smooth muscle relaxation and vasodilatation.

- *Nifedipine:* facial flushing and ankle swelling, headaches and dizziness
- *Verapamil:* headaches and dizziness, constipation, heart block and bradycardia
- *Diltiazem:* Constipation, ankle oedema, flushing, headache.

Drug interactions
Nifedipine can be combined with beta-blockers in angina or hypertension; rarely, the combination may precipitate heart failure. The combination of verapamil with beta-blockers can be dangerous (especially if verapamil is given intravenously) and causes severe hypotension and bradycardia.

3.2 Cardiac failure

Cardiac failure is usually the result of damage to the myocardium, either from ischaemic heart disease, myocarditis or cardiomyopathy. Other causes include poorly controlled hypertension or damage to the valves of the heart, fluid overload, metabolic disease such as thyrotoxicosis, or drugs. Cardiac failure may result in poor perfusion of tissues or vital organs (forward failure) and congestion of the lungs or periphery (backward failure).

The renin–angiotensin–aldosterone axis

Reduced perfusion of vital organs prompts counter regulatory mechanisms to restore perfusion. The sympathetic nervous system causes peripheral vasoconstriction and stimulates the heart directly. The renin–angiotensin–aldosterone system, a physiological means of controlling blood pressure and fluid balance, is activated. Renin is secreted by the juxtaglomerular apparatus in the kidney in response to a fall in renal perfusion. Renin converts angiotensinogen, a protein produced by the liver, to angiotensin I, and angiotensin-converting enzyme (ACE) converts this to the active angiotensin II. Angiotensin II acts at specific receptors (AT receptors) to cause direct vasoconstriction, raising the blood pressure (Fig. 23). It also stimulates release of aldosterone from the adrenal gland, which in turn promotes Na^+ and fluid retention and enhances the actions of the sympathetic system by promoting noradrenaline release.

In cardiac failure, all of these are useful in the short term, but in the long term they increase the load on the failing heart and are ultimately detrimental.

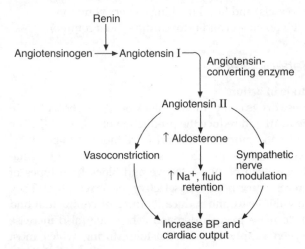

Fig. 23
The renin–angiotensin–aldosterone axis.

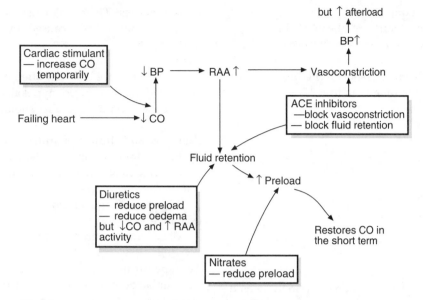

Fig. 24
Treating heart failure. RAA, renin–angiotensin–aldosterone axis.

Treatment of cardiac failure is by reducing the fluid retention by diuretics and reducing the preload or afterload on the heart by using vasodilators, particularly the ACE inhibitors which will also block the renin–angiotensin–aldosterone system (Fig. 24). Drugs which stimulate the heart have only a minor role.

Drugs to treat congestive cardiac failure

- diuretics
- ACE inhibitors
- cardiac stimulants.

Diuretics

Diuretics promote the excretion of water. They can act at different sites in the nephron and in different ways. Diuretics may have effects by mechanisms other than diuresis: for instance, only part of the effect of the thiazides in lowering blood pressure is owing to diuresis and the effect is mostly the result of vasodilatation. There are three major groups:

- thiazides
- loop diuretics
- potassium-sparing diuretics.

Thiazides and related drugs

Mode of action

Thiazides inhibit the absorption of Na^+ and, therefore, of Cl^- at the beginning of the distal convoluted tubule. Water is lost with the Na^+. More Na^+ reaches the distal tubule, where it is exchanged for K^+, and the thiazides also cause K^+ loss. Magnesium is also lost, while Ca^{2+} is retained (Fig. 25).

The maximal hypotensive response to thiazides is reached at relatively low doses, and the thiazides are ineffective in the presence of renal impairment. In the past, thiazides were used in excessively high doses with a high incidence of adverse effects: low-dose thiazides are equally effective in hypertension and cause fewer problems.

Example and clinical pharmacokinetics

Bendrofluazide is well absorbed after oral administration and cause a diuresis in about 1–2 hours, which lasts for up to 12 hours. It is metabolised by the liver.

Therapeutic uses

- Hypertension
- Congestive cardiac failure.

Adverse effects

- Dehydration: a risk in all diuretic use, especially in the elderly
- Hypokalaemia: usually mild and not requiring treatment

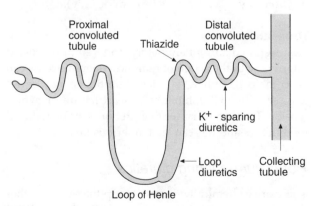

Fig. 25
Sites of action of diuretics.

- Hyperuricaemia/gout
- Impaired glucose tolerance/diabetes mellitus. Insulin resistance occurs, the significance of which is uncertain
- Hypercholesterolaemia: in short-term therapy, but probably not seen in long-term use
- Impotence
- Hypercalcaemia.

Contraindications

- Gout
- Diabetes mellitus
- Renal disease.

Loop diuretics

Mode of action

Loop diuretics inhibit the resorption of Cl^- in the ascending limb of the loop of Henle. This causes loss of Cl^- and its main cation, Na^+, and water follows the electrolytes. The response to loop diuretics is dose related, and they remain effective even in renal impairment, unlike thiazides. The loop diuretics have a greater diuretic effect than the thiazides. When used intravenously in acute pulmonary oedema, the loop diuretics also cause venodilatation and reduce preload before diuresis can start. Like the thiazides, the loop diuretics cause K^+ loss, but unlike them, they also cause Ca^{2+} loss.

Examples and clinical pharmacokinetics

Frusemide or **bumetamide** act within 10 minutes of an intravenous dose. After oral administration, their effects peak at about 1 hour and last about 4–6 hours.

Therapeutic uses

- Congestive heart failure
- Oedema for other reasons.

Adverse effects

- Hypokalaemia
- Renal impairment: resulting from dehydration and from prerenal failure and a direct toxic effect on the kidney
- Ototoxicity, i.e. deafness (frusemide only).

Drug interactions

Non-steroidal anti-inflammatory drugs and probenecid interfere with the action of diuretics. Loop diuretics can be combined with K^+-sparing diuretics to reduce K^+ loss, or with ACE inhibitors in heart failure or hypertension. Lithium (Chapter 6) excretion may be reduced by diuretics and this can lead to serious toxicity.

Potassium-sparing diuretics

These are a chemically diverse group that, unlike other diuretics, retain K^+. They act in the distal convoluted tubule where K^+/Na^+ exchange occurs and are only weak diuretics. Their major use is in treating or preventing hypokalaemia caused by thiazides or loop diuretics. In the past, K^+ supplements were widely used, but very high doses are required, reducing patient compliance. It is not often necessary to prevent or treat diuretic-induced hypokalaemia, but if this is required, K^+-sparing diuretics should be used.

Examples and clinical pharmacokinetics

Spironolactone is an aldosterone antagonist. Aldosterone causes Na^+ retention and K^+ loss, and spironolactone does the reverse.

Triamterene and **amiloride** interfere with Na^+/K^+ exchange.

All are administered orally.

Therapeutic uses

Spironolactone: uses are limited because of concerns about carcinogenicity; they include:

- Ascites resulting from liver disease
- Resistant congestive heart failure (with loop diuretics)
- Primary hyperaldosteronism (Conn's syndrome).

Triamterene/amiloride uses include:

- Diuretic-induced hypokalaemia
- Oedema.

Adverse effects

- Hyperkalaemia
- Gynaecomastia (spironolactone only).

Drug interactions

Combinations with K^+ supplements or ACE inhibitors may lead to dangerous hyperkalaemia.

Other diuretics: osmotic diuretics

These drugs are only used in very restricted circumstances.

Mode of action: these inert compounds are filtered at the glomerulus and excreted. Because of their osmotic effects, they retain water within the tubule and cause a diuresis of water but relatively little loss of electrolytes.

Example and clinical uses: *mannitol* is given intravenously to treat oliguria in incipient renal failure, to lower intracranial pressure and in glaucoma.

Adverse effects: dehydration, hypernatraemia or hyperkalaemia. The increase in the plasma volume may precipitate heart failure.

ACE inhibitors

Mode of action

ACE inhibitors prevent the formation of angiotensin II, preventing its vasoconstrictor effects as well as decreasing aldosterone production and fluid retention. Angiotensin-converting enzyme also breaks down a number of inflammatory peptides, such as bradykinin, and the potentiation of these may contribute to its anti-hypertensive effect. Tachycardia in response to vasodilatation is minor, probably because of the effects of this enzyme.

Angiotensin-converting enzyme is widely distributed in the body; the relative importance of the systemic effects of ACE inhibitors versus their effects on local angiotensin production in tissues is not yet clear.

Examples and clinical pharmacokinetics

Captopril is given orally and is cleared by the kidney. It is given two or three times per day.

Enalapril is also given orally. It is a prodrug and is activated to the active compound, enalaprilat, by the liver. It is cleared by the kidneys. Enalapril is given once per day.

Therapeutic uses

- Cardiac failure: ACE inhibitors clearly reduce mortality
- Hypertension: widely used although not yet proved to reduce the incidence of stroke; ACE inhibitors may be particularly useful in treating hypertension in diabetics, as they may delay the onset of micro-albuminuria
- After myocardial infarction: particularly in patients who have experienced heart failure as a complication, but also in other patients to a lesser extent. The mechanism of the benefit is not entirely clear but seems to involve a reduction in left ventricular enlargement.

Adverse effects

- Severe hypotension: especially in heart failure, on the first dose, or patients on high-dose diuretics. The dose of diuretic should be reduced as much as possible before starting ACE inhibitors
- Hyperkalaemia: because K^+-losing effects of aldosterone are blocked
- Impairment of renal function: through decrease in renal perfusion and intrarenal haemodynamics
- Cough: very common but not serious, probably because of potentiation of bradykinin
- Angioedema: more serious and possibly also caused by potentiation of bradykinin.

Contraindications

- Renal artery stenosis which is often asymptomatic but should be suspected in a patient with hypertension and peripheral vascular disease
- ACE inhibitors should be used cautiously in other forms of renal disease, where they may precipitate a reduction in renal function.

Drug interactions

With K^+-sparing diuretics or K^+ supplements, there is a risk of dangerous hyperkalaemia. ACE inhibitors are very effective in hypertension if used with a diuretic, which increases dependence on the renin–angiotensin system, which is then blocked.

Angiotensin II receptor antagonists

These are a new class of drug which blocks the receptor at which angiotensin II acts rather than blocking its production. Their effects are broadly similar to those of ACE inhibitors, but because they will not affect bradykinin, cough is rare. Other potential benefits, for example maintenance of renal blood flow, are not yet proved. **Losartan** is the first drug of this type, currently only used for hypertension.

Cardiac stimulants: digoxin and other digitalis glycosides

Mode of action

Cellular: digitalis compounds block the exchange of intracellular Na^+ for extracellular K^+ by inhibiting Na^+/K^+-ATPase in the cell membrane; this increases intracellular Na^+ and encourages its exchange for Ca^{2+}, raising intracellular Ca^{2+} and causing increased force of contraction of cardiac muscle (positive inotropic effect) (Fig. 26). These effects cause characteristic changes in the ECG ('reverse tick').

In the body: digitalis compounds also stimulate the vagus and increase vagal tone. This is its mode of action in its main clinical use, which is to slow the heart in atrial fibrillation. The positive inotropic effect may be useful in heart failure, even if the patient is in sinus rhythm, although this is controversial.

Examples and clinical pharmacokinetics

Digoxin can be given orally (well absorbed) or parenterally and is excreted unchanged by the kidneys. Its half-life is 1.5 days but is greatly prolonged in renal impairment. Digoxin has a narrow therapeutic range, and it is useful to monitor plasma digoxin levels. If a rapid effect is required, it is useful to give a loading dose initially, followed by a maintenance dose daily because of the long half-life.

Digitoxin has a longer half-life — about 6 days — and is metabolised by the liver.

Therapeutic uses

- Atrial fibrillation (to slow the ventricular response)
- Congestive heart failure (probably useful even in sinus rhythm, but this is controversial).

Adverse effects

Note: hypokalaemia or hypercalcaemia increase the risk of digitalis toxicity. In severe overdose, hyperkalaemia and hyponatraemia can occur because of the cellular effects.

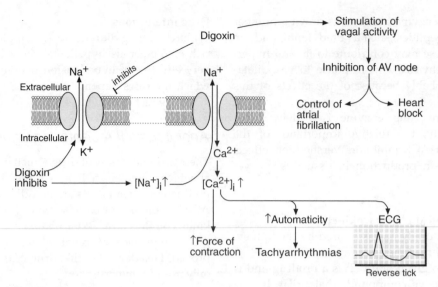

Fig. 26
Actions of digoxin.

Hypothyroidism or old age increase sensitivity to standard doses.

- **Gastrointestinal effects:** anorexia, nausea, vomiting, occasionally diarrhoea
- **Neurological effects:** malaise, fatigue, depression, confusion, insomnia, altered colour vision (yellow/green predominance)
- **Cardiovascular effects:** any cardiac arrhythmia may occur, especially ventricular bigeminy and bradycardias including complete heart block. The ECG may show first-degree heart block at an early stage, but serious arrhythmias may occur without warning
- **Others:** gynaecomastia.

Contraindications

- Acute myocardial ischaemia (may increase oxygen demand)
- Disease of the AV node (may cause heart block)
- Renal impairment (especially digoxin)
- Before electrical cardioversion (may precipitate heart block).

Drug interactions

Diuretics may cause hypokalaemia and worsen digoxin toxicity. Verapamil, amiodarone, and quinidine all increase plasma digoxin levels by reducing its clearance. Cholestyramine may block absorption of digoxin.

Treatment of digoxin toxicity

Treatment depends on severity:

1. Withdraw drug
2. Correct low serum K^+ by intravenous administration
3. Treat ventricular arrhythmias with phenytoin or lignocaine
4. Digoxin-specific antibodies will bind to and inactivate digoxin and can be used in life-threatening cases (very expensive).

3.3 Cardiac arrhythmias

Many minor cardiac arrhythmias do not require treatment; for example, atrial or ventricular ectopics rarely need treatment. Others are more serious and require treatment for termination or prophylaxis. This may include correction of the underlying cause where possible; non-drug treatment, such as carotid sinus massage for supraventricular tachycardias; electrical cardioversion or pacemaking for serious supraventricular or ventricular arrhythmias; and drugs. Antiarrhythmic drugs are usually classified according to the Vaughan Williams system, which is based on the changes in the action potential produced by drugs in isolated cardiac cells. Many drugs have mixed properties and do not fit neatly into any one class. The classification is of limited clinical value.

The action potential

The gradient of electrical charge across the membrane of a resting cardiac cell is –80 to –90 mV. This is maintained by movement of ions through specific ion channels in the membrane. Depolarisation and repolarisation of cardiac cells occurs in the following stages (Fig. 27):

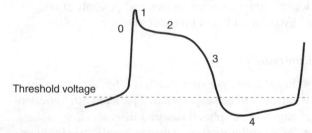

Fig. 27
The action potential in a Purkinje fibre. Cells from the AV node and other fibres show different patterns.

Phase 0: rapid depolarisation caused by entry of Na^+ through the 'fast' sodium channel

Phase 1: early repolarisation, caused by closing of the Na^+ channel and opening of K^+ channels

Phase 2: a plateau where there is a balance between K^+ exit and Ca^{2+} entry; the Ca^{2+} entry is through the opening of 'slow' channels

Phase 3: the late repolarisation phase caused by further K^+ exit and closing of the Ca^{2+} channels

Phase 4: the slow depolarisation phase, the resting potential is restored and Na^+ and K^+ concentrations are restored by exchange pumps. There is a slow entry of Na^+ into the cell decreasing the potential difference until the threshold potential is reached and a new action potential is triggered.

Classes of antiarrhythmic

Class I

Class I block the rapid Na^+ current and slow phase 0. There are three subgroups: Ia, which delay repolarisation and lengthen the action potential; Ib, which accelerate repolarisation and shorten the action potential; and Ic, which have no effect on action potential duration but affect Purkinje tissue to slow conduction and prolong the QRS complex.

Class Ia. *Disopyramide* is the most commonly used in Europe, *quinidine* in the United States. Disopyramide is used to treat atrial and ventricular arrhythmias. It may be given orally (as prophylaxis) or i.v. (for treatment). Its adverse effects include anticholinergic effects (urinary retention, blurred vision, dry mouth) and a negative inotropic effect, leading to hypotension or heart failure. It may precipitate cardiac arrhythmias in some patients.

Class Ib. *Lignocaine* (also used as a local anaesthetic, see Ch. 8) is given i.v. (poorly absorbed orally and subject to first-pass metabolism) to treat acute ventricular arrhythmias, especially after myocardial infarction as it is particularly effective in ischaemic tissue. It is rapidly metabolised by the liver with a half-life of 2 hours during prolonged infusion. Single bolus doses have a much shorter duration of action (5–10 minutes) because of redistribution. Its toxic effects include drowsiness, paraesthesia and convulsions. It has little negative inotropic or proarrhythmic effect. *Mexiletine* is similar but is active after oral administration.

Class Ic. *Flecainide* is used orally or intravenously for atrial or ventricular arrhythmias. It is proarrhythmic and negatively inotropic, and it is usually reserved for very serious arrhythmias. It may also cause dizziness, headache and rashes.

Class II

These are the beta-blockers, which have little effect on intracellular electrical activity except to slow phase 4. They may be given intravenously or orally, especially for atrial or exercise-induced arrhythmias. See above for adverse effects and other uses.

Class III

These drugs prolong the action potential by inhibiting repolarisation (phase 3). Drugs in this class particularly overlap with other classes.

Amiodarone is used to treat atrial and ventricular arrhythmias. It also has Na^+-blocking effects (class I). It has little negative inotropic effect but it lengthens the QT interval and is proarrhythmic. It is difficult to use because it has an exceedingly long half-life, 25–110 days, and because of its adverse effects: serious effects such as pneumonitis and pulmonary fibrosis, hypo- or hyperthyroidism, peripheral neuropathy and hepatitis; minor effects such as corneal microdeposits of the drug (may cause halos around lights) and photosensitivity of the skin and skin pigmentation. There are also drug interactions, with decreased metabolism of warfarin, increased digoxin concentration and risk of arrhythmias in patients given other proarrhythmic drugs, such as tricyclic antidepressants.

Class IV

The calcium antagonists (verapamil mainly, but not dihydropyridines) (see above) are effective in AV nodal arrhythmias, where the action potential largely results from Ca^{2+} entry rather than Na^+ entry. Verapamil is used intravenously or orally to treat supraventricular arrhythmias.

Other drugs used in cardiac arrhythmias

These three drugs do not fit into the classification given above.

Atropine. The anticholinergic drug atropine is used acutely in severe symptomatic bradycardias, as it blocks vagal tone. If long-term treatment is required, an electronic pacemaker is used.

Digoxin. Used for atrial fibrillation (see above).

Adenosine. This purine nucleoside acts on specific adenosine receptors in the sinoatrial node and causes bradycardia. It is used intravenously to treat supraventricular arrhythmias. It has no negative inotropic effects (unlike verapamil) and a very short half-life (less than 2 seconds) and so adverse effects are likely to be only transient; they include wheezing (asthma is contraindication), flushing and hypotension.

Drug of choice in arrhythmias

The **antiarrhythmic drug of choice** depends on speed of response required, presence of other conditions, including heart failure, etc.

- Supraventricular tachycardia (not caused by Wolff–Parkinson–White): adenosine or verapamil
- Arrhythmias caused by Wolff–Parkinson–White: amiodarone, disopyramide, flecainide
- Atrial flutter: drugs generally unsatisfactory, digoxin or disopyramide

- Atrial fibrillation: cardiac glycosides to control the rate; disopyramide or amiodarone to cardiovert back to sinus rhythm
- Ventricular tachycardia: lignocaine, amiodarone.

3.4 **Hypertension**

Hypertension is usually asymptomatic but is associated with increased risks from ischaemic heart disease and cerebrovascular accidents, and, in severe cases, with heart and renal failure. Treating hypertension reduces mortality and morbidity from these conditions, with the possible exception of ischaemic heart disease, where the evidence is equivocal.

Causes of hypertension

The cause is usually unknown ('primary hypertension'), but about 5–10% of cases are secondary, resulting from alcohol abuse, coarctation of the aorta, phaeochromocytoma (a tumour that secretes catecholamines), primary hyperaldosteronism (Conn's syndrome), Cushing's syndrome (excessive glucocorticoids, either endogenous or iatrogenic), or renal disease (including renal artery stenosis).

Diagnosis

Hypertension should be diagnosed by the finding of an elevated blood pressure (160/100) on three or more occasions while the patient is sitting comfortably, over several weeks. The exact level considered as elevated is controversial and must be considered in the light of the patient's overall risk profile and any evidence of damage caused by hypertension.

Treatment

Urgent lowering of blood pressure is rarely necessary (but see below for hypertensive emergencies). Non-pharmacological treatment should be the first approach in mild to moderate hypertension, including weight loss, alcohol and salt restriction, perhaps behavioural therapy, and mild exercise. Other cardiovasular risk factors should be considered also, such as smoking, hyperlipidaemia, etc. If this fails to improve the blood pressure substantially over a period of months, or sooner in patients with more severe hypertension, drug therapy should be considered. The target blood pressure is usually a systolic of less than 160 or a fall of at least 10 mmHg, and a diastolic of 80–85 mmHg, but these, like the level at which to begin treatment, depend on consideration of the patient's risk.

Drugs in hypertension

There are four major classes of drugs used in the treatment of hypertension:

- thiazide diuretics
- beta-blockers
- calcium-channel blockers
- ACE inhibitors.

All these are described above.

Other drugs used in hypertension include alpha-blockers and some drugs used in special circumstances which are considered below. Other drugs are largely obsolete: they include *hydralazine*, an arterial vasodilator; and *methyldopa*, which still has a role in treating hypertension in pregnancy.

Alpha-blockers: these vasodilatate by blocking the α_1-adrenoceptor in peripheral blood vessels; for example *prazosin, doxazosin*. Adverse effects include postural hypotension (particularly a risk after the first dose), headache, urinary frequency and tachycardia.

Choice of drug

In the past the general approach was the use of 'stepped care', i.e. step 1 a thiazide or a beta-blocker; step 2, a thiazide and a beta-blocker; step 3, a thiazide, a beta-blocker and a vasodilator. Today, the 'tailored care' approach is favoured, i.e. tailoring the choice of drug to the individual patient taking into account the total risk factor profile. In this scheme, drugs might be used as follows:

Thiazides. The first choice for most patients, especially the elderly; inexpensive, effective and proved to prevent strokes. But not suitable for patients with diabetes mellitus, hypercholesterolaemia, renal disease or gout.

Beta-blockers. These are also a reasonable first choice, especially in younger patients or patients with angina pectoris. Not suitable for patients with asthma, heart failure or peripheral vascular disease.

Calcium-channel blockers. These tend to have a higher rate of adverse effects, but this is improved by the use of slow-release preparations. Useful in patients with angina, hyperlipidaemia or renal disease. Expensive.

ACE inhibitors. These are the first choice in diabetics but are best avoided in renal disease, need close monitoring of renal function. Expensive.

Alpha-blockers. These are considered a reserve drug in patients who do not tolerate other drugs; possibly suitable particularly for hyperlipidaemics or patients with urinary hesitancy.

Combinations. About 50–70% of patients will respond to any one drug; many patients will need more than one. Appropriate combinations include: thiazide plus beta-blocker; thiazide plus ACE inhibitor; beta-blocker plus calcium-channel blocker; ACE inhibitor and calcium-channel blocker.

Treatment of hypertension in special circumstances
Hypertensive emergencies. Urgent lowering of blood pressure is only indicated in patients with hypertensive

encephalopathy, or hypertension-induced renal or heart failure. These conditions are rare.

High blood pressure readings alone in the absence of these do not warrant urgent blood pressure reduction, which may be dangerous by reducing cerebral or coronary perfusion. If urgent treatment is needed, the patient should be admitted to hospital for rest and very careful monitoring. Oral therapy with beta-blockers, ACE inhibitors or calcium antagonists may be adequate. In rare cases where parenteral therapy is necessary, *sodium nitroprusside* is used by intravenous infusion: it is a very powerful arterial and venous vasodilator. It acts very rapidly and has a very short duration of action: blood pressure rises within a minute of the infusion being stopped. It allows control of the blood pressure while other slower-acting drugs are introduced. If used for prolonged periods (>24 hours),

cyanide, a toxic metabolite, may form. *Labetalol*, a combined alpha- and beta-blocker can also be given intravenously.

Resistant hypertension. Failure to respond to triple therapy with standard drugs should be fully investigated to exclude secondary hypertension. Poor compliance with treatment or 'white coat' hypertension are common and may give the appearance of resistance.

Minoxidil is used in resistant hypertension. It is a vasodilator that causes fluid retention and tachycardia and should be used only with diuretics and a beta-blocker for that reason. A peculiar side effect is the stimulation of male pattern hair growth, and hence it is generally avoided in women.

Hypertension in pregnancy. This is covered in Chapter 19.

Self-assessment: questions

Multiple choice questions

1. Drug combinations used in the treatment of angina include:
   a. Glyceryl trinitrate and salbutamol
   b. Digoxin and verapamil
   c. Nifedipine and isosorbide dinitrate
   d. Diazepam and atenolol
   e. Metoprolol and nifedipine

2. The following drugs are safe to use in patients with congestive cardiac failure:
   a. Propranolol
   b. Carbenoxolone
   c. Enalapril
   d. Amoxycillin
   e. Morphine

3. A patient with an acute myocardial infarction should usually be given:
   a. Thrombolytic therapy
   b. Paracetamol
   c. Diamorphine
   d. Nitrates
   e. Diazepam

4. With regard to the use of nitrates:
   a. Tolerance occurs only to the adverse effects and not to the antianginal effect
   b. Nitrates may have a diuretic effect
   c. Glyceryl trinitrate is given to relieve angina rapidly
   d. The major adverse effects of nitrates are predictable from their pharmacological action
   e. Liver metabolism rapidly terminates the action of all nitrates

5. Beta-blockers:
   a. May be used to treat tachycardia in patients with hypovolaemic shock or congestive cardiac failure
   b. Atenolol does not precipitate asthma
   c. Down-regulation of adrenoceptors may occur in patients who take propranolol long term
   d. Lipophilic beta-blockers are more likely to cause CNS adverse effects
   e. Plasma concentrations are closely related to clinical activity

6. Calcium-channel blockers:
   a. Are negatively inotropic
   b. Are all highly selective for vascular smooth muscle
   c. Nifedipine may sometimes cause angina
   d. Nifedipine may be used in hypertensive crisis
   e. Verapamil is an effective antiarrhythmic for ventricular arrhythmias

7. Drugs that may worsen cardiac failure include:
   a. Corticosteroids
   b. Calcium-channel blockers
   c. Nitrates
   d. Indomethacin
   e. Daunorubicin

8. In congestive heart failure:
   a. Secondary hyperaldosteronism is a feature
   b. Fluid retention is a physiological response to a fall in cardiac output
   c. Positive inotropic drugs are the major treatment
   d. Diuretics prevent activation of the renin–angiotensin–aldosterone system
   e. Thiazides and loop diuretics may have vasodilator effects

9. In diuretic treatment:
   a. Thiazides may cause hypercholesterolaemia
   b. Hyperkalaemia is a common adverse effect of thiazides and loop diuretics
   c. High-dose thiazides are appropriate in severe hypertension
   d. Frusemide acts mainly in the distal convoluted tubule
   e. Potassium-sparing diuretics are the first choice in treating congestive cardiac failure

10. Digoxin:
    a. May be safely used in standard doses in patients with a glomerular filtration rate of 10 ml/min
    b. May cause tachyarrhythmias or bradyarrhythmias
    c. May cause hyponatraemia and hyperkalaemia in overdose
    d. May cause ST elevation on an ECG
    e. If given with diuretics, the serum K^+ should be monitored

11. ACE inhibitors:
    a. Are specific and only block breakdown of angiotensin
    b. Are effective vasodilators
    c. Improve life expectancy of patients with congestive cardiac failure
    d. May increase intrarenal blood flow
    e. Cough is the most common adverse effect

12. The following statements are correct:
    a. Many antiarrhythmics span several classes of the Vaughan Williams classification
    b. Lignocaine is excreted unchanged by the kidney
    c. Many antiarrhythmics have negative inotropic effects
    d. Amiodarone reaches a steady plasma concentration after about 25 days
    e. Adenosine is used to treat supraventricular tachycardias

13. Drugs used in treating hypertension include:
    a. Diuretics
    b. L-Dopa
    c. Oral nitrates
    d. ACE inhibitors
    e. Naproxen

14. In hypertension:
    a. A curable cause is found in most cases
    b. Treatment reduces the risks of stroke
    c. The choice of drug is often dictated by the patient's overall condition
    d. Non-drug therapy has no role
    e. A blood pressure reading of 210/120 with no complications requires urgent intravenous therapy

Case histories

History 1

> A 65-year-old man presents to an A/E department with a history of severe central chest pain for 2 hours and typical ECG changes of an acute inferior myocardial infarction.

1. What drugs should he be given in the absence of any contraindication?
2. What contraindications would make you hesitate about giving each of these?
3. The patient suddenly develops an acute brady-cardia: what drug might you give to correct this?
4. The patient subsequently has an uncomplicated course. What drug therapy would be appropriate for him to continue taking at home after discharge?
5. What advice might you give him?

History 2

> A 60-year-old man who smokes and who has a history of chronic obstructive airways disease (COAD) is diagnosed as having angina on exertion.

1. What drug therapy might he be given?
2. What advice might he be given?
3. What is nitrate tolerance and how can it be avoided?
4. He is also found to be hypercholesterolaemic, with a cholesterol of 8.6. How would you treat this initially?
5. His serum cholesterol fails to respond to your first treatment. What would you consider next?
6. He uses nebulised high-dose salbutamol for his COAD but notices that this tends to bring on an attack of angina: why might this be?

History 3

> A 45-year-old woman develops recurrent supra-ventricular tachycardias. She is treated with several drugs over a period unsuccessfully, and then given amiodarone which seems to control the arrhythmias.

1. What blood tests should be considered before she starts on amiodarone?
2. If she starts taking it at the usual maintenance dose, how long will it be before the plasma concentrations of the drug reach steady state?
3. She is also taking warfarin because of a previous pulmonary embolism: does starting amiodarone pose any problems, and if so, how can the problems be managed?
4. Why was amiodarone not the first choice of antiarrhythmic drug?

History 4

> A 70-year-old man develops dyspnoea and oedema and is found to have mild congestive cardiac failure.

1. What drug or drugs might he be started on?
2. He is also found to be in atrial fibrillation and this is assumed to be chronic: how should this be treated?
3. If he does not respond adequately to your first choice of treatment for his heart failure, what drug or drugs might be added in later?
4. If he develops acute pulmonary oedema, how should this be treated?
5. He complains of knee pain and is prescribed indomethacin: why might this not be wise?

History 5

> A 55-year-old woman is found to have a blood pres-sure of 180/110 on several occasions. No cause is found, although she is obese.

1. What general advice should she be given?
2. She asks why she should be bothered about her blood pressure: what will you tell her?
3. What drug therapy might be considered as a first line?
4. Her blood pressure still is not controlled: what factors might you need to reconsider?
5. What drug therapy might be tried next?
6. She subsequently develops diabetes mellitus: does this alter your choice of drug?

Self-assessment: answers

Multiple choice answers

1. a. **False.** Glyceryl trinitrate is appropriate, but salbutamol is a β_2-agonist.
   b. **False.** Digoxin may increase oxygen demand and worsen ischaemic heart disease. It has no role in angina unless there is also atrial fibrillation. Verapamil is useful in angina and is sometimes combined with digoxin to control difficult cases of atrial fibrillation (because of its effects at the AV node).
   c. **True.** Both of these drugs are used in angina and act by different mechanisms and so can be usefully combined.
   d. **False.** The use of diazepam, a sedative, is inappropriate: it will have no effect on myocardial oxygen balance. Atenolol is valuable in angina. Beta-blockers are sometimes used in anxiety states because they reduce the somatic manifestations (tachycardia, tremor, etc.).
   e. **True.** Both drugs are used in angina and can be combined in more severe cases.

2. a. **False.** Beta-blockers have a negative inotropic effect which may worsen cardiac failure.
   b. **False.** Carbenoxolone is structurally related to aldosterone and may cause fluid retention.
   c. **True.** Enalapril should be used with diuretics as standard therapy in most cases of cardiac failure.
   d. **True.** But some penicillins have a large Na^+ load, e.g. carbenicillin, and should be avoided in cardiac failure.
   e. **True.** Morphine is used for its vasodilatating and sedative effects in addition to diuretics and vasodilators in acute left ventricular failure.

3. a. **True.** Standard treatment unless there is a clear contraindication. A patient who has recently had streptokinase could be given altepase.
   b. **False.** This would be inadequate as analgesia and has no antiplatelet action. Aspirin in contrast has been proven to improve mortality.
   c. **True.** Pain relief is very important, and strong opiates are the drugs of choice.
   d. **True.** Usually in the form of a GTN spray, but some would give them intravenously.
   e. **False.** The patient may understandably be anxious, but this is better treated by pain relief and reassurance.

4. a. **False.** Tolerance occurs to both, although often more to the adverse effects; hence the need for a nitrate-free period when prescribing nitrates.

   b. **False.** Nitrates are effective in heart failure by reducing preload (venous vasodilatation).
   c. **True.** Standard treatment.
   d. **True.** Since nitrates are vasodilators, and the adverse effects are vasodilatatory in nature, this is a definition of a type A adverse effect (see Ch. 21).
   e. **False.** Although true for GTN, this in not true for isosorbide mononitrate.

5. a. **False.** This is likely to kill a patient.
   b. **False.** Even the β_1-specific blockers such as atenolol block β_2-receptors to some extent.
   c. **False.** Up-regulation, i.e. increased number and sensitivity of receptors, occurs.
   d. **True.** Because they cross the blood–brain barrier more readily.
   e. **False.** The clinical activity often lasts longer than might be anticipated from the plasma half-life. The relevant factor is the duration of receptor binding, which is difficult to measure; plasma concentration is only a surrogate for this, which works reasonably well for some drugs but not for beta-blockers.

6. a. **True.** They reduce the force of contraction and may cause cardiac failure. Nifedipine may increase the force of contraction by sympathetic reflex; however, if the patient is beta-blocked, this is prevented and the negative inotropic effects of nifedipine may become more apparent.
   b. **False.** Hence adverse effect like constipation, caused by smooth muscle relaxation in the gastrointestinal tract.
   c. **True.** A paradox, because although used for treating angina, nifedipine may cause a tachycardia and can bring on angina. Nifedipine is, therefore, not first choice for exercise-induced angina, for which beta-blockers should be used.
   d. **True.** But urgent treatment in hypertension is rarely necessary.
   e. **False.** Verapamil is used for supraventricular arrhythmias because the action potential at the AV node is largely Ca^{2+} dependent, unlike the action potential in ventricular muscle which is mainly Na^+ dependent.

7. a. **True.** May cause sodium retention.
   b. **True.** Negative inotropes.
   c. **False.** Frequently used to treat cardiac failure.
   d. **True.** Along with most non-steroidal anti-inflammatory drugs, it may reduce prostaglandin production in the kidney and hence cause fluid retention and reduce the effects of diuretics.
   e. **True.** May cause a cardiomyopathy.

8. a. **True.** May cause Na$^+$ and fluid retention. Secondary hyperaldosteronism may be worsened by diuretic therapy.
   b. **True.** Ultimately it becomes harmful in cardiac failure.
   c. **False.** A very minor part of therapy for heart failure.
   d. **False.** Diuretics may increase activation of the renin–angiotensin–aldosterone system.
   e. **True.** This accounts for some of the action of frusemide in acute pulmonary oedema and for the action of thiazides in hypertension.

9. a. **True.** Probably not a long-term effect.
   b. **False.** Hypokalaemia is common.
   c. **False.** More likely to cause adverse effects with little increase in hypotensive effects.
   d. **False.** Frusemide is a loop diuretic which works mainly in the ascending limb of the loop of Henle.
   e. **False.** Potassium-sparing diuretics are weak and loop diuretics are the first choice.

10. a. **False.** Digoxin is likely to have a very long half-life in a patient with such poor renal function, and the patient would be at risk of digoxin toxicity if usual doses were used.
    b. **True.** Almost any arrhythmia can result from digoxin: heart block or ventricular bigeminy are the most common.
    c. **True.** Because K$^+$ can no longer enter the cell nor Na$^+$ leave the cell as a result of the poisoning of the Na$^+$/K$^+$-ATPase.
    d. **False.** ST depression is the common change seen on ECG in a reverse tick pattern.
    e. **True.** Since diuretics may cause hypokalaemia, and hypokalaemia makes digoxin toxicity more likely.

11. a. **False.** Other peptides such as bradykinin are also affected.
    b. **True.** Hence their value in hypertension and cardiac failure.
    c. **True.** Hence should be widely used in these patients.
    d. **False.** May decrease intrarenal blood flow and cause renal impairment.
    e. **True.** Especially in women.

12. a. **True.** For instance amiodarone, which is mainly type III but also partially type I.
    b. **False.** Lignocaine is metabolised by the liver.
    c. **True.** This poses problems in managing many patients with cardiac disease.
    d. **False.** Steady state will occur after five half-lives — anything up to 500 days for amiodarone.
    e. **True.** Verapamil was in the past the most common first choice but adenosine is more widely used now.

13. a. **True.** Thiazides are the main diuretics used but in patients with resistant hypertension or renal disease, loop diuretics are used.
    b. **False.** L-Dopa is used to treat Parkinsons (see Ch. 6). Methyldopa is sometimes used to treat hypertension.
    c. **False.** Oral nitrates have little effect in hypertension.
    d. **True.** This is their most common use.
    e. **False.** Naproxen is a non-steroidal anti-inflammatory drug, many of which can cause fluid retention and exacerbate hypertension.

14. a. **False.** Only in 5–10% of cases is an underlying and treatable cause found.
    b. **True.** This is the main justification for treating hypertension.
    c. **True.** This is the essence of 'tailored care'.
    d. **False.** Although how effective non-drug therapy is is often debated.
    e. **False.** Blood pressure is often overtreated in this situation. Oral therapy is probably adequate.

Case history answers

History 1

1. Aspirin, GTN, an opiate for pain relief, streptokinase: other drugs proved to be of benefit but less often used include beta-blockers, intravenous nitrates.
2. A history of active peptic ulceration, surgery or cerebrovascular accident within the previous 6 months, allergy to aspirin or streptokinase.
3. Atropine (not isoprenaline which would increase myocardial O$_2$ demands and might worsen his myocardial infarction).
4. GTN to be used as required, aspirin and a beta-blocker or an ACE inhibitor. (The use of aspirin and a beta-blocker together has not been adequately tested yet, although individually they reduce the risk of reinfarction.)
5. Life-style modification, graded exercise (perhaps as part of a rehabilitation programme), stopping smoking, management of acute angina, what to do in the event of further severe pain and what follow-up arrangements are made.

History 2

1. GTN to be used as required; prophylactic therapy: normally a beta-blocker would be the first choice in a patient with exercise-induced asthma. However, in this patient this might not be appropriate because of the COAD. Alternatives are therefore calcium-channel blockers and oral nitrates.
2. Stop smoking, life-style modification, how to cope with attacks of chest pain.

3. Loss of efficacy of nitrates in treating angina, probably the result of depletion of sulfhydryl groups. Avoid by building a nitrate-free period into the drug regimen, e.g. overnight.

4. Diet, management of other risk factors for ischaemic heart disease, exclude liver and thyroid disease and perhaps screen his family.

5. Drug therapy with diet, e.g. cholestyrmine or simvastatin.

6. Salbutamol stimulates beta 1 and beta 2 receptors in the heart and may cause tachycardia, increasing myocardial O_2 demand and possibly precipitating angina.

History 3

1. Thyroid function tests (hyperthyroidism may cause arrhythmias, or TFTs may be affected by amiodarone therapy), electrolytes, liver function tests.

2. A long time! Usually quoted as five half-lives: in the case of amiodarone, this could be between 125 and 500 days. Hence a loading dose is usually given.

3. Amiodarone may prolong the duration of warfarin activity and increase INR. This is best managed by careful regular measurement of INR when amiodarone is introduced and adjustment of the dose of warfarin accordingly.

4. Amiodarone has too many serious long-term effects to be first choice.

History 4

1. A diuretic, e.g. frusemide, in a low dose, possibly but not necessarily with a K^+-sparing diuretic. An ACE inhibitor would be useful in addition.

2. Digoxin and possibly warfarin (patients on diuretics taking digoxin will need careful monitoring of K^+).

3. An ACE inhibitor if not already used (but stop a K^+-sparing diuretic if he has been on one), and possibly digoxin.

4. Intravenous opiate, frusemide and possibly nitrates, O_2.

5. Indomethacin may cause fluid retention and interfere with the effects of the diuretic. It may also not be necessary; why not use a simple analgesic?

History 5

1. Lose weight, reduce alcohol intake, avoid added salt. Consider other cardiovascular risk factors.

2. To reduce risks of CVA and also heart failure and renal failure; possibly to reduce risks of myocardial infarction, although this is uncertain.

3. There are several reasonable choices: thiazides, beta-blockers, calcium-channel blockers or ACE inhibitors are the most widely used. Traditionally, thiazides or beta-blockers are the first choice since they are proved to reduce CVAs, unlike the other drugs, which are not adequately studied.

4. Is she complying with drug and other treatment, does she have white coat hypertension, could she have secondary hypertension; has the blood pressure been measured properly, e.g. large cuff in an obese patient.

5. Usually, one would consider adding a second drug, e.g. thiazides with a beta-blocker.

6. Diabetes and hypertension are associated: thiazides may cause diabetes and should be stopped. ACE inhibitors have specific nephroprotective effects in diabetics and are the best choice.

Drugs and the blood

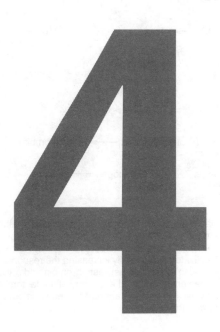

4.1 Coagulation and thrombosis

Conditions where thrombi or emboli are harmful to patients are treated with anticoagulants, which are drugs that inhibit normal clotting.

Thrombosis occurs as a result of the interaction of several clotting proteins in the blood. Many of these are produced by the liver and act as a cascade, amplifying their effect (Fig. 28).

Indications for anticoagulation

- treatment or prophylaxis of thromboembolic disease: deep venous thrombosis or pulmonary embolism
- atrial fibrillation
- mechanical prosthetic heart valve.

Contraindications to anticoagulation

None of these contraindications are absolute; the risks must be weighed against the benefits.

- hypertension
- renal or liver disease
- peptic ulcer disease
- recent surgery or trauma.

Heparin

Mode of action

Heparin is a naturally occurring mucopolysaccharide that binds to antithrombin III, and enhances its anti-

Intrinsic pathway
(e.g. triggered by collagen)

Extrinsic pathway
(e.g. triggered by factor III released from cell membrane)

* Factors where production is decreased by warfarin

Fig. 28
The coagulation cascade. The intrinsic and extrinsic pathways amplify the response of blood damaged tissue. They converge in the formation of thrombin and interact in other ways also. Clotting factors are activated sequentially increasing the response. Heparin enhances interaction between thrombin and antithrombin III, and between antithrombin III and many of the factors in the intrinsic pathway. The proteins are given roman numbers and the activated form is the 'a' form.

coagulant effect, inhibiting the formation of thrombin, factor Xa and other clotting factors. Heparin is active in vitro as well as in vivo.

Clinical pharmacokinetics

Heparin is given parenterally, either subcutaneous (s.c.) or i.v. (usually as an infusion). It has a short half-life and is metabolised by the liver.

Therapeutic uses

Heparin is used where short-term or immediate anticoagulation is required. The degree of anticoagulation achieved is monitored by measuring the APTT (activated partial thromboplastin time), and the dose adjusted, usually until the APTT is two to three times longer than a normal control. There is usually no need to monitor the degree of anticoagulation when subcutaneous heparin is used as prophylaxis. High-dose s.c. heparin is increasingly used instead of i.v. heparin for the treatment of deep venous thrombosis, although not for pulmonary embolism. The duration of heparin therapy is determined by the indication. If it is to be followed by long-term oral anticoagulation, warfarin may be started immediately and heparin discontinued usually within 72 hours.

Adverse effects

The most serious common adverse effect is bleeding, locally at the site of injection or more distantly. Hypersensitivity may occur rarely. Thrombocytopenia may occur (regular platelet counts necessary if used for more than 5 days), and, in long-term use, osteoporosis or hair loss may occur.

Reversal. In the event of bleeding caused by heparin, it may be sufficient to stop the heparin. If a faster reversal is needed, *protamine* can be given intravenously; it binds to heparin and reverses its effects. If given in excessive dose, however, protamine may itself have anticoagulant effects.

Low-molecular-weight heparins

These have been developed for subcutaneous use and are as effective but have a longer half-life than ordinary heparin. Example: *dalteparin.*

Oral anticoagulants

Warfarin is the most widely used. *Phenindione* is also available.

Mode of action

Warfarin competitively inhibits the formation of the vitamin K-dependent clotting factors (II, VII, IX, X). Its onset of action is determined by the time required to clear those factors which are already formed, and warfarin takes 48–72 hours to achieve its full effect. It is only active in vivo.

Clinical pharmacokinetics

Warfarin is given orally. It is heavily protein bound (99%), and is metabolised by cytochrome P450 enzymes of the liver. Drug interactions may occur either by protein displacement or especially by effects of other drugs on liver enzymes (see below).

Therapeutic uses

Warfarin is used for long-term anticoagulation. It is given initially as a loading dose, and later as a maintenance dose adjusted according to its anticoagulant effect. This is measured by the prothrombin time (often expressed as the INR — *International Normalised Ratio* — in which internationally standardised reagents are used) and the dose adjusted to achieve the desired ratio to control: for the treatment of thromboembolic disease, 2–3, for arterial disease, 3–4.5. The INR should be measured daily when therapy is initiated but monthly when stable in long-term use.

Adverse effects

- Bleeding: spontaneous or after minor trauma
- Teratogenetic: should not be given in the first trimester of pregnancy.

Drug interactions

Warfarin is probably the drug most commonly involved in serious drug interactions. Great caution is required when other drugs are coprescribed. Patients must be fully aware of the risks of drug interaction, with both prescribed drugs and with those that may be bought without prescription, and patients should carry an anticoagulant card.

Drugs which inhibit cytochrome P450 enzymes will increase the effects of warfarin: cimetidine, erythromycin, ciprofloxacin, cotrimoxazole, sulphonamides, metronidazole, fluconazole.

Drugs which induce these enzymes will decrease the effects of warfarin: rifampicin, many antiepileptics. These lists are not exhaustive. If a patient has been stabilised on warfarin while taking one of these drugs, its withdrawal may have serious consequences.

Drugs which have an antiplatelet effect, such as aspirin, may enhance the anticoagulant effect of warfarin.

Reversal. The effects of warfarin can be reversed by administration of vitamin K_1. This can be given intravenously, the dose determining whether the reversal is short term or long term. This will take several hours to act, and in urgent cases it may be necessary to replace the deficient clotting factors (usually by giving fresh frozen plasma or factor concentrate intravenously).

Antiplatelet drugs

Aspirin is an effective antiplatelet drug. Its other uses and more detailed pharmacology can be found in Chapter 7.

Mode of action

Activated platelets release thromboxane A_2, a prostaglandin derivative, which activates further platelets and promotes platelet aggregation, as well as causing vasoconstriction. Aspirin, even in low doses, inhibits cyclo-oxygenase, essential for the formation of thromboxane A_2. Aspirin also inhibits the formation of the antiaggregatory prostaglandin, prostacyclin to a lesser extent.

Therapeutic uses

Aspirin is useful in a wide variety of atherosclerotic conditions. There is some controversy over the most appropriate dose of aspirin as an antiplatelet drug, since higher doses may cause more adverse effects and may increase the degree of inhibition of prostacyclin.

Ischaemic heart disease. It reduces the risk of infarction in unstable angina, reduces the number of severe exacerbations in patients with stable angina and reduces mortality in myocardial infarction to a similar extent as thrombolytic therapy (see below). The combination of aspirin and thrombolytic drugs is more effective than either alone.

Cerebrovascular disease. Aspirin is also used to treat transient ischaemic attacks and as secondary prophylaxis to prevent further thrombotic cerebrovascular accidents.

Peripheral vascular disease. It improves the prognosis in peripheral arterial disease.

After cardiovascular surgical procedures. Aspirin also reduces the rate of closure of coronary artery grafts or of restenosis after coronary angioplasty.

Adverse effects

Most important are gastric irritation and bleeding, hypersensitivity.

Thrombolytic drugs

Mode of action

Thrombolysis is a natural breaking down of thrombi, which occurs simultaneously with their formation. There is, therefore, a regulating balance between thrombolysis and thrombosis. Thrombolytics activate plasminogen to plasmin, which then breaks down fibrin and fibrinogen (Fig. 29).

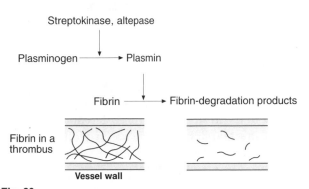

Fig. 29
The action of thrombolytic drugs.

Therapeutic uses

Drugs which promote fibrinolysis are valuable in a variety of cardiovascular conditions, such as venous thromboembolic disease, but are most commonly used in the treatment of myocardial infarction. If given early, they can break down the thrombus that has caused the infarct, allowing reperfusion and limiting the extent of the damage. This has been proven to substantially reduce mortality from myocardial infarction.

Contraindications to thrombolytic therapy

- Active peptic ulcer
- Bleeding condition of any sort
- Severe hypertension
- Recent cerebrovascular accident
- Recent surgery or trauma.

Adverse effects

- Bleeding
- Allergy (streptokinase only).

Streptokinase

Streptokinase is produced from β-haemolytic streptococci and when given in large doses converts plasminogen to plasmin. Patients may have antibodies to streptokinase, from a streptococcal infection or from previous use of streptokinase: when a large dose of streptokinase is given, these antibodies are neutralised. In 1–2% of patients, signs of an allergic reaction will develop: urticaria, wheezing, even hypotension and anaphylaxis. Streptokinase is effective given intravenously as a short infusion and its effects last about 3–4 hours.

Alteplase

Alteplase is the naturally occurring activator of plasminogen in humans, and it can now be produced by genetic recombinant techniques. Since it is not a foreign protein, it does not cause allergic reactions. It is as effective or possibly more effective as streptokinase but may be associated with more haemorrhagic complications, especially cerebrovascular accidents. It is also considerably more expensive than streptokinase and is often reserved for those patients who have already received streptokinase.

Antifibrinolytic drugs

Tranexamic acid impairs the breakdown of fibrin by inhibiting activation of plasminogen. It is used occasionally to try to stop uncontrolled bleeding, e.g. after dental extraction in haemophiliacs (in addition to clotting factors), or after streptokinase overdose or in the treatment of severe menorrhagia.

4.2 Formation of blood

Anaemia is defined as a deficiency of haemoglobin, below the normal for the patient's age and sex. There are many causes, and each case needs careful investigation; anaemia itself is not an adequate diagnosis. This discussion is limited to those anaemias caused by deficiencies which can be corrected pharmacologically.

Iron-deficient anaemia

Iron-deficient anaemia can arise when either the intake of iron is inadequate to meet physiological needs, e.g. in pregnancy or in elderly patients with a poor diet, or when there is loss of iron, e.g. in patients with chronic bleeding. The anaemia is typically a hypochromic microcytic anaemia, and serum iron and iron stores are low.

Iron is well absorbed from the small intestine when there is an iron-deficient state. There are numerous iron salts available.

Ferrous sulphate is inexpensive. Its adverse effects include constipation, epigastric pain and nausea. If these are intolerable, a reduced dose or an alternative preparation should be used. The stools usually darken in patients taking oral iron. Therapy needs to be prolonged — often 3–4 months — to ensure that the anaemia is corrected and stores replenished. Failure to respond to oral iron is usually because of poor compliance (see Ch. 19) but may occasionally be the result of malabsorption or of continued blood loss.

Iron dextran. In occasional patients, no oral forms can be tolerated, and parenteral iron (iron dextran) can be given by intravenous infusion or by deep intramuscular injection. The major risk of the infusion is anaphylaxis, which occurs in rare cases.

Vitamin B$_{12}$ deficiency

Vitamin B$_{12}$ is necessary for the adequate formation of nucleic acids. Deficiency usually arises from an autoimmune disease affecting the gastric mucosa so that a cofactor necessary for the absorption of the vitamin is not produced. The body usually has extensive stores and the anaemia will not arise for some months or years. The anaemia is hypochromic but macrocytic, and the bone marrow contains megaloblasts. In severe cases, the spinal cord may also be damaged.

Treatment is by parenteral vitamin B$_{12}$ (*hydroxycobalamin*), avoiding the need for absorption from the gastrointestinal tract. Life-long treatment will be required, usually with monthly or 2-monthly injections.

Folic acid deficiency

Folic acid is also a cofactor for nucleic acid production, and deficiency also causes a hypochromic macrocytic anaemia. Body stores of folic acid are very limited, and deficiency is usually quickly apparent. Deficiency arises from malabsorption, or from inadequate diet or excessive demand, e.g. in pregnancy or in patients with rapid cell turnover (severe psoriasis or haemolytic anaemia). Folic acid replacement is by mouth, with very high doses being used if malabsorption is the underlying problem.

Other causes of anaemia

Erythropoietin, a glycoprotein released by the kidney, stimulates the bone marrow to produce red blood cells. In renal disease and especially in patients on dialysis, it is deficient and the patient may become anaemic. Erythropoietin can now be synthesised and given parenterally as replacement to treat such patients. Adverse effects are usually the result of its overuse, when an attempt is made to restore haemoglobin levels fully to normal. This may result in severe hypertension with encephalopathy and thrombosis. Most patients are asymptomatic with a haemoglobin of around 10 g/dl and experience no adverse effects.

Colony stimulating factors (CSF) encourage white cell proliferation in the marrow and are increasingly used in patients with neutropaenia, especially after anti-cancer chemotherapy: they may also be used after anti-cancer chemotherapy (see Ch. 15).

Self-assessment: questions

Multiple choice questions

1. Heparin:
   a. Can be taken orally
   b. Activity may be enhanced by drugs that are heavily protein bound
   c. By the subcutaneous route reduces the risk of thromboembolic disease in hospitalised patients
   d. Is antagonised by proteamine
   e. Dosage is monitored by the international normalised ratio (INR)

2. Drugs which may interact with warfarin include:
   a. Phenytoin
   b. Metronidazole
   c. Dextropropoxyphene
   d. Trimethoprim
   e. Gemfibrizol

3. Warfarin:
   a. Is active in vitro
   b. Can be antagonised by vitamin K
   c. Hypersensitivity is a common adverse effect
   d. Should not be given to pregnant women in the first trimester
   e. Is used to treat pulmonary embolism

4. Aspirin:
   a. Inhibits the production of both aggregatory and antiaggregatory mediators
   b. Improves the prognosis in acute myocardial infarction
   c. Increases bleeding time
   d. Low doses may be safely given to patients with allergy to aspirin
   e. Is contraindicated in cerebrovascular disease

5. Thrombolytics:
   a. Depend on the presence of plasminogen
   b. Are contraindicated in patients with active peptic ulcer disease
   c. Dosage is adjusted according to bleeding time
   d. Activity of streptokinase may be decreased in patients with a recent streptococcal infection
   e. Bleeding is a potentially serious complication

6. In treating anaemia:
   a. Oral iron is often poorly absorbed by iron-deficient anaemics
   b. Patients with B_{12} deficiency may present with weakness of the legs
   c. Folate deficiency may occur because of gastro-intestinal bleeding
   d. Erythropoietin is deficient in chronic renal disease
   e. Anaemia should always be treated in the first instance by blood transfusion

7. Drugs which may cause anaemia include:
   a. Indomethacin
   b. Carbimazole
   c. Methotrexate
   d. Penicillin
   e. Morphine

Case histories

History 1

> A 57-year-old man develops an extensive deep venous thrombosis after discharge from hospital where he has recently had a cholecystectomy.

1. Should he be admitted to hospital?
2. What drug or drugs should he receive initially?
3. What drug should he receive for long-term management?
4. How is the dose determined?
5. What interactions must he be warned of?

History 2

> A 25-year-old woman with menorrhagia and a poor diet presents with an iron-deficient anaemia.

1. How should the anaemia be treated?
2. What likely adverse effects of treatment should the patient be warned of?
3. If the patient fails to respond to treatment, what possible explanations should be considered?
4. When would i.v. therapy be considered?

Self-assessment: answers

Multiple choice answers

1. a. **False.** Heparin must be used parenterally.
   b. **False.** Heparin is not itself protein bound and so is unaffected by other drugs in this way.
   c. **True.** Patients who are immobilised in hospital should be considered for subcutaneous heparin.
   d. **True.** Used in overdoses of heparin.
   e. **False.** The INR is used to monitor warfarin. The APTT is the correct test to monitor heparin. Clotting time is an alternative.

2. a. **True.** Liver enzyme induction.
   b. **True.** Liver enzyme inhibition.
   c. **True.** A liver enzyme inhibitor although this is often forgotten.
   d. **False.** No plasma protein binding or enzyme inhibition.
   e. **True.** Plasma protein displacement.

3. a. **False.** It is only active as a result of the inhibition of protein metabolism and so can only act in vivo and only after 1–2 days.
   b. **True.** Warfarin is a competitive antagonist for vitamin K.
   c. **False.** Bleeding is by far the most common adverse effect: hypersensitivity is rare.
   d. **True.** May be teratogenic.
   e. **True.** Although there are many other indications also.

4. a. **True.** Both prostacyclin (antiaggregatory from the endothelium) and thromboxane A_2 (proaggregatory, from the platelets) are affected. In theory, low-dose aspirin inhibits thromboxane more, since platelets have no nuclei and cannot secrete new thromboxane-manufacturing enzymes.
   b. **True.** By as much as streptokinase in some trials.
   c. **True.** Prevents formation of platelet plugs.
   d. **False.** In hypersensitivity, the dosage is usually unimportant in triggering a reaction.
   e. **False.** It is widely used for this indication.

5. a. **True.** Thrombolytics activate plasminogen to plasmin, which then breaks down established clots.
   b. **True.** The risks would seem to outweigh the benefits.
   c. **False.** There is at present no way of adjusting the dose according to need, and all patients receive the same dose.
   d. **True.** Antistreptococcal antibodies may be present and inhibit streptokinase.
   e. **True.** The most common and serious adverse effect.

6. a. **False.** In the absence of a specific malabsorption syndrome, iron is very avidly absorbed by iron deficient patients.
   b. **True.** Lack of B_{12} can cause damage to the spinal cord.
   c. **False.** Folate deficiency is the result of either an inadequate diet or excessive utilisation, e.g. in psoriasis, pregnancy, etc.
   d. **True.** Can now be given to such patients to correct their anaemia.
   e. **False.** Anaemia is a sign, not a diagnosis. Transfusion may interfere with investigations of the underlying cause as well as being potentially hazardous.

7. a. **True.** By gastrointestinal blood loss.
   b. **True.** By marrow suppression.
   c. **True.** By marrow suppression (folate antagonism).
   d. **True.** High-dose penicillins may cause haemolytic anaemia.
   e. **False.** This has never been recorded.

Case history answers

History 1

1. Yes. There is a risk of life-threatening pulmonary embolism.
2. Heparin should be given immediately, usually intravenously.
3. Warfarin will usually be given for 6 weeks to 3 months after a deep venous thrombosis to reduce the risks of recurrence or extension of the clot.
4. Dose of warfarin is determined by its effects on clotting, as measured by the INR.
5. Warfarin is commonly involved in serious drug interactions; there are many examples, including those with liver enzyme inducers and inhibitors (see Ch. 20).

History 2

1. Oral iron, usually ferrous sulphate, for several months both to treat the anaemia and restore iron stores.
2. Constipation, darkening of the faeces and other gastrointestinal symptoms are the most common adverse effects of oral iron preparations.
3. The diagnosis should be reconsidered: if the patient genuinely has an iron-deficient anaemia, then could she be malabsorbing? However, the most likely explanations for failure to respond is either continued heavy blood loss or poor compliance with the medication.
4. Intravenous iron is rarely necessary: perhaps if there was severe malabsorption or if the patient was unable to tolerate a variety of oral iron preparations.

Hyperlipidaemia

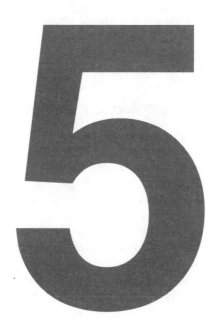

5.1 Risk factors

Hypercholesterolaemia is a risk factor for atherosclerosis. Other treatable risk factors include cigarette smoking and hypertension. Combinations of factors are particularly likely to cause disease. Even the average cholesterol in the UK (5.7 mmol/l) is associated with an increased risk of ischaemic heart disease. Although increasing concentrations of cholesterol are associated with myocardial infarction, the majority of patients with infarction do not have very high cholesterols; this emphasises firstly the need to tackle all risk factors in a patient, and secondly the need for population interventions around diet and education, as well as those aimed at individual patients.

Some forms of hypercholesterolaemia are inherited either as a single gene (usually severe) or more commonly as polygenic traits (less severe). Hypercholesterolaemia may occur as an isolated abnormality, or in association with rises in triglycerides. Isolated hypertriglyceridaemia can also occur.

Cholesterol

Cholesterol is derived from the diet and also manufactured in all cells but mainly by the liver. It is essential for the formation of lipid membranes, steroid hormones, and many other vital bodily functions. Absorbed cholesterol is taken from the intestine in chylomicrons to the liver. Cholesterol and triglyceride are then transported in the blood from the liver in association with lipoproteins, as very low density lipoproteins (VLDL). VLDL are broken down by lipoprotein lipase in peripheral tissues to low density lipoproteins (LDL). LDL carry cholesterol to the cells, and these are cleared by specific receptors on the cells and especially in the liver. LDL cholesterol is particularly associated with atheroma. High density lipoproteins (HDL) carry cholesterol from the tissues back to the liver (reverse transport) and seem to be protective against atheroma.

The role of triglycerides in atherosclerosis is uncertain, but high triglyceride concentrations are associated with pancreatitis.

Value of lowering lipid concentrations

Lowering cholesterol concentrations by diet or drug therapy reduces mortality from one cause, ischaemic heart disease. However, it has not been shown to reduce overall mortality, except in patients with established ischaemic heart disease who are at very high risk. It may be that in patients at low risk, harmful effects of lowering cholesterol (not well defined) outweigh the beneficial effects. There is therefore great controversy over whether active lipid-lowering therapy should be widely applied to asymptomatic patients with modest elevation of cholesterol, or reserved only for those at the greatest risk because of other risk factors, particularly existing ischaemic heart disease, or very high levels of cholesterol; the risk benefit ratio would favour the latter, but is not so clear for the former.

5.2 Treatment of hyperlipidaemia

The decision to treat hyperlipidaemia should not be taken lightly, since therapy is likely to be life-long and is not without risk. At least two readings of cholesterol should be obtained over 2–3 months. Underlying diseases which may cause hyperlipidaemia, such as hypothyroidism or liver disease, should be excluded. The exact cholesterol concentration requiring treatment depends on other risk factors: in a patient with established ischaemic heart disease as low as 5.5 mmol/l would be appropriate, while in otherwise healthy patients, higher levels should be required. The first line of treatment for hyperlipidaemia should always be diet, although in many patients this will be ineffective and in many other patients, compliance with the diet may be poor. Drug therapy may be needed in patients who do not respond to diet alone after several months. Drugs may take several weeks to achieve their effects and frequent changes of drug are not advised. Combinations of drugs are sometimes required.

Drugs used in treating hypercholesterolaemia

Bile acid sequestrants

Mode of action
These are taken orally and are not absorbed but bind to bile acids in the intestines. The bile acids are lost in the faeces, breaking their enterohepatic circulation and reducing the bile acid pool. The liver cells take up more cholesterol from LDL, lowering LDL serum concentrations, to increase its production of bile salts. An example is *cholestyramine*.

Therapeutic uses
Hypercholesterolaemia in the absence of hypertriglyceridaemia. High doses are required. Many patients find them unpleasant to take and compliance may be poor.

Adverse effects

- Constipation
- Abdominal discomfort
- Elevation of triglyceride concentrations.

Drug interactions
Interference with absorption of drugs, such as digoxin and thiazides, and fat-soluble vitamins (especially vitamin K).

Fibrates

Mode of action

Fibrates mainly lower triglycerides, and to a lesser extent LDL cholesterol, while slightly increasing HDL. Their exact actions are unclear but may include inhibition of hydroxymethylglutaryl coenzyme A (HMG CoA) reductase (see below) and activation of lipoprotein lipase. Fibrates are excreted unchanged by the kidney. They are heavily protein-bound and this may interfere with other drugs, e.g. warfarin.

Examples include *gemfibrizol*, proved to lower mortality from ischaemic heart disease, also *bezafibrate* and *fenofibrate*.

Therapeutic uses

- Hypertriglyceridaemia
- Hypercholesterolaemia in combination with hypertriglyceridaemia.

Adverse effects

- Myositis
- Gastrointestinal upset
- Increased gall stone formation.

HMG CoA reductase inhibitors

Mode of action

HMG CoA reductase is an enzyme which controls the rate-limiting step in the synthesis of cholesterol in the liver. If inhibited, the hepatocyte cannot manufacture cholesterol and responds by increasing its uptake of LDL from the blood. This does not interfere with the production of steroid hormones. LDL falls by 25–30%. An example is *simvastatin*.

Therapeutic use

Hypercholesterolaemia, with or without hypertriglyceridaemia, which may also be lowered. These drugs are taken once per day and are usually very well tolerated. They are the most effective cholesterol-lowering drugs currently available. They have been shown to reduce mortality when given to patients with established ischaemic heart disease.

Adverse effects

- Headache
- Abdominal pain
- Transient minor elevations of liver function tests or of creatine phosphokinase are common and resolve spontaneously despite continued therapy
- Myositis.

Nicotinic acid

Mode of action

Nicotinic acid inhibits formation of LDL and VLDL, lowering both cholesterol and triglycerides, while increasing HDL concentrations.

Therapeutic use

The use of nicotinic acid is limited by its adverse effects, which include nausea and vomiting, as well as severe flushing and vasodilatation. The flushing can be prevented by administering aspirin half an hour before the nicotinic acid. A further problem is the need for high doses of nicotinic acid, which requires taking a large number of tablets.

Self-assessment: questions

Multiple choice questions

1. With regard to hypercholesterolaemia:
   a. Patients with an average serum cholesterol are not at risk of myocardial infarction
   b. Lowering serum cholesterol improves life expectancy
   c. Hyperthyroidism may cause hypercholesterolaemia in patients without overt ischaemic heart disease
   d. Cholesterol is a vital part of cell membranes
   e. High HDL cholesterol is associated with an increased risk of atherosclerosis

2. Considering the drugs used to treat hyperlipidaemia:
   a. Simvastatin inhibits drug-metabolising enzymes
   b. Gemfibrizol may cause gallstones
   c. Simvastatin has a long safety record and can be recommended as first-line therapy
   d. Bile acid sequestrants are used for isolated hypercholesterolaemia
   e. Cholestyramine depletes the bile acid pool

3. The following drugs are correctly paired with their adverse effects:
   a. Gemfibrizol and abdominal pain
   b. Simvastatin and renal failure
   c. Cholestyraime and diarrhoea
   d. Simvastatin and Addison's syndrome (adreno-cortical failure)
   e. Nicotonic acid and myositis

Case history

A 45-year-old man who has had a myocardial infarction is found to have a moderately elevated serum cholesterol (6.4).

1. Is this cause for concern?
2. His triglycerides are normal and the LDL cholesterol is the fraction raised. He is given a low cholesterol diet but his serum cholesterol does not improve over the next 3 months. What treatment should be considered now?
3. Should HMG CoA reductase inhibitors be first-choice drugs for hypercholesterolaemia?
4. Will lowering the patient's serum cholesterol substantially reduce the risk of further episodes of ischaemic heart disease?
5. Should all patients with a cholesterol of 6.4 receive drug treatment?

Self-assessment: answers

Multiple choice answers

1. a. **False.** Cholesterol is only one risk factor and, in the UK, the average concentration is associated with ischaemic heart disease.
   b. **False.** Although the risks of ischaemic heart disease are reduced, improved life expectancy has not been proved.
   c. **False.** Hypothyroidism causes hypercholesterolaemia.
   d. **True.** Hence some of the concerns about blocking its production.
   e. **False.** High HDL concentrations seem to be protective against ischaemic heart disease.

2. a. **False.** Its inhibition of HMG CoA reductase is very specific.
   b. **True.** A well-recognised adverse effect.
   c. **True.** Simvastatin has an established safety record and is proved to reduce overall mortality in hypercholesterolaemic patients with ischaemic heart disease.
   d. **True.** They tend to stimulate triglyceride production and are not suitable for mixed lipid disorders.
   e. **True.** This causes the liver to take up cholesterol from the blood.

3. a. **True.** Because of gastrointestinal upsets and gall stones
   b. **False.** No association
   c. **False.** On the contrary, constipation is a problem
   d. **False.** If simvastatin blocks cholesterol synthesis, it might be expected to have an effect on cholesterol based hormonal production, such as cortisol. In fact, this is not a problem.
   e. **False.** Though both HMG CoA reductase inhibitors and fibrates may do this

Case history answer

1. Yes: this cholesterol is raised and is probably a contributory factor in such a young patient having an infarct. If persistently elevated, it should be treated. Other risk factors such as smoking, etc. should also be considered.
2. Drug treatment with simvastatin should be the first choice.
3. HMG CoA reductase inhibitors are highly effective at lowering serum cholesterol, but until recently were regarded as second line drugs because they were relatively new with a short safety record. There were concerns that lowering cholesterol with drug therapy might be harmful. Recently, simvastatin has been proven to reduce overall mortality in patients with ischaemic heart disease; this has never been shown for other classes of lipid drug and hence simvastatin should now be used as the first one drug in patients with hypercholesterolaemia and ischaemic heart disease. HMG CoA reductase inhibitors are also more palatable than the resins, and patient compliance is better.
4. Yes, and will reduce mortality risk.
5. No. This may sound odd, but at this level of cholesterol, treatment should be given only to patients with several risk factors (e.g. hypertension, smoking, bad family history of ischaemic heart disease) or patients who have shown themselves to be at high risk (such as the patient in this case who has already had an infarct). Treating patients at low risk simply because of a high cholesterol would commit many patients to unnecessary treatment with little benefit and potential harm from drug adverse effects.

Drugs used in CNS disease

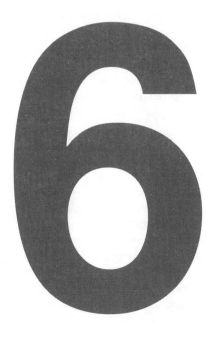

6.1 Anxiety and insomnia

Occasional anxiety is a normal part of life and has beneficial effects, but when persistent or occurring without good reason, it may interfere with normal activity. Similarly, occasional sleeplessness is normal, but persistent insomnia can be disturbing. The management of these problems can be difficult; drugs are not a solution to such complaints, and are usually inadvisable long term because of the risk of developing dependence. However, drugs can be helpful, especially for the short-term management of 'life events' such as bereavement. Drugs of this class are frequently used during medical and dental procedures.

The ideal sedative (or anxiolytic) drug would exert a calming effect with minimal impairment of consciousness, while the ideal hypnotic would induce and maintain natural sleep. In fact, both sedation and hypnosis are produced by all drugs in this class: sedation occurs at lower doses and hypnosis develops at higher dose. All sedatives therefore impair cognitive function and should not be used by drivers, pilots or those in charge of machinery.

The response to sedative/hypnotics declines with continuous exposure. This is termed *tolerance* and may result from receptor down-regulation (Ch. 1). Furthermore, continuous exposure to a sedative drug reduces responses to other sedatives and to alcohol: this phenomenon is termed *cross-tolerance*.

The benzodiazepines

Mode of action

Gamma-aminobutyric acid (GABA) is a major inhibitory neurotransmitter which works by increasing post-synaptic Cl⁻ conductance. Benzodiazepines require the presence of GABA to produce an effect and seem to work by potentiation of this neurotransmitter. Benzodiazepine receptors have been found in many regions of the brain, mainly in GABA-ergic synapses: these receptors are situated close to those for GABA — although the two are not identical (Fig. 30).

The dose–response curve (Ch. 1) of benzodiazepines is shallow, and overdoses tend not to cause life-threatening toxicity other than in patients with respiratory impairment.

Examples and clinical pharmacokinetics

Diazepam is well absorbed when given orally, but absorption is slowed when it is taken with food. The parenteral formulations of diazepam should only be given i.v., as intramuscular (i.m.) absorption is slow and erratic. Diazepam is extensively bound to plasma proteins, but in patients with renal failure or hypoalbuminaemia the extent of binding is reduced, potentiating drug effects. Diazepam is converted to *active* metabolites many of which have very long half-lives: the half-life of diazepam is about 30 hours, but *N*-des-

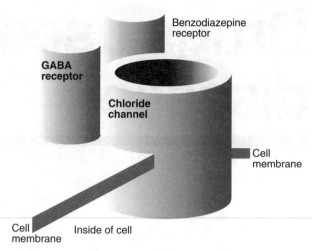

Fig. 30
Schematic representation of the benzodiazepine receptors.

methyl diazepam, a metabolite, can have a half-life up to 200 hours.

Temazepam, itself a metabolite of diazepam, is well absorbed from the gut. It is cleared by conjugation (with glucuronic acid) to an inactive metabolite. Temazepam has a half-life of about 8–12 hours.

Clonazepam too is well absorbed from the gut. A parenteral form is available for i.v. use. Clonazepam is less extensively protein bound than diazepam. The drug is cleared by metabolism, one metabolite having some pharmacological activity.

Midazolam is usually given i.v. It is extensively protein bound: changes in plasma protein concentration can greatly affect the clinical response. The drug is cleared by metabolism, to inactive derivatives, and has a half-life of about 2 hours.

Therapeutic uses

- Anxiety: diazepam is an appropriate choice because of its relatively long duration of action
- Insomnia: temazepam is appropriate because of its relatively short duration of action
- Alcohol withdrawal: in chronic alcoholics withdrawal can induce confusion ('delerium tremens') and seizures; sedatives (commonly diazepam) are given prophylactically and gradually withdrawn
- Seizures: i.v. diazepam is the treatment of choice for status epilepticus; oral clonazepam is used for the prevention of several seizure types (see below)
- Medical procedures: i.v. midazolam is commonly used because of its short half-life.

Adverse effects

- Psychomotor impairment: benzodiazepines can impair memory and interfere with motor skills and intellectual function
- Dependence: psychological or physical dependence (Ch. 18); benzodiazepines with very short half-lives seem particularly prone to inducing dependence

- Sleep disturbance: natural sleep is distinguished by two patterns: non-rapid eye movement (NREM, stages 1, 2, 3 and 4), which accounts for about 75% of sleep time, and rapid eye movement (REM), during which most recallable dreams occur. Hypnotic drugs reduce the time spent in REM and stages 3 and 4 of NREM. The physiological importance of this is not established, but patients may complain that their sleep is not fully satisfactory
- Respiratory depression: patients with respiratory impairment may be worsened by sedative drugs.

Contraindications
Respiratory impairment is the only contraindication.

Drug interactions

- Other sedative drugs, including alcohol, chloral derivatives, barbiturates, phenothiazines, antihistamines and other neuroleptic agents: give additive CNS depression when taken with benzodiazepines
- Cimetidine, a potent enzyme inhibitor: prolongs the half-life of midazolam. The specific benzodiazepine antagonist flumazenil reverses the effect of benzodiazepines and can be used in life-threatening overdoses. Few benzodiazepine overdoses are severe enough to require flumazenil.

Other sedative/hypnotics

The three examples, zopiclone, chlormethiazole and chloral hydrate, are not structurally related: all are thought to enhance the effects of GABA.

Clinical pharmacokinetics
Zopiclone is well absorbed from the gut, with peak concentrations occurring about 1 hour after dosing. Zopiclone is cleared by metabolism to less active derivatives. The half-life is short. The drug is excreted in the breast milk.

Chlormethiazole is rapidly absorbed from the gut but is subject to first-pass metabolism which, though usually extensive, varies between individuals. An i.v. formulation is available. Chlormethiazole is cleared by metabolism to mainly inactive derivatives; its half-life is about 4 hours in healthy subjects, but up to 8 hours in the elderly or those with hepatic dysfunction.

Chloral hydrate is well absorbed, and subject to extensive first-pass metabolism. The drug's effects are mainly via its active metabolite, trichloroethanol. The parent drug has a very short half-life, but that of trichloroethanol is longer.

Therapeutic uses

- Hypnotic: in the elderly chlormethiazole and chloral hydrate are sometimes used rather than benzodiazepines; zopiclone is used for insomnia in young and elderly subjects
- Alcohol withdrawal: chlormethiazole

- Status epilepticus: i.v. chlormethiazole can be useful, but continuous supervision is needed because of the high risk of respiratory depression.

Adverse effects

- Respiratory depression
- Dependence (particularly chlormethiazole)
- Nasal irritation (chlormethiazole)
- Gastric upset (chloral hydrate).

Contraindications

- Respiratory impairment
- Hepatic dysfunction.

Drug interactions
Cimetidine prolongs the half-life of chlormethiazole. Both show additive effects when combined with alcohol and other sedative drugs.

6.2 Epilepsy

Epilepsy can be defined as recurrent episodes of abnormal cerebral neuronal discharge; the resulting seizures are usually clinically obvious. Epilepsy can be caused by a wide range of neurological diseases — ranging from infection and trauma through to infarction and neoplasia — and heredity has an important role (especially in the idiopathic generalised epilepsies). Seizure patterns vary between patients: they can occur spontaneously or may (rarely) be 'triggered' by various stimuli such as flickering light, stress or the onset of a period. The clinical manifestations of seizures are related to the parts of the brain that are involved; this has led to a clinical classification of seizure types which is of practical value since responses to drugs can often be predicted.

Management

The management of epilepsy involves:

1. Supportive care during a seizure: the airway should be protected, the patient should be removed from dangerous situations and nursed in a semi-prone position (in case of vomiting). In children with fever, temperature should be lowered using paracetamol and tepid sponging.
2. Termination of seizures: most seizures occur in the community and stop spontaneously within 5 minutes. However, when major seizures occur in sequence without remission (status epilepticus) the patient is at risk of cardiorespiratory failure. Diazepam (i.v.) is the drug of choice; if a bolus injection fails to terminate status then infusions of diazepam or chlormethiazole may be used. Slow i.v. phenytoin may be useful in status epilepticus.

3. Prophylaxis of seizures; the following guidelines should be borne in mind:
   - the choice of drug should be compatible with the likely seizure type (see below)
   - only one drug should be used at a time if possible
   - the drug should be started at low dose, and doses should be tailored to seizure frequency and adverse effects.

Management in pregnancy: Advising pregnant women with epilepsy can be difficult. In general, drugs should be avoided in pregnancy, especially in the first trimester. However, given the risk to both mother and fetus of discontinuation of anti-epileptic drugs, most physicians advise their continuation. Several anti-epileptic drugs are associated with a substantially increased risk of congenital abnormalities, and this must be discussed with the patient — preferably before pregnancy starts.

Common seizure types

Generalised seizure
Absence (petit mal). Absence seizures have an abrupt onset and cessation, with impaired consciousness, but with normal posture often retained. The EEG shows a typical 'spike and wave' pattern. **First choice drugs:** valproate, ethosuximide.

Tonic/clonic (grand mal). These may be preceded by an 'aura', consciousness is impaired and patient usually falls to the floor. Brief phase of muscle contraction (tonic phase) followed by irregular muscle clonus (clonic phase) and followed by sleep. Incontinence may occur. **First choice drugs:** carbamazepine, valproate.

Myoclonic. Consciousness is usually intact; jerking of single or multiple muscle groups. **First choice drugs:** valproate, clonazepam.

Atonic. Sudden loss of limb tone causes the patient to fall; consciousness is usually intact. **First choice drugs:** valproate, clonazepam.

Partial seizures
Simple partial seizures. Features are determined by the anatomical site of activity, e.g. motor seizures (Jacksonian) result from discharge in the precentral gyrus. Consciousness is usually unimpaired. **First choice drugs:** carbamazepine, valproate.

Complex partial seizures (temporal lobe epilepsy). Consciousness is impaired; seizure may involve complex, often repetitive, actions; may be confused with psychosis. **First choice drugs:** carbamazepine, valproate.

Phenytoin

Mode of action
Phenytoin probably works by maintaining the deactivation of voltage-sensitive sodium channels, thereby blocking the repetitive firing of neurones.

Clinical pharmacokinetics
Phenytoin is usually well absorbed after oral administration, but this is very dependent on formulation. The drug is extensively bound to plasma proteins. Phenytoin is cleared mainly by hepatic metabolism, but this process can be saturated at concentrations readily reached in clinical practice. The relevance of such zero-order pharmacokinetics (Chapter 1) is seen as drug doses are increased: at lower doses, plasma phenytoin concentration correlates well with dose, but at higher doses small dose increments can produce large increases in plasma concentration, leading to toxicity (Fig. 31). The 'half-life' of phenytoin, at therapeutic concentrations, is around 20 hours but is prolonged at high concentration. Phenytoin clearance is reduced in patients with liver disease and is enhanced in pregnancy.

Because phenytoin's therapeutic range is relatively narrow (40–80 µmol/l), and its dose–response relationship is unpredictable, therapeutic drug monitoring is *essential*.

Therapeutic uses
- Partial seizures
- Tonic/clonic seizures: phenytoin is not usually effective against other generalised seizure types
- Status epilepticus: i.v. phenytoin is a second-choice drug after diazepam; it is given as a slow injection while monitoring the ECG and vital signs; it should not be diluted in i.v. fluid, since it readily precipitates.

Adverse effects
- Acute, concentration-dependent effects:
  - diplopia
  - nystagmus
  - ataxia
  - nausea and vomiting
  - sedation (usually only at very high concentration)
- Chronic effects:
  - gingival hyperplasia, hirsutism and coarsening of facial features (these are very common)
  - peripheral neuropathy
  - enhanced vitamin D metabolism causing osteomalacia
  - folate malabsorption causing macrocytosis

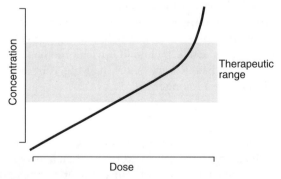

Fig. 31
Relationship between phenytoin dose and steady-state plasma concentration.

- Idiosyncratic effects:
  — fever
  — rashes
  — lymphadenopathy
- Teratogenic effects:
  — associated with increased risk of congenital abnormalities including cleft palate/lip and congenital heart disease.

Contraindications

- Porphyria.

Drug interactions

Phenytoin is an inducer of hepatic enzymes. The following list of interactions is not exhaustive.

- Phenytoin enhances the elimination of:
  — warfarin
  — carbamazepine
  — oral contraceptive steroids
  — theophyllines
- Plasma concentrations of phenytoin may be increased by hepatic enzyme inhibitors including:
  — sulphonamides
  — some sulphonylureas
  — ketoconazole
  — cimetidine
- Plasma concentrations of phenytoin may be reduced by:
  — carbamazepine
  — antacids.

Carbamazepine

Mode of action

Carbamazepine shares many of the cellular effects of phenytoin. Like phenytoin, carbamazepine blocks Na^+ channels. However, carbamazepine appears to have no effect on GABA.

Clinical pharmacokinetics

Absorption of carbamazepine is slowed by giving it with food. Unlike the tricyclics, to which it is structurally related, carbamazepine has a small volume of distribution. Carbamazepine is cleared largely by hepatic metabolism, and one of its metabolites possesses anticonvulsant activity. The half-life is about 36 hours after the first dose but, because it is a potent inducer of hepatic enzymes, with chronic dosing the half-life can fall by up to 50%.

Therapeutic uses

- Partial seizures
- Tonic/clonic seizures: carbamazepine is not effective against other generalised seizure types
- Chronic pain: including trigeminal neuralgia.

Adverse effects

Concentration-dependent CNS adverse effects are similar to those of phenytoin. Other dose-related adverse effects include hyponatraemia leading to water intoxication. Idiosyncratic responses to carbamazepine are uncommon and include: aplastic anaemia, agranulocytosis, rashes and hepatic dysfunction. Carbamazepine carries a risk of causing spina bifida.

Contraindications

- Hypersensitivity
- Porphyria
- Carbamazepine may worsen myoclonic seizures.

Drug interactions

Carbamazepine is a potent inducer of liver enzymes.

- Carbamazepine reduces the plasma levels of:
  — oral contraceptive steroids
  — warfarin
  — phenytoin
- Carbamazepine levels have been reported to rise when it is combined with:
  — dextropropoxyphene
  — sodium valproate.

Sodium valproate

Mode of action

The mode of action is unknown, but valproate's effects include: (a) increase of CNS GABA levels; (b) potentiation of GABA; (c) changes in K^+ conductance.

Clinical pharmacokinetics

Valproate is rapidly and extensively absorbed when given orally. It is cleared by hepatic metabolism with a half-life of 10–20 hours. At high concentration, the clearance of valproate becomes zero order, like that of phenytoin.

Therapeutic uses

- Absence seizures
- Myoclonic seizures
- Tonic/clonic seizures
- Partial seizures.

Adverse effects

- Symptomatic:
  — indigestion, nausea and reflux
  — weight gain
  — alopecia
- Idiosyncratic:
  — hepatotoxicity, particularly in children (often those with multiple handicap)
  — thrombocytopenia
- Teratogenicity:
  — increased risk of spina bifida and other congenital abnormalities.

Contraindications

Liver disease.

Drug interactions

Valproate can inhibit the metabolism of other anti-convulsants including phenytoin, phenobarbitone and carbamazepine. Valproate can also displace phenytoin from plasma protein binding, thereby increasing its efficacy and toxicity.

Phenobarbitone

Mode of action

Phenobarbitone, like the other barbiturates, potentiates the effects of GABA (although the two have separate receptors), but whether this is the mechanism of its anticonvulsant activity is unclear. Phenobarbitone also antagonises the effects of the excitatory transmitter glutamate.

Clinical pharmacokinetics

Phenobarbitone may be given orally, i.m. or by slow i.v. injection. The therapeutic range is 40–120 µmol/l, in the short term; patients on long-term treatment develop tolerance and often have higher levels, above 120 µmol/l. Most of a dose of phenobarbitone is excreted as pharmacologically inactive metabolites, but about 40% is excreted unchanged. This becomes relevant after overdosage, where raising urinary pH (alkaline diuresis) increases the drug's clearance (Ch. 1).

Therapeutic uses

This is not a first-choice drug for epilepsy since better drugs are available and phenobarbitone is sedative; because of low cost it is commonly used in developing countries. Indications remain:

* Partial seizures
* Tonic/clonic seizures
* Prevention of febrile convulsions.

Adverse effects

* Sedation
* Respiratory depression.

Contraindications

* Porphyria.

Drug interactions

Phenobarbitone is an inducer of liver enzymes and increases the clearance of many drugs including warfarin, carbamazepine, oral contraceptive steroids and folate. Phenobarbitone has additive effects with other sedative/hypnotic drugs.

Other antiepileptics

Ethosuximide. Absorption of ethosuximide from the gut is rapid, and it is cleared mainly by metabolism to inactive derivatives. The therapeutic range is about 60 to 100 mg/l. Ethosuximide is used for generalised seizures (mainly absence) in children, but it is less frequently used than valproate because gastrointestinal adverse effects (nausea, vomiting and abdominal pain) are common.

Vigabatrin. Vigabatrin works by inhibiting enzymic breakdown of GABA and thereby increasing CNS concentrations of this inhibitory neurotransmitter. The drug is currently used in combination with other antiepileptic drugs as supplementary therapy for refractory seizures — particularly complex partial seizures. The main adverse effect is sedation.

Lamotrigine. Lamotrigine works by inhibiting the release of excitatory amino acid neurotransmitters (principally glutamate) which may be involved in the generation of seizure activity. Lamotrigine is used in combination with other antiepileptic drugs as supplementary therapy in refractory seizures. The adverse effect profile of this drug is not yet fully known, but it has, rarely, been associated with severe illness including multi-organ failure.

6.3 Depression and hypomania

Sadness is a normal reaction to many life events. Usually this abates with time, but the term depression is used for abnormally protracted or severe sadness. Depression is common and, if ignored, may result in anorexia, 'retardation' (which indicates slow mental processes) and inability to work. Suicide may be attempted, and suicidal ideas should be enquired about when assessing such patients. Hypomania is a less common, but equally disruptive, overactivity of mentation; it may alternate with depression in so-called 'bipolar affective disorder'.

The possibility that depression results from a 'depletion' of monoamine neurotransmitters (5-hydroxytryptamine serotonin, 5-HT and noradrenaline) has been at the centre of antidepressant drug development for many years: drugs that interfere with monoamine release or storage, such as reserpine (a disused antihypertensive), can cause depression, while drugs that release monoamines can relieve it. This 'amine hypothesis' has been questioned recently.

Tricyclics are the antidepressants most commonly used, while newer generation agents include the selective 5-HT-reuptake inhibitors (SSRI); patients with bipolar affective disorder often benefit from lithium.

Tricyclics

Mode of action

Tricyclics block the reuptake into the presynaptic neurone of noradrenaline and 5-HT, thereby increasing their availability to the postsynaptic membrane (so-called uptake I; Fig. 32). The tricyclics also have anti-

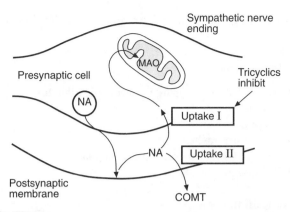

Fig. 32
Mode of action of tricyclics. NA, noradrenaline; MAO, monoamine oxidase; COMT, catechol-O-methyl transferase.

muscarinic properties, which can cause unwanted effects, especially in overdosage.

Examples and clinical pharmacokinetics
Imipramine is well absorbed but subject to extensive first-pass metabolism; the principal metabolite, desipramine, is active (and is itself used as a drug). Both imipramine and desipramine have large volumes of distribution (relevant after overdose, see Ch. 17). The half-life of the drug is about 12 hours, while that of the metabolite is about 24 hours.

Amitriptyline is also well absorbed and has extensive first-pass metabolism. Like imipramine, and other tricyclics, amitriptyline's principal metabolite, nortriptyline, is active (nortriptyline is also marketed as a drug).

Therapeutic uses

- Depression: there is a delay of about 2 weeks before benefit is seen
- Chronic pain: neuralgias may be improved by tricyclics or the antiepileptic carbamazepine.

Adverse effects

- Anticholinergic effects
- Tachyarrhythmias and QT prolongation, especially in overdose
- Postural hypotension
- Sedation, particularly with amitriptyline
- Weight gain
- Hepatotoxicity and blood dyscrasias (both are unusual)
- Exacerbation of epilepsy.

Contraindications

- Glaucoma
- Prostatic hypertrophy
- Immediately after a myocardial infarction.

Tricyclic poisoning
Overdose with tricyclics is common and may be life-threatening. Features include CNS depression, causing

impaired consciousness, seizures and tachyarrhythmias (Ch. 17). There is no antidote, and drug elimination cannot be increased; management is supportive.

Drug interactions
Tricyclics should not be combined with monoamine oxidase inhibitors (MAOI) because of a rare, but potentially fatal, hyperthermia syndrome.

Imipramine clearance can be reduced by cimetidine and chlorpromazine.

Selective 5-HT-reuptake inhibitors (SSRI)

Mode of action
Selective inhibition of 5-HT reuptake by postsynaptic nerve terminals (unlike the tricyclics which inhibit the uptake of both noradrenaline and 5-HT).

Examples and clinical pharmacokinetics
Fluoxetine is among the commonest antidepressants in use. Fluoxetine is well absorbed from the gut, and is metabolised to an equipotent metabolite. Both parent drug and active metabolite are very slowly eliminated and may accumulate in patients with severe liver or kidney disease.

Sertraline, in contrast, has a shorter elimination half-life and is not metabolised to active derivatives.

Therapeutic uses
Depression. Like the tricyclics, there is considerable delay between starting treatment and the onset of benefit. Unlike the tricyclics, SSRIs do not have marked sedative hypotensive or anticholinergic effects, have less effect on cardiac conduction and do not cause weight gain. In overdose, the SSRIs appear to be better tolerated than tricyclics.

Adverse effects

- Vasculitis rash: a rare but serious reaction to fluoxetine
- Seizures: fluoxetine (like the tricyclics) can exacerbate seizures, and is commonly reported to cause (dose-related) anorexia and agitation
- Sexual dysfunction: may be caused by fluoxetine.

Drug interactions

- Fluoxetine, like the tricyclics, can produce a fatal hyperthermia syndrome if combined with MAOIs
- The combination of lithium with fluoxetine may increase the risk of seizure.

Non-selective monoamine oxidase inhibitors (MOAI)

Mode of action
Noradrenaline and 5-HT are metabolised by monoamine oxidase after they are taken up from the

synaptic cleft; MAOIs inhibit this enzyme and thereby potentiate these neurotransmitters.

Tranylcycpromine, an example of this group, is well absorbed from the gut and cleared mainly by metabolism to active derivatives.

Therapeutic uses
MAOIs are used for depression and other psychiatric disorders; they are employed less frequently than tricyclics because of the risk of drug interactions (below).

Adverse effects

* Weight gain
* Nausea
* Anticholinergic effects
* Bizarre adverse reactions including hepatitis and agranulocytosis occur rarely but can be serious.

Contraindications

* Liver disease
* Cerebrovascular disease, because of the risks of hypotension or increased cerebral blood flow.

Drug interactions
Foods containing tyramine and dopamine are contraindicated because of the risk of severe hypertension; these foods include ripe cheese and pickled herring. Likewise nasal decongestants, which contain sympathomimetics, and L-dopa combinations should be avoided. MAOIs reduce opiate clearance, and opiate doses should be much lower than those usually required.

Reversible inhibitors of monoamine oxidase-A (RIMA)

There are two subtypes of monoamine oxidase: A and B. MAO-A metabolises noradrenaline and 5-HT and is, therefore, relevant to depression, while MAO-B metabolises dopamine. Specific MAO-B inhibitors have been available for some time for the treatment of Parkinsonism (see below). Specific inhibitors of MAO-A, such as moclobemide, are now becoming available for depression. Unlike older MAO inhibitors (above), RIMA drugs do not produce the risk of hypertensive crises with sympathomimetics.

Lithium

The mode of action of lithium, which is used for the prophylaxis and treatment of bipolar affective disorder, is unknown. It is well absorbed orally and is excreted by the kidney; its clearance is reduced in patients with renal impairment. Lithium's therapeutic range (0.75–1.25 µmol/l) is generally accepted and therapeutic monitoring is mandatory.

Exceeding the upper limit of the therapeutic range is dangerous and a serum lithium concentration, 12 hours postdose, greater than 3.5 µmol/l can be life threatening.

Adverse effects

* Renal damage causing nephrogenic diabetes insipidus
* Hypothyroidism
* Acneiform rashes
* Weight gain and peripheral oedema
* Teratogenicity.

Contraindications

* Renal impairment, because of the risk of accumulation
* Psoriasis, because this rash may be worsened.

Drug interactions
Diuretics and NSAIDs can cause accumulation of lithium.

6.4 Schizophrenia

Schizophrenia is the most common psychosis and probably results from overactivity of dopaminergic neurones, particularly in the mesolimbic system. This 'dopamine hypothesis' is based on the observation that all neuroleptics block dopamine receptors, and drugs which potentiate CNS dopamine can induce schizophreniform psychoses. These is no succinct definition of psychosis but most are characterised by full orientation, but marked thinking disturbance, which commonly includes delusions and auditory hallucinations.

Neuroleptic drugs

Examples include chlorpromazine, haloperidol and flupenthixol.

Mode of action
Neuroleptics (otherwise known as 'major tranquilizers') are structurally heterogeneous drugs that abolish or reduce the thought disorder which characterises schizophrenia. All act by blocking dopamine D_2 receptors, primarily in the mesolimbic system. Antagonism of D_1 receptors does not contribute therapeutically but may cause dystonic reactions. The role of other neurotransmitter receptors is less clear: many of these drugs block receptors to 5-HT, histamine (H_1) acetyl choline (muscarinic receptors) and noradrenaline (α_1-receptors).

Clinical pharmacokinetics
Chlorpromazine is incompletely absorbed from the gut and subject to first-pass metabolism giving it a bioavailability of about 10%. Parenteral formulations are also available. Chlorpromazine is extensively metabo-

lised, and some derivatives may have pharmacological activity.

Depot preparations. Other neuroleptic drugs are available as depot i.m. preparations, which allow a reduction in the frequency of dosing.

Therapeutic uses

- Schizophrenia and related disorders
- Severe organic psychosis.

Adverse effects

Psychological. Neuroleptics can exacerbate or cause depression and can cause a lack of motivation.

Neurological. Blockage of D_1 receptors may result in Parkinsonism and other extrapyramidal reactions including akathisia (severe restlessness), and acute dystonic reactions (including torticollis). All these syndromes may respond to anticholinergic drugs. Tardive dyskinesia, the late onset of choreoathetoid movements, may occur in up to 40% of patients; it is probably caused by dopamine receptor up-regulation and can be very difficult to treat.

Autonomic effects. Neuroleptics have antimuscarinic effects (see Ch. 2) and block α_1-adrenoceptors; this may result in postural hypotension, premature ejaculation, visual disturbance, dry mouth, retention of urine and constipation. Differing drugs can produce different degrees of each autonomic effect, so swapping to another compound can be beneficial.

Idiosyncratic. Jaundice, rashes and agranulocytosis are rare with most neuroleptics.

Miscellaneous. Hyperprolactinaemia can result from chronic dopamine antagonism and may cause gynaecomastia. Weight gain is common. Neuroleptic malignant syndrome is a rare but serious reaction to all these drugs, comprising hyperpyrexia and muscle rigidity.

Contraindications

- Hypersensitivity
- Glaucoma
- Parkinson's disease
- Impaired consciousness.

Drug interactions

Most of the interactions are pharmacodynamic and predictable from a knowledge of the receptor groups blocked by the drugs. Additive effects are seen between neuroleptics and other antidopaminergic, antimuscarinic, antihistaminergic and antiadrenergic drugs.

6.5 Parkinsonism

Parkinsonism comprises bradykinesia (or difficulty initiating movement), coarse tremor, rigidity and disordered posture. There are many causes, but idiopathic disease and neuroleptic-induced Parkinsonism are the most common. Other causes include encephalitis, a variety of CNS degenerative conditions, poisoning and metabolic problems.

In idiopathic disease, the normally high concentration of dopamine in the substantia nigra is markedly reduced; this reduces the inhibition of excitatory cholinergic fibres. Neuroleptic drugs, by comparison, upset the 'balance' by blocking dopamine receptors.

The aim of therapy is to restore the 'balance' between dopamine and acetyl choline, either by increasing the concentration of dopamine in the basal ganglia or by blocking the effects of cholinergic fibres.

Levodopa

Mode of action

Levodopa (dihydroxyphenyl-L-alanine; L-dopa) is the precursor of dopamine, which, unlike the latter, can cross the blood–brain barrier. Both within the CNS, and elsewhere in the body, L-dopa is metabolised (by decarboxylation) to dopamine; it is the 'peripheral' synthesis of dopamine which results in many of the adverse effects of L-dopa. To offset this, L-dopa is combined with a decarboxylase inhibitor (either carbidopa or benserazide); peripheral decarboxylation is reduced but, as carbidopa and benzeraside do not cross the blood–brain barrier, decarboxylation in the CNS is unaffected.

The clinical response to L-dopa combinations is usually good initially but declines with time. Although L-dopa does not prevent the progression of the disease, there is some evidence that starting the drug early reduces mortality. In some patients, the response to L-dopa may be lost altogether, while in others the dose must be reduced to diminish adverse effects which develop on long-term therapy. L-Dopa is of no value in neuroleptic-induced Parkinsonism, where dopamine receptors are blocked by the neuroleptic drug.

Clinical pharmacokinetics

L-Dopa is absorbed by a facilitated carrier mechanism and, since certain other amino acids compete for transport, its absorption is reduced after meals. The drug is subject to extensive first-pass metabolism and has a bioavailability of about 33%. Even when combined with a decarboxylase inhibitor, only about 10% of the L-dopa dose enters the brain. L-Dopa is largely cleared by metabolism to dopamine and other derivatives.

Adverse effects

- Nausea and vomiting: dopamine is the principal neurotransmitter of the vomiting centre in the brainstem, and dopamine agonists can cause nausea; this is reduced by combination of L-dopa with a decarboxylase inhibitor
- Dyskinesias: seen in 80% of patients with prolonged use, including facial choreoathetosis, hemibalismus, dystonia, tics and myoclonus
- Cardiovascular: postural hypotension is common but some patients develop hypertension; tachyarrhythmias may occur

- Erratic response: marked variation in drug response occurs in a high proportion of patients after several years of treatment; in some, several bradykinesia is seen several hours after dosing (end of dose phenomenon) while in others the fluctuation in response seems unrelated to drug doses and periods of severe bradykinesia alternate with periods of dyskinesia (on–off phenomenon).

Contraindications

- Glaucoma
- Psychosis.

Drug interactions

L-Dopa should not be given to patients on a non-selective MAO inhibitor, because of the risk of severe hypertension.

Dopamine agonists

Mode of action

Bromocriptine, lysuride and pergolide are structurally different from dopamine but are direct agonists at dopamine receptors. Amantadine is an antiviral drug (Ch. 14) which promotes the release of dopamine and, therefore, acts as an indirect agonist. Its effects are less potent than those of L-dopa.

Clinical pharmacokinetics

Bromocriptine, lysuride and pergolide are subject to extensive and variable presystemic metabolism and are cleared mainly by hepatic metabolism to inactive derivatives. Amantadine is well absorbed from the gut and mainly excreted unchanged; it should, therefore, be used with caution in patients with renal failure.

Therapeutic uses

Bromocriptine, lysuride and pergolide. As adjuvants to L-dopa therapy, particularly where responses to L-dopa are diminishing. Also used in hyperprolactinaemia and acromegaly.

Amantadine. Amantadine is used infrequently because of the availability of more potent alternatives.

Adverse effects

Bromocriptine, lysuride and pergolide. Nausea, dizziness, visual disturbance, vivid dreams and postural hypotension are among the commoner symptomatic reactions; these may improve if the drug is continued. Idiosyncratic reactions are very rare.

Amantadine. Dose-dependent CNS adverse effects, including seizures and confusion, can occur and the drug may exacerbate heart failure.

Selegiline

Selegiline selectively inhibits MAO-B, which metabolises dopamine, thereby potentiating it. Hypertensive crises in response to sympathomimetic compounds are not a major problem with MAO-B inhibitors. Selegiline is given by mouth and is well absorbed. The drug is cleared largely by metabolism to pharmacologically active derivatives.

Therapeutic uses

- In combination with L-dopa either to restore the clinical response to the latter where this has been lost or in patients with 'on–off' symptoms (see above)
- As sole therapy in early Parkinson's disease, selegiline may slow disease progression.

Adverse effects

Mild gastrointestinal effects.

Anticholinergics

Mode of action

Depletion of striatal dopamine, as in idiopathic Parkinsonism, or blockade of dopamine receptors, as seen with neuroleptics, reduces inhibition of excitatory cholinergic neurones. This balance may be restored using antimuscarinic drugs (Ch. 2).

Examples and clinical pharmacokinetics

Benztropine is well absorbed from the gut, and cleared by hepatic metabolism to inactive derivatives. Its half-life is about 4 hours.

Procyclidine is available in oral and i.v. forms, which can be very useful in acute dystonic reactions to neuroleptics. It is completely absorbed from the gut but subject to first-pass metabolism. Its half-life is about 12 hours.

Therapeutic uses

- Drug-induced Parkinsonism
- Idiopathic Parkinsonism: rarely used nowadays.

Adverse effects

Systemic antimuscarinic effects (Ch. 8).

Contraindications

- Glaucoma
- Prostatic hypertrophy
- Tardive dyskinesia.

Drug interactions

Anticholinergics may exacerbate dystonic reactions to L-dopa.

6.6 Migraine

5-HT is a vasoactive amine which is normally released

from platelets as blood clots and is vasoconstrictor in most parts of the body (therefore aiding haemostasis). Three main receptor subgroups have been identified, but the complicated classification of these is beyond the scope of the present chapter. The main organ-specific effects of 5-HT are:

- cardiovascular: vasoconstrictor in all sites except in skeletal muscles and heart where it is vasodilator; 5-HT is also venoconstrictor, which causes a marked cutaneous flush if blood levels are markedly raised (as with carcinoid tumours)
- gastrointestinal: increases peristalsis
- platelets: 5-HT causes platelet aggregation.

Migraine is probably caused by the abnormal release of 5-HT within intracranial blood vessels (both in meninges and brain). The underlying defect is unknown, but it involves release of 5-HT with resulting vasoconstriction; it is this which causes the typical 'aura' which may involve visual disturbance, speech abnormalities or even temporary hemiparesis. Vasodilatation, possibly caused by 5-HT depletion, then follows and it is this which is associated with the headache, which is severe, classically unilateral and often causes prostration and nausea.

Migraine is common, particularly in adolescents, is often familial and tends to decrease in frequency as age advances. Most cases show some response to simple analgesics, which should be tried first. Where these fail, attacks may be *treated* by ergotamine or sumatriptan (which are both 5-HT agonists), and where attacks are common they may be *prevented* by beta-blockers, pizotifen, tricyclics or methysergide (which is a 5-HT antagonist).

Ergotamine

Ergotamine is a naturally occurring ergot alkaloid, which is an α-adrenoceptor antagonist, and a partial agonist for 5-HT$_2$ receptors. The therapeutic benefit of ergotamine in migraine probably results from vasoconstriction, which opposes the vasodilatation responsible for the headache.

Clinical pharmacokinetics
Ergotamine may be given by inhalation, sublingually, orally, subcutaneously or i.m. The bioavailability of the non-parenteral routes is very low, probably because of presystemic metabolism. The drug is cleared mainly by hepatic metabolism, and metabolites are excreted in the bile.

Therapeutic uses
Ergotamine should be taken during the prodromal illness, before the onset of headache; taken later it is less effective. Although the drug's plasma half-life is short, its vasoconstricting effects are long lasting: thus once the maximum daily dose (about 6 mg) has been taken, no further ergotamine should be taken for 4 days.

Parenteral administration should be reserved for use in hospital. Ergotamine is inappropriate for the prophylaxis of migraine.

Adverse effects
- Arterial vasoconstriction: causing gangrene, myocardial infarction and renal failure
- Retroperitoneal fibrosis: this is rare, and complicates long-term use
- Headache: if used frequently.

Contraindications
- Vascular disease.

Drug interactions
- Beta-blockers and oral contraceptives: increased risk of vascular occlusion
- Methysergide: ergotamine doses should be reduced.

Sumatriptan

Sumatriptan is a specific 5-HT$_1$ agonist which, like ergotamine, opposes the vasodilatation responsible for the headache.

Clinical pharmacokinetics
The drug is formulated for oral and subcutaneous administration. Sumatriptan is well absorbed from both sites but is subject to presystemic metabolism when taken orally. It is cleared by hepatic metabolism to inactive derivatives.

Therapeutic uses
- Acute migraine and cluster headache.

Adverse effects
- ECG changes and chest pain after subcutaneous administration
- Drowsiness, nausea and vomiting.

Contraindications
- Ischaemic heart disease
- Uncontrolled hypertension.

Drug interactions
Because it causes drowsiness, sumatriptan should probably not be taken in combination with sedatives.

Methysergide

Methysergide is a potent, semi-synthetic 5-HT$_2$ antagonist; its prophylactic effect probably results from antagonism of platelet-derived 5-HT. Methysergide should be used with great caution under hospital supervision because of the high risk of serious adverse effects. It should be reserved for those patients with debilitating migraine who have not been helped by other drugs. Methysergide is given to prevent attacks, but therapy should be gradually withdrawn and stopped, for at lease 4 weeks, every 6 months.

Clinical pharmacokinetics

Methysergide is given orally and is well absorbed. It is cleared by both hepatic metabolism and renal excretion.

Adverse effects

- Fibrotic reactions in about 1:5000 patients: these most commonly manifest as retroperitoneal fibrosis with ureteric obstruction, but lung and pericardial fibrosis can also occur
- Vasoconstriction: may exacerbate angina.

Contraindications

- Vascular disease
- Renal impairment.

Other drugs used for migraine

Pizotifen: Pizotifen is a 5-HT antagonist used to prevent migraine attacks; in addition, it has antihistaminergic and anticholinergic effects. Pizotifen is well absorbed from the gut and cleared mainly by hepatic metabolism. It causes mild sedation and weight gain, and can cause dryness of the mouth. Pizotifen gives additive sedation if combined with alcohol or sedative drugs.

Beta-blockers and tricyclic antidepressants. These classes of drug are effective in the prophylaxis of migraine. For more detail of their pharmacology, see Chapter 3.

Self-assessment: questions

Multiple choice questions

1. Diazepam:
   a. Causes sedation which is abolished by the elimination of the drug
   b. Interacts adversely with amitryptilline
   c. Can prove useful in very anxious asthmatics during an attack
   d. Can be given orally, over prolonged periods, to prevent seizures
   e. Is a suitable choice for the sedation of outpatients undergoing endoscopy

2. Chlormethiazole:
   a. May be given to alcoholics regularly to reduce their alcohol intake
   b. Has a relatively flat dose–response curve
   c. Causes sedation which is abolished by the renal excretion of the drug
   d. May be used for status epilepticus
   e. Causes exaggerated sedation in alcohol-dependent patients

3. Carbamazepine:
   a. Is an appropriate choice to treat a patient with absence seizures (petit mal)
   b. Can be considered to be a prodrug
   c. Induces its own metabolism
   d. May be eliminated from the body after overdose using haemodialysis
   e. Potentiates the effects of warfarin

4. Sodium valproate:
   a. Is the treatment of choice for atonic seizures
   b. Induces the metabolism of warfarin
   c. Should be withdrawn if a woman is trying to become pregnant
   d. Is the anticonvulsant of choice in patients with cirrhosis
   e. Potentiates phenytoin

5. Amitriptylline:
   a. Enhances the uptake of catecholamines by the presynaptic neurone (uptake I)
   b. Can be expected to lift mood within 2 days
   c. Is contraindicated in patients with glaucoma
   d. Is free of sedative effects
   e. Is the treatment of choice for someone who has become depressed following a myocardial infarction

6. Monoamine oxidase A inhibitors:
   a. Reduce noradrenaline metabolism
   b. Reduce 5-HT metabolism
   c. Predispose to hypertensive crises
   d. Are safely combined with tricyclics in the treatment of depression
   e. Are safely combined with L-dopa

7. Chlorpromazine:
   a. Should always be combined with an anticholinergic antiparkinsonian drug
   b. Works by enhancing the effect of dopamine at D_2 receptors
   c. Often improves depressive symptoms in patients with psychosis
   d. Is the treatment of choice for confusion in the elderly
   e. Is potentiated in chronic liver disease

8. L-Dopa:
   a. Has a high oral bioavailability
   b. Should be given at higher dosage in Parkinsonism if facial tics develop
   c. Should be withdrawn without delay if the 'on–off' phenomenon develops
   d. May be combined with MAO-B inhibitors
   e. Is converted to dopamine by MAO-B

9. In the management of migraine:
   a. During an acute attack, as much ergotamine should be used as needed to abolish headache
   b. Methysergide is an alternative to ergotamine for the treatment of an attack
   c. Sumatriptan may be used in patients with ischaemic heart disease
   d. Beta-blockers can give effective prophylaxis
   e. Most patients can be managed with simple analgesics like paracetamol

Case histories

History 1

An 80-year-old woman is given diazepam to help her sleep at night. After 2 weeks, neighbours discover her in a state of self-neglect. She is taken to hospital where she is found to be somnolent and confused.

1. Why was diazepam a bad choice of drug in this case?
2. How should she be treated in hospital?

History 2

A woman with epilepsy, on phenytoin, on 200 mg per day, continues to have seizures at an unacceptable rate. The drug level is measured and found to be 30 µmol/l (therapeutic range 40–80 µmol/l), so the dose is increased to 400 mg daily. After 1 week, the patient has nystagmus and cannot walk because of ataxia.

What has happened?

History 3

> A 19-year-old man has gastroenteritis and is given metoclopramide. He develops acute torticollis (involuntary spasm of the neck muscles) 2 days later, which is very painful.

What is the likeliest diagnosis and what should be done?

History 4

> A 60-year-old woman with schizophrenia has been on haloperidol for many years, and has been well controlled. However, her doctor thinks that her control is 'slipping' as she has recently started to move very strangely: when doing nothing, her arms writhe continuously in a rather jerky but semi-purposeful way.

What is the likeliest diagnosis and what should be done?

History 5

> A patient with long-standing idiopathic Parkinsonism finds that she is no longer getting so much benefit from her L-dopa/carbidopa combination. Specifically, she finds that she is unable to rise from a chair because of stiffness well before her next dose is due.

1. What is the problem, and what should be done?

> The same patient had her dose of L-dopa increased; her Parkinsonism was improved marginally, but after a couple of months she complains that shortly after taking the drug she suffers an hour of uncontrollable facial grimacing.

2. What is the problem, and what should be done?

> The same lady develops nausea and dizziness, from an intercurrent illness, and is started on prochlorperazine.

3. What is the principal risk?

History 6

> A 40-year-old woman, who smokes cigarettes, suffers from frequent migraine headaches. She takes propranolol as prophylaxis for migraine and uses ergotamine for the treatment of acute attacks.

What adverse drug reactions and interactions are likely to occur?

History 7

> A 65-year-old childless man is given amitriptylline because of prolonged grief following the death of his wife. He is a cigarette smoker and suffers from angina pectoris. He is admitted to hospital 2 weeks later with noisy confusion. He is dehydrated, his pulse is irregular at 140 beats per minute and he is anuric.

Advance some possible causes of his problems.

Essay questions

1. Discuss the clinical pharmacology of the drugs used for the treatment of (a) status epilepticus, and (b) complex partial seizures.
2. Discuss the modes of action, disposition and adverse effects of the drugs used in the treatment of depression.
3. Predict the possible effects of chronic renal disease on response to the following drugs:
   a. phenytoin
   b. lithium.

Matching item question

Theme: The clinical pharmacology of anti-Parkinsonian drugs.
Options

A. It stimulates dopamine receptors
B. It crosses the blood–brain barrier
C. It blocks the metabolism of dopamine
D. It inhibits conversion of DOPA to dopamine in the CNS
E. It doesn't cross the blood–brain barrier
F. It blocks acetyl-choline [ACh] receptors, thereby restoring the dopamine/ACh balance
G. Because drug-induced parkinsonism results from the blocking of dopamine receptors by neuroleptics [so-called 'major tranquilizers'].
H. Because drug-induced parkinsonism results mainly from excess acetyl-cholinergic activity in the CNS.

For each of the brief case histories below choose the most appropriate answer. Each option may be used once, more than once or not at all.

i. Why is dopamine not used for idiopathic parkinsonism?
ii. Carbidopa, with which levo-DOPA is formulated, is a DOPA-decarboxylase inhibitor [it blocks the conversion of DOPA to dopamine]: so why doesn't it abolish the therapeutic effect of levo-DOPA?
iii. Why is levo-DOPA contra-indicated in drug-induced parkinsonism?
iv. How does selegiline work?

Self-assessment: answers

Multiple choice answers

1. a. **False.** Diazepam is converted to pharmacologically active metabolites which persist in the body after the parent drug has been eliminated.
   b. **True.** Amitriptylline has marked sedative effects; were diazepam taken simultaneously, the two sedatives would produce additive sedation.
   c. **False.** Diazepam may well kill asthmatics during an attack by causing respiratory depression. Anxiety in an asthmatic is appropriate and should be treated by tackling the asthma.
   d. **False.** Though diazepam can be used to stop a seizure, it has no proven preventative efficacy.
   e. **False.** Diazepam's effects are too long lived; a more appropriate choice would be midazolam.

2. a. **False.** Chlormethiazole can rapidly induce a state of dependence, compounding the patient's problem.
   b. **False.** The dose–response curve is steep, and chlormethiazole causes dangerous respiratory depression at high dose.
   c. **False.** Chlormethiazole's pharmacological effect is terminated by hepatic metabolism.
   d. **True.** Chlormethiazole is not the first-choice drug for status but can be helpful if i.v. diazepam has failed. Chlormethiazole is given as an i.v. infusion.
   e. **False.** Because of cross-tolerance between alcohol and chlormethiazole, the latter is less effective in alcohol-dependent patients, and doses need to be greater.

3. a. **False.** Carbamazepine is indicated for partial seizures; it is useful for tonic/clonic seizures, but for no other generalised seizure types.
   b. **False.** Though carbamazepine does have a pharmacologically active metabolite, the parent drug possesses anticonvulsant activity.
   c. **True.** Carbamazepine is a potent enzyme inducer, and with chronic therapy, this enhances the elimination of the drug.
   d. **True.** Though structurally similar to the tricyclic antidepressants, carbamazepine has a small VD and can be removed by dialysis (this topic is more fully covered in Ch. 6).
   e. **False.** Carbamazepine induces the metabolism of warfarin and, therefore, reduces its effects.

4. a. **True.** Atonic seizures are not common; they are characterised by sudden loss of muscle tone causing the patient to collapse. Consciousness is often retained. Valproate is the drug of first choice.
   b. **False.** Valproate is a selective enzyme inhibitor; furthermore, it does not interact with warfarin.
   c. **False.** Standard advice for women on anti-epileptic drugs is that treatment should continue during pregnancy despite the relatively small risk to the fetus.
   d. **False.** Valproate is contraindicated in patients with chronic liver disease because of the increased risk of drug-induced hepatic dysfunction.
   e. **False.** Valproate probably does not have clinically relevant effects on phenytoin.

5. a. **False.** Tricyclics block uptake I.
   b. **False.** No therapeutic response is usually seen within the first 2 weeks.
   c. **True.** The anticholinergic effects of tricyclics raise the intraocular pressure.
   d. **False.** Amitriptylline is a potent sedative and is usually given at night for this reason.
   e. **False.** Tricyclics are contraindicated immediately after a myocardial infarction because of their effects on the QT interval, and their anticholinergic effects.

6. a. **True.** MAO-A metabolises noradrenaline; MAO-B metabolises dopamine.
   b. **True.** MAO-A metabolises 5-HT.
   c. **True.** Sympathomimetics, as occur naturally in some foods and are the active ingredients in some proprietary cough mixtures, can cause severe hypertension in patients on MAO-A inhibitors.
   d. **False.** The combination of tricyclic plus an MAO-A inhibitor may cause 'malignant hyperthermia'.
   e. **False.** The combination of L-dopa plus an MAO-A inhibitor may cause severe hypertension.

7. a. **False.** Not all patients develop Parkinsonism, and there is no benefit starting therapy until they do.
   b. **False.** Neuroleptics are dopamine antagonists.
   c. **False.** Neuroleptics frequently exacerbate depression.
   d. **False.** Although neuroleptics may be indicated in organic psychosis, confusion in elderly patients is often worsened by sedative drugs.
   e. **True.** Chlorpromazine is metabolised in the liver.

8. a. **False.** L-Dopa is subject to extensive first-pass metabolism.
   b. **False.** L-Dopa may cause dyskinesias like tics.
   c. **False.** Sudden withdrawal of antiparkinsonian drugs may cause life-threatening deterioration; drugs must be withdrawn slowly in hospital.

   d. **True.** Selegiline may be combined with L-dopa to restore the clinical response to the latter where this has been lost.

   e. **False.** L-Dopa is metabolised by dopa decarboxylase.

9. a. **False.** Ergotamine is a potent vasoconstrictor and may cause severe peripheral ischaemia if recommended doses are exceeded.

   b. **False.** Methysergide is used prophylactically.

   c. **False.** Sumatriptan contraindicated in patients with ischaemic heart disease because it may exacerbate angina.

   d. **True.** But caution is needed if ergotamine is used for acute attacks.

   e. **True.** The majority of patients gain relief from paracetamol.

Case history answers

History 1

1. Diazepam itself is slowly eliminated, as are its active metabolites, and impaired hepatic or renal function slow their rate of elimination further. The elderly often have subclinical renal or hepatic impairment, and benzodiazepines accumulate causing a so-called 'hangover effect'. With continued use confusion may develop.

2. The benzodiazepine should be stopped even though confusion may initially become worse. A specific benzodiazepine antagonist such as flumazenil is indicated in respiratory failure after overdose but not in the present circumstances. Prescription of further sedative drugs, e.g. in the event of noisy confusion at night, should be avoided.

History 2

The relationship between the dose of phenytoin and its plasma concentration is not linear (as it is with most drugs): relatively small dose increases frequently lead to a large rise in blood level. Doubling the dose, as here, can cause major toxicity.

History 3

This is an involuntary movement disorder induced by the antidopaminergic actions of the drug. Acute reactions, as in this patient, are common with neuroleptics and antiemetics (see Ch. 11) and may come in the form of akathisia (inability to sit still) or acute dystonias such as torticollis (as here) or retrocollis. The last two may be painful and may compromise breathing. The pharmacological basis of the reaction is not clear, but anticholinergic drugs such as benztropine or procyclidine are indicated; as the latter may be given i.v., it is probably indicated here because of the pain. After i.v. dosing improvement should occur within about 5 minutes.

History 4

This patient's symptoms illustrate tardive dyskinesia. This complicates chronic neuroleptic use in about 40% of cases. Elderly women are the most common group affected, though it can occur in either sex and at any age. Tardive dyskinesia also complicates use of anti-dopaminergic antiemetics such as metoclopramide. The movements described are typical: so-called choreo-athetoid movements. Early recognition is advisable as neglected cases can be more difficult to treat. The current hypothesis is that there is increased sensitivity to dopamine, possibly receptor up-regulation, resulting from the chronic use of an antagonist. Most doctors would reduce the neuroleptic dose (and stop the drug if possible), even though this may worsen the dyskinesia in the short term; diazepam is often helpful to control symptoms.

History 5

1. This unfortunate patient has developed a common problem in late Parkinson's disease referred to as 'end of dose akinesia'. She may be helped by increasing the frequency of her L-dopa doses.

2. She has gone on to develop 'on–off' effects where the high concentration of L-dopa shortly after dosing induces acute diskinesia; such patients 'see-saw' between akinesia and dyskinesia with only brief spells of normal movement. This can be difficult to treat: the dose of L-dopa should probably be reduced, and a supplementary drug such as bromocriptine or selegiline started. In the worst cases, the patient may need admission to hospital to allow gradual withdrawal of all drugs, a 'drug holiday'; when reintroduced, the benefit from L-dopa is restored, but this is usually only temporary.

3. Prochlorperazine is a neuroleptic drug (though it is not used for schizophrenia) which works by blocking dopamine receptors: the patient's Parkinsonism would be made acutely worse, and this could be very serious.

History 6

This woman is at risk from atheroschlerosis caused by smoking. Both the beta-blocker propranolol (see Ch. 3) and ergotamine are vasoconstrictor and might exacerbate peripheral vascular disease. She would be at particular risk should she exceed the recommended dose of ergotamine during an attack, for its effects accumulate.

History 7

At this man's age, a degree of prostatic hypertrophy can be expected. Tricyclics have anticholinergic effects, which tend to increase the tone of the sphincter while reducing the tone of the bladder wall: this can cause acute retention of urine. His bladder should be easily palpable. Acute retention is painful and causes tachycardia and confusion. He should be catheterised and the tricyclic should be stopped. However, it sounds as if this patient either has atrial fibrillation, which may have been precipitated by the anticholinergic effects of the drug, or else multiple ectopic beats. The possibilities of myocardial infarction and of tricyclic overdose should be considered.

Essay answers

1. a. Status epilepticus (multiple seizures without recovery of consciousness in between episodes) is life-threatening because it causes hypoxia, and it may damage the brain independently of hypoxia. Diazepam (given slowly i.v.) or clonazepam (given as an i.v. infusion) are the drugs of first choice. If these fail to stop seizures, then phenytoin (given as a very slow i.v. injection) is the next choice. Deal with the modes of action and toxicity of each of these drugs.
    b. Complex partial seizures (temporal lobe seizures) respond to carbamazepine, phenytoin and sodium valproate. The modes of action and adverse effects of these should be described.
2. a. Modes of action. For the tricyclics, describe the fate of noradrenaline after release into the synaptic cleft, mention uptake 1 and uptake 2. For SSRIs, the role of blockage of the reuptake of 5-HT into the neurone is not fully understood, but 5-HT may modulate noradrenaline release. For MAO inhibitors, describe the substrates of MAO-A (noradrenaline and 5-HT) and MAO-B (dopamine). Mention that MAO inhibitors selective for MAO-A are now available.
    b. Disposition. Tricyclics are mostly well absorbed from the gut. All have large volumes of distribution (this is relevant to the overdose situation, they are not dialysable). Most are metabolised to active metabolites.
        SSRIs. Fluoxitine is well absorbed, metabolised to an equipotent metabolite and eliminated slowly. Most MAO inhibitors are well absorbed and metabolised to active derivatives.
    c. Adverse effects. Mention the antimuscarinic properties of tricyclics, which may, therefore, exacerbate glaucoma, retention of urine, constipation and tachyarrhythmias. Mention weight gain, sedation (especially amitriptylline) and idiosyncratic reactions.
        For SSRIs, mention vasculitis, anorexia and exacerbation of seizures.
        Mention weight gain, anticholinergic effects and gastrointestinal upset with MAO inhibitors. Mention the risk of hypertensive crisis with sympathomimetic compounds found in cough medicines, cheese and red wine; this is not a problem with RIMAs.
3. Chronic renal diseases may alter drug response either by changing their plasma protein binding (albumin concentrations may fall, and waste products may compete for binding sites) or by reducing their clearance. (This subject is dealt with more fully in Ch. 20.)
    a. Phenytoin is extensively bound to albumin but cleared by hepatic metabolism to inactive derivatives. Hypoalbuminaemia or uraemia cause the unbound drug fraction to rise: at a given total plasma concentration the drug, therefore, seems to be more effective and more toxic. Phenytoin doses should be reduced
    b. Lithium is a metallic ion which is distributed in body water and unbound to plasma proteins. It undergoes no metabolism but is cleared unchanged by the kidney. Renal impairment causes drug accumulation.

Matching item answers

i. E
    Levodopa crosses the blood–brain barrier, where it is metabolised to the neurotransmitter dopamine. Dopamine itself cannot easily cross the blood–brain barrier.
ii. E
    Carbidopa doesn't easily cross the blood–brain barrier, so its effects are confined to the extra-cerebral metabolism of levadopa [which is responsible for many of the drug's adverse effects].
iii. G
    It would be illogical to give levodopa in this setting. Instead, the acetylcholinergic system is antagonised using drugs like benztropine and benzhexol.
iv. C
    Selegiline is an inhibitor of the enzyme monoamine oxidase-b [MAO-b], which metabolises dopamine. MAO-a metabolises noradrenaline and 5-hydroxy-tryptamine.

Analgesics

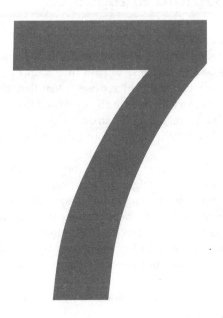

7.1 Pain

Pain is defined as 'An unpleasant sensory and emotional experience associated with actual or potential tissue damage, or described in terms of such damage'.

Somatic pain can arise from damage of any kind, to skin, joints, bone, tendons, fascia, meninges, peritoneum, gonads, pleura and teeth. Somatic pain is usually well localised; the sensory modality is conducted to the CNS along small myelinated *delta* fibres and non-myelinated *C-fibres*.

Visceral pain can arise from damage to heart, gut, and bladder, but not brain, liver, lung and spleen. Visceral pain is often poorly localised and may be *referred* to a distant site. It is not transmitted to the CNS by specific fibres but rather by changes in the rate of discharge of afferent autonomic fibres.

Neurogenic pain can result from damage to the CNS itself: such *neurogenic pain* is felt in the periphery. A classical example is damage occurring to the thalamus (e.g. from infarction) causing contralateral chronic, severe pain in the arm, leg, face or all three. Such pain can also result from disseminated sclerosis, paraplegia, syringomyelia, syphilis, or can be idiopathic as in *trigeminal neuralgia*. Neurogenic pain tends not to respond to the drugs described below: but tricyclic antidepressants or antiepileptic drugs, particularly carbamazepine, may be useful (see Ch. 6).

Analgesic drugs

Analgesics are classified according to their mode of action, into opioids, non-opioids, and non-steroidal anti-inflammatory drugs (NSAIDs). As suggested by their name, this last group has the additional therapeutic property of reducing inflammation (Ch. 9).

7.2 Opioid analgesics

Mode of action
Endogenous analgesic compounds, called *endorphins*, are released in response to pain in certain parts of the CNS. Many endorphins have been identified: they vary widely in structure but are all peptides. Opioid analgesics, which are alkaloids structurally quite different from the endorphins, are agonists at endorphin receptors.

The main receptor subtypes are μ, κ and σ. The μ-receptor causes analgesia at a supraspinal level and is also responsible for drug-induced euphoria, respiratory depression and drug dependence. κ-receptors cause analgesia at a spinal level and also induce miosis and sedation. The σ-receptors seem to have no clinically useful properties but cause dysphoria and hallucination.

With continuous exposure to opioids, larger doses are required to produce the same effects: this is called *tolerance*. Addiction is a risk if opioids are used regularly for long periods: withdrawal then causes an unpleasant, but not clinically serious, reaction (Ch. 18).

The effects of opioids on specific organs are as follows:

CNS. Opioids impair the perception of pain, both somatic and visceral. They also alter the subject's response to pain: the patient may feel 'at ease' even though pain is still perceived. This latter may in part be the result of the drug-induced *euphoria*, which is the main sensation sought by addicts (though some subjects experience unpleasant restlessness and malaise, termed *dysphoria*). *Sedation* is a dose-dependent effect, which may lead to respiratory depression. Other CNS effects include cough suppression, nausea and miosis (small pupils).

Gastrointestinal tract. Opioid receptors are present in the gut; partly by stimulation of these and partly through CNS effects, opioids cause a reduction in gut motility leading to constipation. In the biliary tree, tone may be increased, and the sphincter of Oddi may contract.

Cardiovascular system. Opioids cause peripheral arteriodilatation and venodilatation, possibly as a result of effects on the vasomotor centre in the CNS. The blood pressure may fall in subjects with reduced blood volume.

Examples and clinical pharmacokinetics
Morphine, like other members of the group, is well absorbed from i.m. and s.c. sites but is subject to extensive first-pass metabolism in the liver, if given orally. Morphine is widely distributed and crosses the blood–brain barrier readily. The drug is metabolised in the liver, mainly by glucuronidation. While it is unusual for drug conjugates, which are water-soluble, to retain pharmacological activity, morphine 6-glucuronide retains analgesic properties. The duration of analgesia after a therapeutic dose of morphine is about 4 to 6 hours.

Diamorphine is more potent than morphine, possibly because it crosses the blood–brain barrier more readily. Its pharmacokinetic properties are similar to morphine and it is metabolised in part to morphine. The duration of analgesic action of diamorphine is 4 to 6 hours.

Pethidine is a synthetic opioid with a shorter duration of action (2–4 hours) than morphine or diamorphine and a lower potency.

Codeine has a higher bioavailability than morphine but is less potent.

Buprenorphine is a synthetic opioid with both agonist and antagonist effects. It may precipitate a withdrawal reaction in opiate addicts. Its oral bioavailability is low, and buprenorphine is given either sublingually or parenterally. Buprenorphine has a long duration of action (4–8 hours) but is less potent than morphine.

Fentanyl is a potent synthetic opioid mainly used in anaesthesia.

Dextropropoxyphene is about as potent as codeine and is used in compound analgesics.

Therapeutic uses

Analgesia. Diamorphine and morphine are the most potent analgesics currently available, pethidine is less potent, while codeine and buprenorphine are the least potent. Opioids are useful for both somatic and visceral pain. They are, however, contraindicated in biliary colic (see above) and are useless against neurogenic pain. The severe visceral pain of myocardial infarction is treated with morphine or diamorphine, usually by slow intravenous injection, accompanied by an anti-emetic. The same drugs are commonly used for the somatic pain that follows major trauma, or surgery. In terminal disseminated cancer, constant-rate subcutaneous infusions can be very useful, and oral slow-release preparations are available. Pethidine is commonly used for postoperative pain relief, and is commonly given i.m. While codeine and buprenorphine are less potent than the other examples, they are more effective analgesics than non-opioids such as paracetamol.

In pulmonary oedema. Morphine or diamorphine are commonly used in this medical emergency, in combination with loop diuretics. The opioid acts partly by relieving respiratory distress and partly by reducing venous return.

Diarrhoea. Opioids can be useful in diarrhoea, though the priority is maintenance of hydration, especially in children.

Cough suppression. Opioids are used for cough suppression, especially in terminally ill subjects.

Adverse effects

- Respiratory depression: after overdose (Ch. 17), especially in patients with chronic respiratory disease
- Nausea
- Constipation.

Contraindications

- Acute or chronic respiratory disease: patients with chronic retention of CO_2 caused by type II respiratory failure (e.g. caused by chronic obstructive bronchitis) are particularly at risk
- Acute, chronic or acute-on-chronic hepatic failure: opioids, even codeine, may cause fatal coma in such patients and are absolutely contraindicated
- Head injury: opioids cause respiratory depression, which leads in turn to CO_2 retention, a cause of cerebral vasodilatation which may exacerbate intracranial hypertension.

Drug interactions

Opioids produce additive sedation when given with other sedative drugs or alcohol.

Opioid antagonists

Naloxone is the main antagonist in widespread use for opioid overdose. Opioid effects are dramatically reversed within 2 minutes of i.v. naloxone. However, naloxone has a short half-life and must sometimes be given repeatedly to those who have taken large overdoses.

7.3 Paracetamol (acetaminophen)

This is one of the most common 'over-the-counter' medications in use for mild pains. Though its mode of action seems similar to the NSAIDs, paracetamol is without anti-inflammatory effects.

Mode of action

The pathophysiology of common pains is poorly understood, but injection of certain prostaglandins induces headache and hyperalgesia. Paracetamol probably works by inhibiting the enzyme prostaglandin synthetase within the CNS. Furthermore, inhibition of prostaglandin E_2 synthesis in the hypothalamus accounts for the drug's *antipyretic* effects (though it does not lower a normal body temperature). Little inhibition of prostaglandin synthesis is seen peripherally — hence the lack of anti-inflammatory properties.

Clinical pharmacokinetics

Paracetamol is well absorbed from the gut. It is cleared mainly by the liver, to form a sulphate and a glucuronide. In overdosage (Ch. 17) these pathways become saturated, and the drug is metabolised by oxidation, forming a toxic derivative.

Therapeutic uses

- Analgesia
- Antipyretic effect.

Adverse effects

In therapeutic doses the drug is virtually without adverse effects.

7.4 Non-steroidal anti-inflammatory drugs

Aspirin and ibuprofen are available as simple analgesics without prescription in the UK. Other NSAIDs require a prescription, and are usually reserved for inflammatory conditions (see also Ch. 9).

Therapeutic uses

- Analgesia: aspirin and ibuprofen are widely used

for common pain, such as headache and dysmenorrhoea

- Analgesia in bone metastases: in the terminal care of patients with bone metastases NSAIDs can be a useful adjunct to opioids
- Antipyretic: aspirin used to be a common remedy for childhood fevers, but fears about its role in Reye's syndrome have caused a switch to paracetamol for paediatric use.

7.5 Compound analgesics

Many such drug combinations are marketed: they are often expensive, are rarely more potent than use of a single drug and are dangerous in overdosage. Examples include:

Co-proxamol: paracetamol plus dextropropoxyphene.
Co-codamol: paracetamol plus codeine.
Co-codaprin: aspirin plus codeine.

Self-assessment: questions

Multiple choice questions

1. The following are appropriate choices of drug:
   a. Diamorphine for pulmonary oedema
   b. Pethidine for biliary colic
   c. Paracetamol for arthritis
   d. Aspirin for dyspepsia
   e. Morphine for joint pain in haemophiliacs

2. Paracetamol plus dextropropoxyphene (co-proxamol):
   a. Is safe in patients with severe renal failure
   b. Is safe in patients with liver failure
   c. Is as potent an analgesic as morphine
   d. Can induce addiction
   e. If taken in overdose, may cause both CNS and hepatic dysfunction

3. In patients with painful bony metastases:
   a. Oral morphine may be used
   b. The combination of an opioid with a non-steroidal anti-inflammatory drug (NSAID) is beneficial
   c. Opioids do not produce important adverse effects in such patients
   d. When using parenteral morphine (via an infusion pump) it is important that the rate of infusion is not controlled by the patient
   e. Carbamazepine of tricyclics may have better analgesic effects than opioids

Essay question

Contrast the modes of action, disposition, clinical use and adverse effects of aspirin and paracetamol.

Matching item question

1. Theme: Prescribing the best drug.
Options

a. Paracetamol
b. Dihydrocodeine
c. Aspirin
d. Ibuprofen
e. Methysergide
f. Indomethacin

For each of the following cases prescribe the best drug for the patient. Each option may be used once, more than once or not at all.

i. A thirty year old man with unilateral headache, which was preceded by visual disturbance and is accompanied by nausea and prostration.
ii. A sixty five year old woman with osteoarthrosis and reflux oesophagitis.
iii. A young woman with tendonitis.

2. Theme: Predict the adverse effects of analgesics.
Options

a. Liver damage
b. Kidney damage
c. Gastro-intestinal bleeding
d. Coma
e. Respiratory arrest
f. Angioedema
g. Shock
h. Rash

For each of the following cases predict the most likely adverse reaction to the named drug. Each option may be used once, more than once, or not at all.

i. A fifty year old with alcoholic cirrhosis is admitted with mild confusion. He complains bitterly of severe back pain, and the doctor prescribes *dihydrocodeine*.
ii. A woman with a past history of peptic ulcer disease is given diflunisal for dysmenorrhoea.
iii. An 80 year old man with severe chronic bronchitis suffers a nasty fall and is admitted 24 hours thereafter with pneumonia. The partial pressure of oxygen in his arterial blood is found to be very low, while that of carbon dioxide is markedly elevated. He is in a great deal of pain from two broken ribs, and this is making physiotherapy very difficult. The doctor gives him an injection of *diamorphine*.

Self-assessment: answers

Multiple choice answers

1. a. **True.** Diamorphine reduces anxiety and breathlessness and is vasodilator, thereby reducing venous return.
   b. **False.** Pethidine can cause smooth muscle contraction and may exacerbate biliary colic.
   c. **False.** Paracetamol has no anti-inflammatory properties.
   d. **False.** Aspirin may exacerbate peptic ulcers and, because of its effects on clotting, may cause gastrointestinal bleeding. However, proprietary effervescent antidyspeptics may contain aspirin.
   e. **False.** Haemophilia is a life-long problem which causes repeated painful intra-articular bleeds. Frequent use of opioids may lead to addiction.

2. a. **False.** The effects of dextropropoxyphene are enhanced in renal failure; paracetamol, however, is safe.
   b. **False.** Opioids undergo extensive liver metabolism and, in the presence of hepatic failure, may induce fatal coma. The role of paracetamol in severe liver disease is more contentious; in theory the patient may be more prone to toxicity, but in practice many physicians are forced to use the drug because alternatives are usually less safe.
   c. **False.** This drug combination is probably no more potent than paracetamol alone.
   d. **True.** Dextropropoxyphene does induce dependence.
   e. **True.** Co-proxamol is particularly dangerous when taken in large doses: the opioid effects are clinically obvious (depression of consciousness and respiration) but those of the paracetamol may be missed unless drug levels are assayed.

3. a. **True.** Although morphine has a low bioavailability, it is given in a slow-release formulation which can easily be used in the community.
   b. **True.** The NSAID is often a very effective addition to the opioid.
   c. **False.** Constipation is the main problem encountered, and this is often very distressing to the dying patient. It needs to be tackled vigorously.
   d. **False.** Current practice is to give limited control of infusion rates to the patient: doses of drug are often found to be lower, and many patients find analgesia improved.
   e. **False.** Terminally ill patients may need antidepressants, but these drugs have 'analgesic' properties only in neurogenic pain.

Essay answer

Modes of action. Both inhibit prostaglandin synthe-tase, paracetamol weakly and aspirin relatively more strongly. Aspirin has anti-inflammatory, analgesic and antipyretic effects; paracetamol is analgesic and antipyretic but has no significant anti-inflammatory properties.

Disposition. Both drugs are well absorbed from the gut. Aspirin is hydrolysed, by tissue esterases, into salicylic acid and acetate. Both drugs are extensively bound to plasma proteins. Paracetamol is eliminated by hepatic metabolism (conjugation reactions at therapeutic doses; in overdose, paracetamol is oxidised to a reactive, and toxic, metabolite). Salicylate is mainly eliminated by conjugation in the liver, but a clinically relevant fraction is excreted unchanged by the kidney: renal clearance of salicylate is increased by alkalinisation of the urine.

Clinical use. Both drugs are available without prescription in the UK. Paracetamol is used to treat mild pain (including headache and dysmenorrhoea) and to lower temperature, especially in young children at risk of febrile seizures. Aspirin should not be given to young children because of the possible association with Reye's syndrome; otherwise, aspirin is used for mild pain. Few patients can tolerate the doses of aspirin required for anti-inflammatory effects, and alternative NSAIDs are usually employed. Recently, aspirin has become standard for the secondary prevention of myocardial infarction and is becoming increasingly used for the secondary prevention of non-haemorrhagic stroke.

Adverse effects. At therapeutic doses, it is unusual for paracetamol to cause adverse effects, but aspirin causes gastrointestinal bleeding even at therapeutic doses. Aspirin may exacerbate peptic ulcer. In patients with haemophilia or von Willebrand's disease, aspirin should be avoided because of its antiplatelet effects. In overdose, paracetamol causes concentration-dependent liver damage, which can develop into fulminant hepatic failure; aspirin overdose is characterised by metabolic acidosis.

Matching item answers

Problem 1
  i. A, paracetamol.
     The brief description is typical of migraine, which is usually relieved by simple analgesics. Methysergide [see chapter 6] is used for the *prevention* of migraine as a drug of final resort [because of the frequency of severe adverse effects]. Indomethacin [chapter 9] can cause headache and is not indicated in migraine. Dihydrocodeine may exacerbate nausea, as may aspirin and [to a lesser extent] ibuprofen.
  ii. A or B, paracetamol or dihydrocodeine.
     This is a difficult, but common, problem. The pain

of osteoarthitis can be very disabling, but the various NSAIDs exacerbate oesophageal reflux or peptic ulcer. Some doctors might give NSAIDs while also giving either an H_2-antagonist [e.g. ranitidine] or a proton pump inhibitor [e.g. omeprazole]. However paracetamol and dihydrocodeine, either separately or in combination, may give adequate pain relief.

iii. D, ibuprofen.
   This will be better tolerated than aspirin by most patients. Indomethacin may be used for severe cases, but adverse effects are much more common.

Problem 2

i. D, coma.
   Opioids, even mild ones, are absolutely contraindicated in patients with liver failure.

ii. C, gastrointestinal bleeding.
   Diflunisal [which you may have needed to look up in the British National Formulary] is one of the many commonly-used NSAIDs. GI bleeding is a common adverse effect.

iii. E, respiratory arrest.
   This man has type II respiratory failure [see chapter 10] in that he has carbon dioxide retention. All sedative drugs, including opioids which cause marked sedation, are contraindicated.

Drugs used in anaesthesia

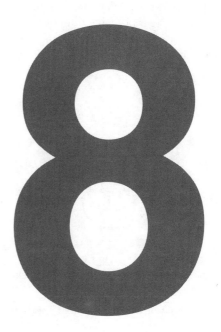

8.1 Pain prevention

While analgesics are used to control pain, anaesthetics are used to prevent it, for a limited period, during surgery. This has long been attempted with drugs, probably since prehistory: alcohol or opioids were the (unsatisfactory) mainstay until the discovery of ether, other inhaled drugs and cocaine.

Broadly, surgery may cause two types of pain: *somatic*, which is produced by cutting skin, peritoneum or other ectodermal structures; and *visceral*, which is produced by traction on organs or omentum. Local anaesthetic agents (LA) are extensively used for both minor and major procedures: instilled locally they prevent somatic pain and abolish much tactile sensation; instilled epidurally, they allow abdominal surgery, though visceral pain may not be entirely prevented. The state of general anaesthesia is complex but includes loss of consciousness, amnesia, analgesia and impairment of sensory and autonomic function. General anaesthetics (GA) may be given i.v. — most frequently for *induction* of anaesthesia — and by inhalation — for *maintenance* of anaesthesia.

Even with GA, much surgery would be technically difficult because of the high tone of abdominal and other muscles. Skeletal muscle relaxants are widely used during major surgery and during mechanical ventilation.

8.2 Local anaesthetic agents

Mode of action
At the molecular level. In the resting state, axons maintain a potential of about –90 mV across their membranes; when the membrane is stimulated sodium channels open and Na$^+$ rapidly diffuses into the cell from the higher extracellular concentration. The membrane then achieves a potential of about +44 mV. With the sodium channels shut, potassium channels open and this ion diffuses out of the cell returning the trans-

membrane potential to –90 mV. Active pumping of Na$^+$ and K$^+$ out/in returns the ionic gradients to the resting state. LAs reversibly block activated sodium channels (Fig. 33) by binding to receptors situated 'within' the channel, close to the intracellular end. LAs seem to have low affinity for the receptor when the channel is resting (Fig. 33a) and bind mainly to activated and inactivated channels (Fig. 33b,c).

LAs are mainly ionised at physiological pH, but only the unionised fraction is capable of crossing the cell membrane. This fraction may gain access to the receptor either by ionisation inside the cell followed by diffusion in aqueous solution or by diffusing through the lipids of the cell membrane in the unionised state.

At the neurone level. LAs block the conduction of impulses along axons (and other excitable membranes such as cardiac muscle, see Ch. 3). The threshold for action potential is increased, the rate of rise of the action potential is slowed and the amplitude of the action potential is decreased. These effects are more marked in rapidly firing neurones than in resting fibres because of the higher affinity of the drug for the receptor in the active state. Furthermore, the effects of LAs vary between differing neurones: in general, small diameter fibres (e.g. those carrying pain modalities) with little or no myelination are more susceptible than large extensively myelinated fibres (such as motor neurones). The sensory modalities which 'convey' pain are, therefore, particularly susceptible, as are autonomic fibres. Motor neurones and proprioceptive sensory neurones are relatively insusceptible.

Examples and clinical pharmacokinetics
Lignocaine. This is perhaps the most commonly used LA. The drug achieves local anaesthesia when applied to conjunctiva and mucous membranes. It is most often used as a local injection, in which case anaesthesia is terminated by drug absorption. Lignocaine may be formulated with adrenaline to cause local vasoconstriction and slow absorption, but gangrene results if this preparation is used for 'ring block' of a digit. Lignocaine is extensively metabolised to inactive derivatives (see also Ch. 3).

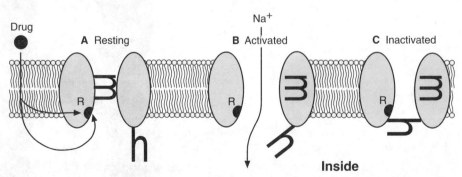

Fig. 33
Effect of local anaesthetic agents on sodium channels. **A.** When resting, the 'm' gate is shut and Na$^+$ cannot diffuse. **B.** On activation, the 'm' gate opens and the 'h' gate begins to shut. **C.** When inactivated, the 'h' gate has interrupted the influx of Na$^+$ and energy must be expended to return the channel to its resting configuration. LAs must access their receptors (R) from within the cell or from within the membrane; they have no direct access from outside the cell. LAs have greater affinity for activated and inactivated channels.

Cocaine. Cocaine is mainly used topically in ENT surgery. It need not be formulated with adrenaline because it prevents the uptake of catecholamines and, therefore, produces vasoconstriction. It is extensively metabolised.

Bupivacaine. This drug, which is more lipophilic than lignocaine, has a longer duration of action than other LAs.

Adverse effects

- CNS: in the doses used for minor local procedures, serious CNS toxicity is rare; high plasma drug concentrations, resulting from incautious or accidental i.v. use, may result in seizures
- Cardiovascular system: the antiarrhythmic and proarrhythmic effects of LAs have been described in Chapter 3.
- Allergy.

8.3 Inhaled general anaesthetic agents

Inhalation general anaesthetics (GAs) have few structural elements in common, but are all capable of inducing the state of general anaesthesia.

Mode of action

At the molecular level. The lack of structural similarity has given rise to the concept that no specific receptor is involved in their mode of action. Rather, it is thought that these lipophilic drugs interact with the lipid of the cell membrane and thereby 'distort' membrane ion channels.

At the clinical level. If anaesthesia is induced using inhalational agents, which is rarely done nowadays, patients pass through four stages:

- I: analgesia without amnesia (e.g. nitrous oxide, N_2O, is used frequently to achieve analgesia during the second stage of labour)
- II: excitation, which is accompanied by irregular breathing and amnesia (the duration of this stage is kept minimal)
- III: surgical anaesthesia, indicated by lack of blepharospasm upon brushing the eyelashes; breathing is regular in this stage
- IV: respiratory depression and hypotension leading to death unless compensated for.

The i.v. induction nowadays in use is so swift that the stages are not recognisable. However, they do indicate an important point about the action of GAs, which is that different neurones manifest different sensitivity: the dorsal horn cells of the spinal cord are particularly sensitive to inhaled GAs, whereas brainstem neurones are fairly resistant.

Examples and clinical pharmacokinetics

To achieve their effects, GAs must pass from the alveolar air into the blood and thence into the CNS. The extent and rate at which these happen depend upon:

1. The concentration (or partial pressure) of the GA in the inspired air.
2. The solubility of the GA in the blood. Drugs with high blood solubility take longer to achieve high partial pressure in the blood and vice versa: so nitrous oxide, which is relatively insoluble in blood, reaches high arterial tension quickly, whereas halothane equilibrates more slowly.
3. Pulmonary physiology. The arterial tension of highly soluble drugs, such as halothane, is very dependent on ventilation. Similarly, pulmonary blood flow changes the arterial tension of very soluble GAs. For example, in patients with low cardiac output, the reduced blood volume exposed to the drug steepens the rise in arterial tensions.

Elimination of a GA from the body is mainly by transfer from tissues to blood and from blood to alveolar air. Some hepatic metabolism also occurs to a degree that varies between drugs. The rate at which consciousness returns after ceasing drug administration depends mainly on:

- the relative solubility of the drug in CNS and blood. For example, nitrous oxide, which is relatively insoluble, is 'washed out' rapidly, whereas halothane is more soluble, and recovery takes longer
- in the case of soluble GAs, the duration of the anaesthetic is important since, after long exposure, drug may accumulate in diverse tissues and clear from them slowly.

GAs are often used in combination to minimise the 'weakness' of one particular drug (e.g. the relatively low potency of nitrous oxide) while taking full advantage of their 'strengths'.

Nitrous oxide. This drug, which is a gas at room temperature, has a rapid onset of action and recovery because of its low solubility (see above). It is not metabolised.

Halothane. Halothane, which is a volatile liquid at room temperature, is more soluble than nitrous oxide and, therefore, has slower onset and recovery rates; it is more potent than nitrous oxide. The drug is mainly eliminated via the lungs, but the fraction metabolised in the liver may be important to the adverse effect profile: the processes are complicated, but involve production of free radicals within the liver.

Isoflurane and enflurane. These drugs are volatile liquids at room temperature; their solubility and potency is somewhere between those of nitrous oxide and halothane. Enflurane undergoes a degree of hepatic metabolism, but that of isoflurane is negligible.

Adverse effects

Cardiovascular. Halothane, enflurane and isoflurane all reduce the blood pressure, mainly by lowering cardiac output, though isoflurane also reduces systemic vascular resistance. Nitrous oxide has little effect on blood pressure.

CNS. All inhaled GAs, with the exception of nitrous oxide, reduce tidal volume and depress responses to CO_2. This is not usually a practical problem as ventilation is under careful control during general anaesthesia. More of a problem is the increase in intracranial pressure induced by all GAs (nitrous oxide the least), especially in the setting of head injury.

Liver. Halothane frequently causes asymptomatic elevation of transaminases and may infrequently cause severe hepatitis.

Uterus. Halothane, isoflurane and enflurane relax uterine muscle. This is a problem if vaginal delivery is in progress but can be used therapeutically if uterine contraction needs to be inhibited.

Malignant hyperthermia. This is a rare, but potentially fatal adverse reaction to halothane, resulting from violent muscle fasciculation.

8.4 Injected general anaesthetic agents

Thiopentone

This is a barbiturate that enhances the effect of the inhibitory transmitter GABA. Thiopentone is given as an i.v. injection. The drug readily crosses the blood–brain barrier, and, at standard doses, surgical anaesthesia is achieved after the lapse of one circulation time. However, thiopentone diffuses out of the brain rapidly and is redistributed to other tissues. This distribution phase has a half-time of about 3 minutes and terminates the anaesthetic effect; the drug's elimination half-life is about 9 hours and has little bearing on the clinical effects. Elimination is mainly by hepatic metabolism.

Thiopentone is used for induction of anaesthesia. It is a potent respiratory depressant, but in the setting of controlled ventilation this is not usually an issue. Thiopentone does not increase intracranial pressure.

Propofol

The mode of action of propofol is unknown. Propofol is given i.v. and rapidly crosses the blood–brain barrier. Like thiopentone, the effect of propofol is terminated by redistribution of the drug from the brain, rather than by elimination. Propofol is an anaesthetic induction agent. The drug may cause pain on injection and may cause tremors.

Ketamine

This is an antagonist of the excitatory neurotransmitter glutamic acid. Ketamine is given i.v. and rapidly crosses the blood–brain barrier. It is eliminated by hepatic metabolism. Ketamine is not used as an induction agent. The drug produces a state called 'dissociative anaesthesia' in which the eyes remain open, and spontaneous respiration is maintained. Pain is not appreciated, and the patient is amnesic. The anaesthesia can be maintained for around 15 minutes after a slow i.v. injection, which is sufficient to allow redressing of burns or similar short-duration procedures.

Ketamine is not used much in adult medicine because there is a high incidence of unpleasant nightmares during emergence from anaesthesia; this is less of a problem with young children. The drug induces salivation, and the airway must be carefully protected. Heart rate, blood pressure and intracranial pressure are all increased.

8.5 Skeletal muscle relaxants

Somatic motor neurones terminate at specialised parts of the cell membrane of striated muscle fibres termed *motor end plates*. The transmitter acetyl choline is released into the synaptic cleft and binds to *nicotinic acetyl choline* receptors on the motor end plate. This causes the opening of cation channels in the cell membrane and depolarisation; if sufficient acetyl choline is released, then a wave of depolarisation spreads through the fibre which goes on to contract. Acetyl choline is removed from the motor end plate partly by **acetylcholinesterase**, an enzyme present in the cleft, and partly by diffusion.

Contraction of skeletal muscle can be prevented by *antagonists* of acetyl choline at the nicotinic receptor (non-depolarising drugs) and also, paradoxically, by *agonists* at the same receptor (depolarising drugs).

Non-depolarising drugs (acetyl choline antagonists)

Mode of action
These non-depolarising agents, which structurally resemble acetyl choline, are competitive antagonists at nicotinic acetyl choline receptors. During GA, they paralyse muscles capable of rapid depolarisation, such as the extra-ocular muscles, at low concentration and the diaphragm at higher concentration.

Examples and clinical pharmacokinetics
Tubocurarine. This is given i.v. after induction of anaesthesia but usually before endotracheal intubation. The drug is eliminated unchanged via the kidneys with a long terminal half-life. The effects are usually reversed using an anticholinesterase such as neostigmine (see below).

Pancuronium. This drug is mainly excreted unchanged with a shorter elimination half-life than that of tubocurarine. It has a slow onset of action, and its effects are usually reversed using an anticholinesterase.

Vecuronium and atracurium. These are short-acting drugs preferred for brief procedures.

Adverse effects
Hypotension. Many non-depolarising drugs cause histamine release with consequent vasodilatation; at higher doses they may block autonomic nicotinic receptors.

Contraindications
Non-depolarising drugs have more potent effects in patients with myasthenia gravis (Ch. 20).

Drug interactions
- GAs: enhance the effects of non-depolarising drugs
- Aminoglycosides: have nicotinic antagonist properties and may enhance non-depolarising drugs.

Depolarising drugs

Mode of action
Like the non-depolarising drugs, these compounds also resemble acetyl choline structurally. Having bound to the nicotinic receptor, they stimulate it (i.e. they are *agonists*) and sodium channels open; this causes transient muscle contraction. Thereafter, though the end plate remains depolarised, the muscle fibre membrane fails to respond, and the muscle becomes flaccid. It is also possible that the drug is able to enter activated sodium channels of the motor end plate, bind at an 'internal receptor' and thereby block further channel opening.

Succinyl choline

This is the only example in common use. It has an extremely short duration of action because it rapidly diffuses away from the end plate and is then metabolised by a plasma enzyme *butyryl cholinesterase* (also called pseudo cholinesterase). It is given i.v. and has a half-life of about 5 minutes.

Succinyl choline is used preoperatively for muscle relaxation. Because its duration of action is short, it can be useful for brief procedures; it is usually given as an i.v. infusion. Unlike non-depolarising agents, succinyl choline does not need to be reversed with neostigmine.

Adverse effects

- *Atypical butyryl cholinesterase*: about 1:2800 patients inherits a butyryl cholinesterase with markedly reduced activity; the drug should be avoided in such patients because of its markedly prolonged duration of action
- *Arrhythmias*: succinyl choline can produce life-threatening bradyarrhythmias
- *Malignant hyperthermia*: this is a rare, but potentially fatal, adverse reaction resulting from violent muscle fasciculation

- *Hyperkalaemia*: can be a problem, particularly during the anaesthesia of trauma victims.

8.6 Anticholinesterases

These act by inhibiting acetylcholinesterase, thereby prolonging the duration of acetyl choline and increasing muscle tension.

Examples and clinical pharmacokinetics
Neostigmine is a polar compound which is poorly absorbed. Its duration of action is mainly determined by the length of time it remains covalently bonded to acetylcholinesterase, rather than by pharmacokinetic processes such as elimination: doses are needed every 2 to 4 hours. Neostigmine does not readily cross the blood–brain barrier.

Pyridostigmine is similar to neostigmine but longer lasting: doses are needed every 3 to 6 hours.

Physostigmine is well absorbed from most sites and crosses the blood–brain barrier well because it is more lipid soluble than its cogeners.

Edrophonium (Tensilon) is a very short-acting anticholinesterase used in diagnostic tests: intravenous injection rapidly produces short-lived improvement of muscle weakness in myasthenia gravis.

Therapeutic uses

- Reversal of depolarising skeletal muscle relaxants
- Myasthenia gravis is an uncommon autoimmune disorder caused by autoantibodies to acetyl choline receptors. Patients have excessive muscle fatigue (because of effects on skeletal nicotinic receptors) and, if neglected, may ultimately develop respiratory failure. Neostigmine and analogues improve muscle function. Excessive doses of anticholinesterases, however, produce paradoxical muscle weakness by depolarisation: it can sometimes be difficult to tell whether the patient is on too high or too low a dose. Edrophonium is useful in this circumstance: clinical improvement with edrophonium suggests underdosage while deterioration/lack of improvement suggests overdosage
- As antidotes to anticholinergic drugs: particularly ingestion of Deadly Nightshade berries by children and overdose with tricyclic antidepressants by adults. Physostigmine is often preferable as it crosses the blood–brain barrier.

Adverse effects

- Heart: the effects of both sympathetic and parasympathetic systems are potentiated, but the parasympathetic predominates and the heart rate and stroke volume fall
- Muscular weakness: at high dosage.

Self-assessment: questions

Multiple choice questions

1. Anticholinesterases:
   a. Markedly reduce the peripheral vascular resistance
   b. Are negatively chronotropic
   c. Can cause muscle weakness in myasthenia gravis
   d. All cross the blood–brain barrier well
   e. Have their effects reversed by edrophonium

2. Local anaesthetic drugs:
   a. Diffuse across the cell membrane in their unionised (uncharged) form
   b. Bind to receptors on the external surface of the cell membrane
   c. Block sodium channels
   d. May be potentiated locally by combination with vasoconstrictor drugs
   e. Cause seizures at high plasma concentration

3. Nitrous oxide:
   a. Is very soluble in blood compared with other inhaled anaesthetics
   b. Is very soluble in brain tissue compared with other inhaled anaesthetics
   c. Works by binding to specific receptors on neurones
   d. Has potent analgesic properties
   e. Depresses respiration

4. Halothane:
   a. Is a liquid at room temperature
   b. Is eliminated from the body mainly by hepatic metabolism
   c. Lowers the cardiac output
   d. Increases the intracranial pressure
   e. Crosses the placenta

5. Succinyl choline:
   a. Is mainly metabolised in the liver
   b. Has a long duration of action
   c. Causes depolarisation of motor end plates
   d. Causes histamine release
   e. Is reversed by neostigmine

Essay question

Discuss the uses of thiopentone, nitrous oxide, halothane, pancuronium and neostigmine in general anaesthesia (GA). What are their modes of action, and adverse effects?

Self-assessment: answers

Multiple choice answers

1. a. **False.** Modest vasodilatation may occur.
   b. **True.** By opposing the breakdown of acetyl choline, these drugs increase the effects of the vagus at the SA node.
   c. **True.** Paradoxically, if too much anticholinesterase is used, patients develop weakness.
   d. **False.** Only physostigmine crosses extensively into the brain.
   e. **False.** Edrophonium is a short-acting anticholinesterase used in myasthenia gravis to distinguish weakness caused by excessive anticholinesterase dosage from that caused by the disease.

2. a. **True.** In common with all drugs, the unionised fraction is lipid soluble.
   b. **False.** The receptors are internal.
   c. **True.**
   d. **True.** Cocaine needs no vasoconstrictor, since it stimulates release of catecholamines.
   e. **True.** Especially when used i.v. (e.g. to treat arrhythmias, see Ch. 3).

3. a. **False.** Nitrous oxide is relatively insoluble.
   b. **False.** Because nitrous oxide is relatively insoluble, it has a rapid onset of action and recovery.
   c. **False.** GAs are thought to act by induction of changes to neuronal membranes.
   d. **True.**
   e. **True.** In common with all GAs.

4. a. **True.**
   b. **False.** Although halothane is partly eliminated by hepatic metabolism, this is a minor pathway, most is exhaled.
   c. **True.** It, therefore, lowers BP.
   d. **True.** A particular problem after head injury, where intracranial pressure is already raised.
   e. **True.** May cause apnoea in the neonate.

5. a. **False.** Succinyl choline is metabolised by a plasma enzyme.
   b. **False.** It acts for about half an hour in normal subjects.
   c. **True.**
   d. **False.** This is an adverse effect of the non-depolarising drugs.
   e. **False.**

Essay answer

Thiopentone is an intravenous GA agent with a very rapid onset of action and a short duration of activity; it is used for the induction of GA. Nitrous oxide and halothane are inhaled anaesthetics, used for the maintenance of GA. Pancuronium is a muscle relaxant, an essential class of drug for abdominal surgery. Neostigmine is used to terminate the effects of pancuronium.

Thiopentone is a barbiturate. Mention its effects on the GABA receptor, its steep dose–response curve and its depressant effect on respiration. Mention that its effects are terminated by distribution rather than elimination.

Describe the solubility of inhaled GAs like nitrous oxide in lipid membrane, and mention the current hypothesis that it is this property which explains their activity. Nitrous oxide has a rapid onset of action (though not enough for its pleasant use as an induction agent) and recovery. It has relatively few adverse effects and is widely used with other GA gases; however, nitrous oxide is not very potent when used alone.

Halothane has a slower onset of action and recovery than nitrous oxide, but is more potent. Halothane reduces the blood pressure and can be hepatotoxic if used repeatedly for the same patient.

Describe the mode of action of non-depolarising agents like pancuronium. Pancuronium is excreted more rapidly than tubocurarine but even so is usually reversed using an anticholinesterase.

For neostigmine describe the breakdown of acetyl choline by acetylcholinesterase in the cleft between the motor end plate and the motor neurone. Explain that this is not confined to nicotinic receptors on striated muscle but extends to nicotinic receptors of the autonomic nervous system too (parasympathetic effects predominate and the heart rate and stroke volume fall).

Drugs for arthritis

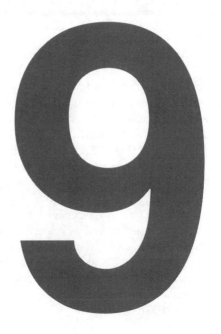

9.1 Arthritis

The term arthritis denotes joint *inflammation* (redness, local heat and loss of function) and not simply joint pain (which is termed arthralgia). The most common causes of non-suppurative arthritis are rheumatoid disease, osteoarthritis and gout. The treatment of each differs, but the non-steroidal anti-inflammatory drugs (NSAIDs) are used in all three.

Rheumatoid arthritis

Rheumatoid arthritis (RA) is the result of disordered immune function. It is a chronic inflammatory condition principally involving the joints but often also involving lung, heart, eye, blood vessels and spleen. RA causes a symmetrical polyarthritis, usually of small peripheral joints (hands, wrists and feet) though any joint may be involved. The disease has a very long course of relapses and remissions and may cause gross deformity. Treatment of RA usually involves NSAIDs and may require disease-modifying drugs (penicillamine or gold), corticosteroids (locally as injections, and systemically) and/or other immunosuppressing agents (see Ch. 15).

Osteoarthritis

Osteoarthritis (OA) is usually the result of 'wear and tear' and so often involves large, weight-bearing joints (vertebral column, hips and knees). Fractures that involve an articular surface and damage caused by other joint diseases predispose towards OA. In some patients OA is a familial trait. Treatment usually involves NSAIDs and may require local steroid injections; joint replacement may become necessary.

9.2 Non-steroidal anti-inflammatory drugs (NSAIDs)

Mode of action

At a cellular level, the inflammatory response involves the release of mediator substances that attract further inflammatory cells to the locality and increase vascular permeability. Many of the mediator substances are synthesised from phospholipid in membranes of the endoplasmic reticulum, through the intermediate substance *arachidonic acid* (Fig. 34). Corticosteroids oppose inflammation by inhibiting phospholipase A_2 (Ch. 15) whereas NSAIDs inhibit *prostaglandin synthetase* (*cyclo-oxygenase*). This enzyme is effected both in peripheral tissues and in the CNS, and NSAIDs have true anti-inflammatory properties as well as being analgesic and lowering body temperature in the presence of fever (antipyretic effects). NSAIDs also reduce the synthesis of thromboxane A_2, which promotes platelet aggregation and is vasoconstrictor (Ch. 7). Aspirin is the most potent NSAID in this regard.

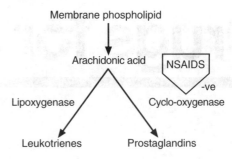

Fig. 34
Site of action of NSAIDs.

Examples and clinical pharmacokinetics

Aspirin (acetylsalicylic acid) is well absorbed from the stomach and small bowel. It is extensively bound to albumin. Aspirin is converted to salicylate, an active metabolite, in the tissues. Salicylate is partly excreted unchanged and is partly conjugated; its half-life is about 4 hours.

Ibuprofen is well absorbed and extensively metabolised in the liver. Its half-life is about 2 hours.

Naproxen has a longer half-life (about 12 hours) and is excreted as an inactive glucuronide.

Indomethacin is well absorbed and is extensively bound to plasma proteins. It is partly excreted unchanged and partly as inactive metabolites.

Therapeutic uses

Anti-inflammatory. Although aspirin is a NSAID at high dose, at usual doses its effects are confined to its analgesic and antipyretic effects; anti-inflammatory doses of aspirin are often poorly tolerated because of gastrointestinal effects. Ibuprofen too lacks significant anti-inflammatory effects at usual doses. Naproxen is used as a NSAID in the treatment of RA, OA, gout and other inflammatory conditions. Indomethacin is the most potent NSAID generally available, though it is also prone to common adverse effects. Many other structurally heterogeneous NSAIDs are available. Generally, the newer NSAIDs have fewer gastrointestinal adverse effects than aspirin and many have more convenient dosage schedules; they are, however, usually more expensive.

Antiplatelet. Aspirin reduces the risk of myocardial infarction, and of stroke in patients with symptomatic carotid atheroma.

Analgesia. This is covered in Chapter 7.

Adverse effects

- **Gastrointestinal effects:** all NSAIDs can cause peptic ulceration and bleeding; this may manifest as dyspepsia, iron-deficiency anaemia, haematemesis and melaena or ulcer perforation
- **Sodium and water retention:** a particular problem in patients with heart failure
- **Renal impairment:** all may cause papillary necrosis if taken regularly over a long period; acutely, all may reduce the glomerular filtration rate, particu-

larly when combined with certain other drugs (below)

- **Asthma** attacks may be precipitated by NSAIDs, most commonly aspirin; the mechanism may involve excess production of leukotrienes because of inhibition of prostaglandin synthetase (Fig. 34)
- **Indomethacin:** headache, dizziness and confusion are common causes of discontinuation
- **Indomethacin:** hepatitis and blood dyscrasias are rare but important adverse effects.

Contraindications

- Peptic ulcer
- Renal failure
- Haemophilia: aspirin worsens the bleeding diathesis, but ibuprofen and indomethacin are usually safe
- Asthma.

Drug interactions: aspirin

- Warfarin and other coumarin anticoagulants: these are potentiated; the interaction is mainly pharmacodynamic — through inhibition of platelet aggregation — and partly pharmacokinetic because of displacement of warfarin from protein binding
- Probenecid and sulphinpyrazone: at low dose, aspirin opposes their uricosuric effects.

Drug interactions: all NSAIDs

- Diuretics: NSAIDs cause salt retention and reduce the potency of diuretics; less commonly the combination of potent diuretic (e.g. frusemide) and a NSAID may precipitate or worsen renal impairment
- Lithium: clearance of lithium reduced
- Aminoglycosides, semi-synthetic penicillins and cephalosporins: acute renal failure may occasionally be precipitated.

9.3 Immunosuppresive drugs

Glucocorticoids

This group of drugs (see Ch. 12) is used for its anti-inflammatory properties in many diseases, including RA and gout (see below).

Methotrexate

This anticancer drug (Ch. 15) can be used as an immunosuppressant in diseases such as RA.

Azathioprine

This is a derivative of the anticancer drug 6-meraptop-urine (Ch. 15). Azathioprine is used in severe cases of RA and other inflammatory diseases (such as systemic lupus erythematosus) but is more commonly employed to prevent graft rejection (e.g. renal transplants). The chief toxicity, which is dose dependent, is bone marrow suppression.

Cyclosporin A

This drug is the mainstay of treatment to prevent graft (kidney, bone marrow, heart/lung and liver) rejection. It is given orally on a daily basis. Its adverse effects include hair growth, liver dysfunction and nephrotoxicity. In common with all drugs that suppress immunity over long periods of time, cyclosporin A increases the risk of malignancy (particularly lymphoma). Cyclosporin A does not produce much bone marrow suppression.

9.4 Rheumatoid arthritis

Drugs which slow disease progression

Although NSAIDs are the mainstay of treatment in RA, they do not alter the natural history of the disease. Gold, penicillamine and sulphasalazine slow disease progression.

Gold (sodium aurothiomalate)

The mode of action is unknown, though gold concentrates in synovial membranes and seems to inhibit lysosomal enzymes.

Sodium aurothiomalate is given as i.m injections; an oral dosage form is available but is incompletely absorbed. Gold salts accumulate in the tissues, particularly the renal tubules.

Therapeutic uses

Gold is reserved for patients with active and progressive RA who have not been controlled by more conservative means. The drug is usually given as a weekly injection until a total of 1 g has been given or a response has been seen (though this may take several months). Thereafter, the dose interval is lengthened.

Adverse effects

About one third of patients develop adverse reactions:

- Skin reactions: dermatitis, and mucosal lesions, may be severe, and is often aggravated by light
- Nephritis: proteinuria is common
- Blood dyscrasia: aplastic anaemia, thrombocytopenia and agranulocytosis may occur.

Contraindications

- Hypersensitivity
- Pregnancy
- Pre-existing blood dyscrasias.

Penicillamine

The mode of action is unknown: penicillamine induces changes in white cells and alters immune function. Penicillamine is also a chelating agent for copper. Little is known about the drug's disposition because of difficulties in assay; it is incompletely absorbed from the gut, but absorption is enhanced if the drug is taken after food.

Therapeutic uses

Penicillamine is used when RA is not controlled by more conservative means and when gold has failed. The drug is given orally for prolonged periods. Features of improvement may take months to become apparent.

Separate from its use in RA, penicillamine is used to chelate copper in Wilson's disease.

Adverse effects

Severe adverse effects occur in about 40% of patients and limit this drug's usefulness.

- Nephropathy: proteinuria is common, and some patients develop immune-complex nephritis
- Blood dyscrasia: most deaths from penicillamine result from aplastic anaemia; thrombocytopenia and agranulocytosis also occur
- Skin reactions: most common adverse effect and may respond to dose reduction
- Loss of taste: may lead to anorexia
- Autoimmune diseases: a variety of conditions including autoimmune haemolytic anaemia and thyroiditis may be seen.

Sulphasalazine

This molecule is mainly unabsorbed until it reaches the colon: microorganisms then split the molecule to produce 5-aminosalacylic acid (5ASA) and sulphapyridine, both of which are absorbed. In RA it is the sulphonamide component, not the 5ASA, which has disease-modifying activity. (See also Ch. 11). Adverse effects are common (see Ch. 11) and include severe skin reactions and blood dyscrasias.

9.5 Gout

Gout results from excess tissue levels of uric acid, which is the end product of purine metabolism. While the cause of hyperuricaemia is usually unidentifiable, it may result from metabolic diseases or occur during treatment of malignancy (where sudden necrosis of the malignant clone during chemotherapy increases purine turnover). Acute attacks of gout typically present as monoarthritis affecting a first metatarso–phalangeal joint. Any joint, apart from those of the axial skeleton, may become involved. *Treatment* of acute attacks aims to reduce the agonizing inflammation as quickly as possible, usually with NSAIDs, occasionally with colchicine; systemic steroids are sometimes required. *Prevention* of further attacks may be directed at reducing urate synthesis (using allopurinol) or at increasing its urinary excretion (using a uricosuric drug).

Colchicine

Colchicine binds to the microtubulin protein within cells of the immune system, interfering with its polymerisation and inhibiting cellular migration and division. The synthesis of leukotriene B_4, a potent chemo-attractant for neutrophils, is also inhibited by colchicine. Colchicine is rapidly absorbed from the gut and is metabolised in the liver. An intravenous formulation is also available.

Therapeutic uses

Colchicine is used only for gout and lacks other anti-inflammatory or analgesic properties. However, because of its common adverse effects (particularly diarrhoea) NSAIDs have largely supplanted it. Colchicine remains useful (a) in patients with acute gout and peptic ulcer, and (b) in patients where there is diagnostic difficulty.

Adverse effects

- Diarrhoea
- Nausea and vomiting
- Hair loss: rare
- Dose-dependent bone marrow suppression: rare with standard doses.

Uricosuric agents

Mode of action

Uric acid, being a small molecule, is filtered by the glomerulus but, in common with other relatively strong acids and bases, is subject to both reabsorption and secretion in the proximal tubule. These latter processes are active. Reabsorption predominates, so that uric acid clearance is reduced.

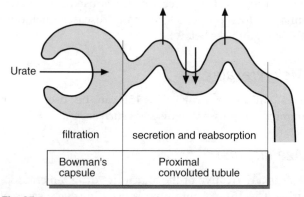

Fig. 35
Uric acid excretion.

Uricosuric drugs interfere with active tubular reabsorption and secretion of strong acids: at **low** doses they mainly inhibit **secretion**, and uric acid may be retained (and gout may worsen), but at **high** doses they inhibit **reabsorption (and are, therefore, used as prophylaxis)**. Similarly, low doses of aspirin cause renal retention of urate and may worsen gout: even though high doses of aspirin can effectively control an acute attack, the drug is avoided for this reason.

Examples and clinical pharmacokinetics
Probenecid: was developed to reduce penicillin clearance when that drug was expensive. Probenecid is well absorbed from the gut and extensively metabolised by the liver. Its elimination is impaired by both liver and renal disease.

Sulphinpyrazone: is well absorbed from the gut and eliminated partly as the parent drug and partly as metabolites; elimination is impaired by renal disease.

Therapeutic uses
The prophylaxis of acute attacks of gout and the treatment of patients with large accumulations of uric acid in their tisues (chronic tophaceous gout). Urinary levels of this relatively insoluble acid are increased, and precipitation may occur — especially in small urinary volumes and low pH.

Adverse effects

• Exacerbation of acute attacks: uricosuric drugs should not be given to treat acute gouty arthritis and should only be started 3 weeks or more after the attack. When first given, uricosurics tend to increase plasma uric acid levels and may exacerbate or precipitate gout; some physicians routinely start treatment under the 'cover' of a NSAID or colchicine
• Gastrointestinal upset
• Formation of uric acid stones in the urinary tract
• Allergic rashes.

Contraindications

• Previous urinary tract stones
• Impaired renal function
• Recent acute gout.˙

Allopurinol

Mode of action
Allopurinol inhibits the enzyme xanthine oxidase (Fig. 36), thereby interrupting purine metabolism at hypox-

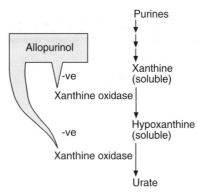

Fig. 36
The mode of action of allopurinol.

anthine — a much more soluble compound than uric acid. Hypoxanthine does not cause arthritis and is readily excreted. However, early in treatment, when uric acid is being withdrawn from tissue deposits, its plasma concentration may rise.

Clinical pharmacokinetics
Allopurinol is given orally but is incompletely absorbed. It is metabolised by xanthine oxidase to a derivative which retains the ability to inhibit the enzyme.

Therapeutic uses
Allopurinol is used for the prophylaxis of gout, particularly in patients with renal stones or renal impairment, and in those with allergy to uricosurics. It is also used during the chemotherapy of haematological malignancy to prevent renal dysfunction from the massive uric acid excretion which results from the death of the malignant clone.

Adverse effects

• Gout may be precipitated or exacerbated because of the early rise in uric acid concentration; the drug should not be used until 3 weeks after an acute attack. As with the uricosurics, some physicians start allopurinol under 'cover' from a NSAID
• Gastrointestinal effects are common
• Allergic rashes.

Drug interactions

• 6-Mercaptopurine and azathioprine: both potentiated; they are structurally similar to allopurinol and are metabolised by xanthine oxidase
• Warfarin: potentiated.

Self-assessment: questions

Multiple choice questions

1. Aspirin:
   a. Should be avoided in patients taking warfarin
   b. Commonly causes gastrointestinal bleeding
   c. Is the drug of first choice for RA
   d. Should be avoided in asthmatics
   e. Is excreted unchanged

2. Indomethacin:
   a. May be used to treat headache
   b. Causes few gastrointestinal adverse effects
   c. Is less likely than aspirin to interact adversely with warfarin
   d. Reduces the clearance of lithium
   e. Is relatively contraindicated in heart failure

Case histories

History 1

An 84-year-old woman takes a NSAID for OA; she is also on frusemide and captopril for heart failure. Following a fall, she breaks her hip and receives emergency surgery, where a prosthetic joint is implanted. The surgeons start her on ceftazidime as prophylaxis against infection. Post-operatively her renal function declines alarmingly.

What may account for her renal failure, and what should be done?

History 2

A 40-year-old man with mild hypertension presents with arthritis, which is diagnosed as gout. He takes bendrofluazide for his BP. His urea and creatinine concentrations are elevated, suggesting renal impairment.

1. It would be correct to start the following treatments:
   a. Indomethacin and allopurinol
   b. Indomethacin and probenecid
   c. Indomethacin alone, and allopurinol after 1 week
   d. Aspirin alone
   e. Allopurinol alone

He gets better from the acute attack, and remains on the thiazide for his hypertension, and allopurinol for gout prophylaxis. Over the next year he has six further bad attacks of gout.

2. In what way would you alter his drugs?
3. His renal impairment is found to be caused by glomerulonephritis: what potential drug interaction should be avoided?

Essay questions

1. Discuss the drug treatment of acute and chronic gout.
2. Discuss the drug treatment of severe, progressive rheumatoid disease.

Self-assessment: answers

Multiple choice answers

1. a. **True.** Aspirin increases the bleeding time by its effects on platelet function; furthermore, by causing gastrointestinal bleeding diatheses, all NSAIDs may induce life-threatening bleeds in patients with prolonged prothrombin times.
   b. **True.**
   c. **False.** Aspirin needs to be given at high dose to induce an anti-inflammatory effect. Many patients cannot tolerate these high doses.
   d. **True.** Aspirin may precipitate asthma in some patients; this is thought to occur through its inhibition of prostaglandin synthetase.
   e. **False.** Aspirin (acetylsalicylic acid) is hydrolysed to salicylate (phase I metabolism) and thereafter conjugates (phase II).

2. a. **False.** Indomethacin is a potent NSAID, which is not used as a simple analgesic but for its anti-inflammatory properties; indomethacin may cause headache.
   b. **False.** It is very prone to gastrointestinal effects.
   c. **True.** Although warfarin is displaced from plasma protein binding, this is not clinically important; indomethacin has less potent anti-platelet effects and interacts little with warfarin.
   d. **True.** See Chapter 6.
   e. **True.** Indomethacin may cause pronounced salt and water retention.

Case history answers

History 1

It is possible that her blood pressure may have fallen as a result of the fracture or the anaesthetic, but her drugs are probably responsible. NSAIDs, frusemide, captopril and ceftazidime are all nephrotoxic, and their effects are additive. The necessity for antibiotic prophylaxis needs to be reconsidered, the captopril should probably be stopped and the NSAID should certainly be stopped. The patient's state of hydration and the risk of withdrawal of frusemide (acute pulmonary oedema) need to be carefully considered. Specialist advice would certainly be required.

History 2

1. a. **False.**
   b. **False.**
   c. **True.**
   d. **False.**
   e. **False.**
   Most physicians would start a NSAID alone for immediate therapy: this should begin to control symptoms within 2 days, but failure to improve may necessitate addition of glucocorticoid. Aspirin would not be a good choice because it causes retention of urate when first started. Any NSAID may worsen control of hypertension, but this can be compensated for by increasing antihypertensive doses. When symptoms have resolved, a prophylactic drug may be started (under NSAID cover to begin with). Uricosurics are less effective in the presence of renal impairment, but more importantly there is the risk of worsening renal function through production of stones. Starting either allopurinol or a uricosuric alone will worsen the gout.
2. Thiazide diuretics elevate plasma urate and should be changed to an alternative drug.
3. Azathioprine is an immunosuppressant which is often used in glomerulonephritis; it is potentiated by allopurinol.

Essay answers

1. The urgent priority in acute gout is relief of symptoms using an anti-inflammatory drug. The usual choices are indomethacin, naproxen or ibuprofen, although any NSAID may be used. In the presence of peptic ulcer disease, or recent upper gastrointestinal haemorrhage, treatment becomes more difficult. Colchicine may be used but generally causes severe diarrhoea. Patients with severe gout may require systemic steroids as well as NSAID treatment.

   NSAID should be continued until the arthritis has subsided; most physicians would continue to give NSAID during the introduction of allopurinol or uricosuric therapy.

   The treatment of chronic gout aims to reduce the risk of further acute arthritis, to preserve renal function and to avoid formation of gouty tophi. Patients who have had more than one clinical attack of gout should probably be offered treatment. Uricosuric drugs (probenecid or sulphinpyrazone) increase the renal clearance of uric acid; they are contraindicated in patients with renal failure because: (a) there is the risk of uraic acid stone formation, which may further worsen renal function, and (b) uricosurics work less well in the presence of renal impairment. Allopurinol inhibits the enzyme xanthine oxidase and reduces the formation of uric acid; it is preferable in patients with renal failure (although doses should be reduced, as the risk of adverse effects increases in renal failure).

   A summary of the main adverse effects of NSAIDs, colchicine, uricosurics and allopurinol should be given.

2. The usefulness and limitations of NSAIDs should be covered: NSAIDs reduce inflammation and help symptoms but do not change the rate of disease progression. The principal adverse effects of NSAIDs should be discussed (gastrointestinal bleeding, gastrointestinal ulceration, dyspepsia, antiplatelet effects, salt retention and exacerbation of heart failure, exacerbation of renal impairment). The use of gold, penicillamine and sulphasalazine should be covered: indications, route of administration, course of therapy, adverse effects.

Respiratory disorders and hypersensitivity

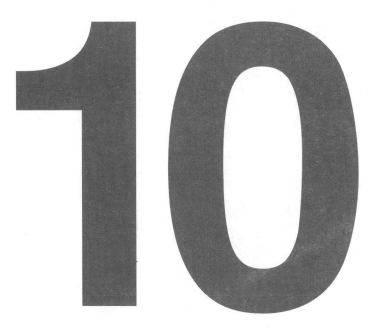

10.1 Asthma

This common condition is characterised by inflammation, which causes recurrent, reversible episodes of obstruction of small bronchi. Obstruction results from mucous membrane oedema, contraction of bronchial smooth muscle and thick mucus plugs that may obstruct the lumen altogether (Fig. 37). The principal symptoms are cough, wheeze and shortness of breath. Most attacks are mild, but asthma still kills round 2000 people in the UK annually, despite available drugs.

Asthma results from *inflammation* of the small airways, which may be caused by type I hypersensitivity The antigen (most commonly the excreta of the house dust mite, or a pollen) is usually inhaled. However, asthmatics also have attacks in response to non-allergic stimuli including exercise, emotion and viral respiratory infection; in many cases (often where symptoms have come on in later life), no allergy can be demonstrated. The role of the autonomic nervous system (Ch. 2) in reactions to increased bronchial responsiveness is not fully understood either, but it is clear that adrenergic (principally β_2-receptors) and cholinergic (muscarinic) receptors are present within bronchial smooth muscle and mucous membrane. Stimulation of β_2-receptors causes relaxation of bronchial smooth muscle, while stimulation of muscarinic receptors causes contraction.

Management of acute severe asthma

An attack of asthma in an adult should be considered severe if any of the following are present:

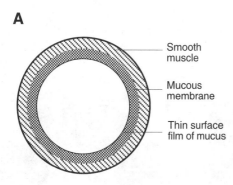

A

- Smooth muscle
- Mucous membrane
- Thin surface film of mucus

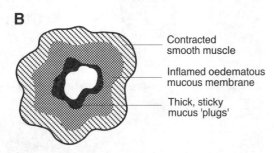

B

- Contracted smooth muscle
- Inflamed oedematous mucous membrane
- Thick, sticky mucus 'plugs'

Fig. 37
Airways obstruction in asthma. **A.** Normal airway. **B.** Airway during an asthma attack.

- the patient is unable to complete sentences in one breath
- respiratory rate is greater than 25 per minute
- heart rate is greater than 110 per minute
- peak expiratory flow rate (PEFR) is less than 50% of the predicted value.

An attack should be considered to be life threatening if any of the following features develop:

- PEFR is less than 33% of predicted value
- there is a silent chest on auscultation
- cyanosis
- Feeble respiratory effort
- bradycardia
- hypotension
- exhaustion, confusion or coma.

The patient must be admitted to hospital, and given a high concentration of O_2 to breathe. High doses of inhaled β_2-agonist should be given (as a nebuliser), and high doses of systemic steroid should start at once (since onset will be delayed). If the patient fails to improve over the next few hours, or has life-threatening features, then nebulised ipratropium and i.v. theophylline should be added. Caution should be used if the patient takes theophylline regularly. In the case of failure to improve or clinical deterioration, referral for mechanical ventilation should be considered. At all times, sedative drugs are contraindicated, and respiratory stimulants are not usually helpful. *It is important to be aware that further deterioration can occur despite initial good response to treatment.* Severe asthma is a medical emergency, and patients need careful observation even though they seem to respond rapidly.

Management of chronic asthma

Many patients can be managed with occasional use of a bronchodilator, but if this is required more than once daily, regular inhaled anti-inflammatory (steroids or disodium cromoglycate) drugs are needed. Some patients need high doses of inhaled steroids and regular use of bronchodilators. A very small minority of patients need regular oral steroid. Though β_2-agonists are well tolerated by individual patients, there has been concern about rising mortality rates among asthmatics in certain parts of the world. This seems to be linked to frequent use of high doses of β_2-agonists.

10.2 Chronic obstructive bronchitis (COB)

Chronic bronchitis is very common and is defined as a cough productive of sputum for more than 3 months in 2 consecutive years. Colonisation of the lower airways by *Haemophilus influenzae* and *Streptococcus pneumoniae* is usual. Chronic bronchitis is usually accompanied by airways obstruction, similar to asthma (sometimes indistinguishable) but usually only partly reversible. The most common cause of this syndrome is cigarette smoking. The drugs used to treat it are the same as those used for asthma, but patients with COB usually require antibiotics in addition.

10.3 Anti-inflammatory drugs

Glucocorticoids

The preferred route of administration is by inhalation: high local concentrations of steroid can then be achieved with small doses, which minimises adverse effects. *Beclomethasone* and *budesonide* are formulated for inhalation via several different devices. The mode of action, pharmacokinetics and adverse effects of steroids are dealt with in Chapter 21.

Therapeutic uses

Inhaled glucocorticoids are useful for the *prevention* of attacks by the reduction of bronchial inflammation. Inhaled steroids are not indicated for acute attacks, but systemic steroids are life-saving drugs under such circumstances.

Sodium cromoglycate

Mode of action

Cromoglycate appears to inhibit the influx of Ca^{2+} which occurs in mast cell membrane after specific antigen has reacted with surface IgE. The influx of Ca^{2+} seems to be necessary for degranulation and formation of leukotrienes and prostaglandins. Recent evidence suggests that cromoglycate also inhibits local neuronal reflexes.

Clinical pharmacokinetics

Because cromoglycate is so insoluble in water it is not absorbed when given orally. Instead, the drug is formulated as an aerosol which is inhaled; sufficient drug enters solution within the airways to achieve an effect.

Therapeutic uses

This is an anti-inflammatory drug which *prevents* asthma attacks; it is useless in the treatment of an attack. Cromoglycate reduces bronchial response to inhaled antigens and to non-specific triggers such as exercise; it is of most use in atopic asthmatics, though non-topic patients may also benefit. Used regularly, it seems to reduce inflammation and may abolish bronchial hyperreactivity. Different formulations of the drug are also used for seasonal rhinitis (hay fever). Cromoglycate is useless in COB.

Adverse effects

These result from laryngeal irritation and comprise sore throat and hoarseness of the voice.

10.4 Bronchodilators

Beta-agonists

Mode of action

The non-specific agonists adrenaline and isoprenaline have been used for asthma in the past, but have been superseded by selective β_2-agonists, which give fewer cardiac effects. See Chapter 2 for details of adrenoceptor classification and function.

Examples and clinical pharmacokinetics

Salbutamol. This drug is well absorbed when given orally but is subjected to extensive first-pass metabolism. Peak drug concentrations are achieved after about 6 hours. More usually, the drug is given as an inhaled powder or aerosol: only about 10% of the drug is inhaled, and the rest is swallowed, but it is the inhaled fraction that gives therapeutic benefit (plasma concentrations are low). If salbutamol is given as a nebulised solution, or in intermittent positive pressure breathing (IPPB) devices, then high concentrations are achieved in the lungs. Salbutamol may be given intravenously in an emergency. **The elimination half-life is short**, and the drug is mainly eliminated by metabolism.

Terbutaline. Terbutaline too is well absorbed from the gut but is subject to first-pass metabolism. The drug may be given topically as a metered-dose inhaler or as nebulised solution; in emergency a parenteral formulation is available. Terbutaline has a **long elimination half-life** of about 14 hours; it is eliminated mainly by metabolism.

Salmeterol. This is a long-acting β-agonist.

Therapeutic uses

Acute severe asthma (status asthmaticus). Nebulised β_2-agonists, such as salbutamol or terbutaline, will usually give rapid symptomatic improvement; both may be given i.v., but this is rarely necessary. Salmeterol is *not* an appropriate choice of drug in this circumstance.

Maintenance of symptomatic asthma. Most physicians recommend the use of inhaled β_2-agonists for the symptomatic relief of wheeze, cough and dyspnoea; some asthmatics need regular drugs but most take 'as required'. Salmeterol can be useful for patients with bad asthma who need regular treatment with a β_2-agonist.

Chronic obstructive bronchitis. Acute exacerbations of COB can be as severe as acute–severe asthma and require very similar management. Again β_2-agonists are used in the maintenance of those with COB, for relief of wheeze and dyspnoea.

Adverse effects

- Tachycardia: these drugs are usually well tolerated; sinus tachycardia is a common adverse effect, but does not usually necessitate a change in therapy;

symptomatic tachyarrhythmias are recorded, but are unusual

- Tremor: fine tremor is a frequent finding but is rarely severe enough to warrant changing therapy
- Change in arterial O_2: a transient fall can occur in acute–severe asthma treated with β_2-agonists.

Anticholinergics

Stimulation of the bronchi by the parasympathetic fibres of the vagus nerves causes bronchoconstriction and secretion of mucus. Muscarinic antagonists, such as *ipratropium*, oppose these effects. Ipratropium is poorly absorbed from the gut and must be used topically as an aerosol. Very little drug is absorbed systemically after topical use. Ipratropium is used both for asthma and COB. It is usually given in conjunction with a β_2-agonist.

Adverse effects

Because little of the drug is absorbed, systemic effects are few. Local absorption in the mouth may result in diminished salivary flow. Rarely, ipratropium may exacerbate glaucoma.

Theophylline

Mode of action

The mode of action is unknown; several hypotheses are advanced.

Inhibition of phosphodiesterase. Cyclic AMP is metabolised by phosphodiesterase to AMP, terminating its effects. Theophyllines inhibit phosphodiesterase and may work by increasing intracellular cyclic AMP concentrations. However, more potent phosphodiesterase inhibitors than theophyllines lack therapeutic properties.

Antagonism of the effects of adenosine. There are adenosine receptors on the surface of bronchial smooth muscle which, when stimulated, inhibit adenyl cyclase. Theophyllines may act as antagonists for adenosine. However, some theophyllines lack this property and are still potent bronchodilators.

Increased force of diaphragmatic contraction. It has recently been suggested that most of the benefit given by theophyllines is related to diaphragmatic effects, rather than bronchodilatation.

Clinical pharmacokinetics

The active drug *theophylline* is very insoluble, and various salts are more commonly used.

Aminophylline. This is the most frequently used salt. Aminophylline may be given orally, rectally or i.v. Oral absorption is good, and the drug is not subject to first-pass metabolism. Aminophylline is mainly cleared by hepatic metabolism (to inactive derivatives); the elimination half-life is short but sustained release formulations allow less frequent dosing (once or twice daily). The **therapeutic range** of theophylline is 27 to

110 µmol/l, and therapeutic drug monitoring is recommended, given the drug's adverse effects at high concentration.

Therapeutic uses

Acute severe asthma. Theophylline is not a first-choice agent but may usefully be combined with β_2-agonists. Aminophylline is usually given as a *slow* i.v. loading dose (given over about 10 min) followed by constant-rate infusion until improvement is seen. *Caution* is needed if the patient takes oral theophylline preparations, as toxicity is more likely.

Control of asthma and COB. Regular doses of oral theophylline may be needed in addition to other bronchodilators.

Adverse effects

- Seizures: at very high theophylline concentrations; seizures are most common when the drug is given i.v.
- Tachyarrhythmias: may be life-threatening and occur at high theophylline concentrations; most common when the drug is given i.v.
- Tremor
- Nausea
- Insomnia.

Drug interactions

Because theophylline is mainly cleared by biotransformation, its effects are enhanced by enzyme inhibitors and opposed by enzyme inducers (see Ch. 21). In addition, pharmacodynamic interaction with sympathomimetics causes enhanced cardiac effects.

10.5 Oxygen therapy

Oxygen therapy is indicated for hypoxaemic patients, those in shock and in carbon monoxide poisoning. Where hypoxaemia is accompanied by normal or low partial pressure of CO_2 (type I failure), the inspired oxygen concentration should be as high as is needed to normalise the arterial partial pressure. Oxygen masks deliver up to 80%, depending on mask design and flow rate, while nasal cannulae will deliver up to 35%. In adult respiratory distress syndrome, even 80% O_2 will often be inadequate, in which case positive-pressure ventilation is needed. In acute type II failure, high inspired oxygen concentrations worsen CO_2 retention, cause acidosis and may lead to death. In this circumstance, 24 to 28% inspired O_2 is usually recommended; if the patient remains unacceptably hypoxaemic, then respiratory stimulants (or ventilation) may be considered.

Chronically hypoxaemic patients benefit from long-term O_2, which should be breathed for more than 15 hours of each day. Such 'domicillary oxygen' can be delivered as cylinders, or by using more cost-effective oxygen concentrators.

10.6 Respiratory stimulants

Respiratory failure is defined as an arterial partial pressure of O_2 less than 8.0 kPa while breathing air at sea level; in type I respiratory failure, the partial pressure of CO_2 is normal, but in type II failure it is elevated.

Type I failure is commonly seen in severe pneumonia, adult respiratory distress syndrome, pulmonary oedema and acute severe asthma. It results from ventilation/perfusion mismatch and is appropriately treated with *high* concentrations of inspired O_2 or by intermittent positive-pressure ventilation in the severest cases.

Type II failure is often caused by hypoventilation and may result acutely from drug overdose or stroke; COB is frequently complicated by type II failure, typically during bacterial lower respiratory tract infections. Respiratory stimulants can be helpful in the acute management of infective exacerbations of COB complicated by type II failure. Bronchodilators, broad-spectrum antibiotics and physiotherapy should all continue while the respiratory stimulant is in use.

Doxapram is the only drug in regular use. It produces a concentration-related increase in neuronal activity in the respiratory centre; this causes tidal volume to rise, partial pressure of O_2 to rise and that of CO_2 to fall. Though doxapram is absorbed from the gut, it is given by i.v. infusion in clinical practice. The drug is eliminated by hepatic metabolism and has a short half-life. One of the metabolites of doxapram has pharmacological activity. Doxapram is appropriate for short-term support in type II respiratory failure; however, where this occurs as a result of drug overdose, mechanical ventilation is preferable. The benefit achieved by doxapram is short lived and the drug should be regarded as 'buying time' to allow more fundamental problems, such as infection, to be addressed. At high doses, doxapram may induce seizures.

10.7 Hypersensitivity

Hypersensitivity can be classified into four groups based on the response of the immune system.

Type I (immediate) (Fig. 38)

Drugs are often too small to function as antigens, but they may be capable of binding to protein forming an antigenic complex: the drug is then termed a hapten. Exposure stimulates production of antigen-specific IgE antibodies by plasma cells and these become attached to the membrane of mast cells and basophils. Repeat exposure results in recognition of the antigenic drug–protein complex by IgE, and the release by the mast cells and basophils of preformed mediator substances (stored in granules) and the rapid synthesis of others. Preformed mediators include histamine, kinins and 5-HT; leukotrienes and prostaglandins are synthesised from membrane phospholipid at the time of mast cell stimulation. The net effects of the mediators are mucosal inflammation, increased capillary leakiness, secretion of mucus and contraction of smooth muscle.

Drugs commonly producing type I reactions are *penicillins* and *cephalosporins*.

Clinical features

- **Anaphylaxis:** a rare, but life-threatening, adverse drug reaction comprising shock (low blood pressure caused by venodilatation) and bronchospasm
- **Asthma:** is common, may be life threatening (see above) and may be caused by drug allergy
- **Angioedema:** oedema of the face and pharynx, which may cause asphyxia
- **Rhinitis/conjunctivitis (Hay fever):** commonly the result of exposure to environmental allergens such as pollen; trivial but common
- **Eczema:** an itchy rash which may be caused by allergens including drugs.

Type II (autoimmunity)

Drugs may induce immune responses to 'self'. The mechanisms are incompletely understood but include: (a) covalent binding of the drug to a cell surface, so that the cell becomes haptenated; (b) binding to a circulating protein, producing a hapten that resembles a cell antigen; and (c) alteration of cell metabolism so that cellular antigens change and become recognised by the immune system as foreign. In all cases the immune system is activated, and cell damage occurs.

Clinical features

Systemic lupus erythematosus (SLE): SLE is a common autoimmune disease with features that include arthritis, vasculitis (inflamed small blood vessels), nephritis and rashes. *Hydralazine* (Ch. 3) *isoniazid* (Ch. 13) and *procainamide* can induce an SLE-like syndrome; this is usually reversible when the drug is stopped.

Blood dyscrasias. *Alpha-methyl-dopa* can induce auto-antibodies towards erythrocytes causing haemolytic anaemia. Similarly, *quinidine* (Ch. 3) can cause thrombocytopenia. Some drugs may induce auto-immunity towards bone marrow precursor cells causing pancytopenia (in which all cell series are affected) or agranulocytosis (in which the granulocyte series is affected): these syndromes may prove irreversible when the drug is stopped and can be fatal.

Type III (immune-complex)

This form of hypersensitivity is characterised by the formation in the circulation of large antigen–antibody complexes, and their subsequent deposition on basement membranes. Attraction of cells of the immune system and local activation of complement cause tissue damage.

Drugs commonly producing the type of reaction are *penicillins* and *sulphonamides*.

Clinical features

- **Serum sickness:** commonly seen with incompatible blood transfusions; comprises urticaria (hives), fever and arthralgia
- **Vasculitis:** may cause severe, occasionally life-threatening, skin reactions (e.g. erythema multiforme) and impaired renal function.

Type IV (delayed)

Whereas type I responses are seen within minutes of exposure, and those of type II and III usually within hours, type IV responses can take days to evolve. Antigens have to be phagocytosed by macrophages, transported to local lymph nodes and presented to lymphocytes; the lymphocyte clone must then proliferate and travel to the site of antigen delivery before inflammation begins. The classical example of a class IV reaction is that towards tuberculin injected into the skin as a Mantoux test, where inflammation takes 72 hours to develop. Contact dermatitis is the only common adverse drug reaction of this class; it may result from many skin preparations and from nickel salts.

Treatment of anaphylaxis/angioedema

The suspected drug should be stopped (mainly relevant to i.v. infusions), and the airway maintained. If the blood pressure is low, then the feet should be elevated to increase venous return. Adrenaline should be given i.m. at once and repeated every 10 minutes if necessary (judged by response of blood pressure). Histamine H_1 antagonists (see below) should be given parenterally. Glucocorticoid should be given, but is of secondary importance because of the delay in its onset of action.

Treatment of seasonal rhinitis

An atopic individual is one prone to seasonal rhinitis/conjunctivitis, asthma and eczema. Seasonal rhinitis is common and, though not medically serious, is a frequent cause of time off school and work. The classical pathogenesis is illustrated in Figure 38. Symptoms are maximal in the summer months when pollen counts are high and comprise rhinorrhoea, sneezing and sore eyes. Treatment is with systemic antihistamines and topical sodium cromoglycate and steroids.

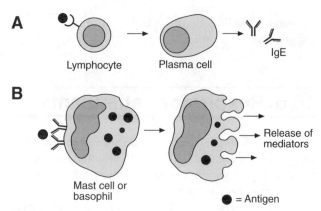

Fig. 38
Type I hypersensitivity. **A.** First exposure. **B.** Re-exposure.

Histamine type I receptor antagonists

As in asthma, histamine is one of the mediators released by activated mast cells. There are at least two classes of histamine receptor: those on mucus-secreting cells and capillaries in the mucous membranes of the upper airways are designated H_1 receptors, and those on gastric oxyntic cells are H_2 (see Ch. 2). Stimulation of H_1 receptors causes vasodilatation, increased capillary leakiness and mucus secretion. Competitive antagonists oppose these effects.

Examples and clinical pharmacokinetics

Chlorpheniramine. This is well absorbed from the gut, but subjected to variable first-pass metabolism. Chlorpheniramine readily crosses the blood–brain barrier. The drug is eliminated 50% as metabolites and 50% as the unchanged drug. The half-life is about 15 hours.

Terfenadine. The drug's clinical effects are the result of an active metabolite. Unlike chlorpheniramine, terfenadine and its active derivative do not readily cross the blood–brain barrier.

Therapeutic uses

These drugs are used for seasonal rhinitis and other allergic reactions including urticaria and angioedema. If a sedative effect is required, e.g. in the management of a child with sleep disturbance because of urticaria, then a drug like chlorpheniramine is preferred. More usually sedation is an undesirable effect, because it impairs skills such as driving and the use of machinery; under these circumstances a drug like terfenadine, which produces less sedation, is indicated.

Adverse effects

- Sedation: patients should be warned not to combine their antihistamine with alcohol, and not to drive if drowsy
- Antimuscarinic effects: many antihistamines have antimuscarinic properties and may cause dry mouth, exacerbation of glaucoma and urinary retention.

Self-assessment: questions

Multiple choice questions

1. Salbutamol:
   a. Takes about 1 hour to produce bronchodilatation
   b. Is an agonist at B_1-receptors
   c. Should be stopped if it causes tremor
   d. Must be taken regularly
   e. May be valuable for acute left ventricular failure

2. Ipratropium:
   a. Is a nicotinic antagonist
   b. May cause intraocular pressure to rise
   c. Is of no value in the treatment of acute severe asthma
   d. Causes a dry mouth
   e. Encourages oral candidiasis

3. The following statements are true:
   a. Doxapram is preferable to mechanical ventilation for young asthmatics with severe respiratory failure
   b. In acute severe asthma, the inhaled O_2 concentration should be low (24 to 28%)
   c. Ciprofloxacin has no effect on the disposition of theophylline
   d. Glucocorticoids potentiate the effects of salbutamol
   e. Antihistamines have no place in the treatment of acute severe asthma

4. Inhaled sodium cromoglycate:
   a. Is beneficial in chronic bronchitis
   b. Is beneficial in acute severe asthma
   c. May cause hoarseness
   d. Is beneficial in allergic conjunctivitis
   e. Is anti-inflammatory

5. Drug hypersensitivity reactions:
   a. May involve more than one hypersensitivity mechanism
   b. May cause renal failure
   c. Should always be treated with systemic steroids
   d. May cause joint pain
   e. Usually occur upon first drug exposure

6. Histamine H_1 antagonists:
   a. Have a major role in the treatment of asthma
   b. Have a major role in the prevention of asthma
   c. Should not be combined with alcohol
   d. Have a major role in the treatment of anaphylaxis
   e. May cause dyskinesia

Case histories

History 1

A 20-year-old non-smoker with severe asthma presents as an emergency. She is given nebulised salbutamol, i.v. hydrocortisone and i.v. ampicillin, and nursed in a side room of the observation ward overnight. Later that night her breathing is no better and she is exhausted and sweaty but cannot sleep because of breathlessness. The doctor gives her temazepam because of her obvious agitation and insomnia.

What is likely to happen next? What comments do you have on her management?

History 2

A 50-year-old smoker with COB takes salbutamol, ipratropium and theophylline. He presents to his doctor with an infective exacerbation of his bronchitis; as he is allergic to penicillin the doctor starts erythromycin.

What is the potential risk?

History 3

A woman takes cotrimoxazole for a urinary tract infection. On the third day she feels unwell and shivery and complains of joint pains; subsequently she loses consciousness briefly. In hospital she is found to have a temperature of 38°C and lymph node enlargement. A diagnosis of bacteraemia is made and the cotrimoxazole is continued.

1. What alternative diagnosis should have been considered?

On the fourth day she is very unwell and develops a generalised rash plus ulceration of her buccal mucosa.

2. What should be done?

Essay question

Describe the modes of action, adverse effects and clinical use of drugs employed in the management of chronic asthma.

Self-assessment: answers

Multiple choice answers

1. a. **False.** The effect is almost immediate.
   b. **True.** Although salbutamol has greater affinity for β_2-receptors, β_1-receptors are stimulated especially at high drug concentration. This may lead to tachycardia.
   c. **False.** Tremor is common but rarely bad enough for drug withdrawal.
   d. **False.** Salbutamol is usually taken when needed for wheeze and dyspnoea.
   e. **True.** Given i.v. salbutamol induces marked vasodilatation (β_2) as well as bronchodilatation. It is not a first-choice drug for LVF but can be useful.

2. a. **False.** It is a muscarinic antagonist.
   b. **True.** This may result from systemically absorbed drug, but it is more likely that part of the aerosol reaches the conjunctiva and is absorbed locally. Antimuscarinics cause the pupil to dilate (mydriasis) and this may occlude entry to the canal of Schlemm; this is only relevant if the patient has closed-angle glaucoma.
   c. **False.** See the therapeutic overview at the start of this chapter.
   d. **True.** Like atropine.
   e. **False.** Inhaled steroids do this.

3. a. **False.** Doxapram is occasionally useful in patients with type II respiratory failure and allows inhaled O_2 concentrations to be kept high without worsening hypercapnia. Young asthmatics with severe respiratory failure will rarely benefit from doxapram, and its use will waste valuable time: such patients need to be ventilated.
   b. **False.** Oxygen concentrations should be high (40%) to try to correct hypoxia; caution is only needed in patients with chronic type II respiratory failure. Blood gases should be measured in all cases of severe respiratory distress to help resolve this issue.
   c. **False.** Ciprofloxacin (Ch. 13) is an enzyme inhibitor and reduces the clearance of theophylline.
   d. **True.** Glucocorticoids interact with β_2-agonists pharmacodynamically, by up-regulating the expression of receptors.
   e. **True.** Their use confers no additional benefit.

4. a. **False.** Chronic bronchitis is secondary to mucosal damage, usually from smoking, and exacerbations are caused by infection.
   b. **False.** Cromoglycate is only of prophylactic value.
   c. **True.**

   d. **True.**
   e. **True.** Though the exact mode of action is unclear.

5. a. **True.** The division into types I, II, III and IV hypersensitivity is convenient, but adverse reactions can involve more than one mechanism.
   b. **True.** Drug allergy may cause renal damage by inducing vasculitis or 'interstitial nephritis'.
   c. **False.** Systemic steroids may be needed for life-threatening disease, but most drug reactions settle quickly upon withdrawal of the drug.
   d. **True.** Arthralgia and arthritis may both be a consequence of types II or III hypersensitivity.
   e. **False.** Previous exposure is usually required.

6. a. **False.**
   b. **False.** Antihistamines are of little use in either setting.
   c. **True.** Antihistamines are sedative.
   d. **True.** After adrenaline has been given subcutaneously, an antihistamine, such as chlorpheniramine, should be given i.v.
   e. **True.** This is not a common adverse reaction, but is well documented.

Case history answers

History 1

This patient has been very badly managed and may die because of the sedative. She was correctly given a β_2-agonist and early systemic steroid, but someone as ill as this ought to have been admitted and not nursed in a side room of the observation ward. Antibiotics were not required. Exhaustion and sweating are features of life-threatening disease, and sedatives are absolutely contraindicated.

History 2

Erythromycin is an inhibitor of drug-metabolising enzymes and potentiates theophylline: drug levels will rise. Commonly this induces nausea, headache and insomnia; arrhythmias and seizures are less common but more serious.

History 3

1. Cotrimoxazole is a compound preparation of trimethoprim and sulphamethoxazole. Women may suffer urinary tract infections frequently and cotrimoxazole is a common prescription; sensitisation to the sulphonamide is therefore very likely. Although this woman did not initially have a rash,

hypersensitivity should have been considered — particularly in view of the arthralgia. Her loss of consciousness was probably simple syncope.

2. Continuation of the drug has worsened her condition, and it now sounds as if she is developing a severe skin reaction, like erythema multiforme. Cotrimoxazole should be stopped, and systemic steroids are indicated.

Essay answer

In very mild cases, occasional doses of inhaled β_2-agonist may be sufficient. If this is needed more than once daily, then an anti-inflammatory drug should be given regularly. In adults, inhaled steroid is probably the drug of first choice, but disodium cromoglycate is preferred as drug of first choice in children. If asthma is not adequately controlled by low-dose inhaled steroid, then doses should be increased (high-dose aerosols and other delivery systems are available). Regular oral steroids are reserved for the most severely compromised patient. Aminophylline (oral) and ipratropium bromide (inhaler) may be needed in addition by some patients to control symptoms.

This question, therefore, calls for the above overview, plus a summary of the clinical pharmacology of inhaled B_2-agonists, cromoglycate, ipratropium, inhaled and oral steroids and aminophylline.

Drugs and the gastrointestinal system

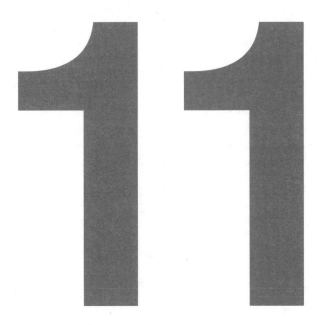

11.1 Peptic ulcer disease

Peptic ulcers (gastric and duodenal) are common. Their aetiology is not yet completely certain. There are two main identified associations: that with *Helicobacter sp.* infection and that with the use of NSAIDs. Smoking increases the risks of developing peptic ulcer disease and the difficulties of healing it.

Helicobacter pylori

Duodenal ulcers are usually associated with infection with *Helicobacter pylori*. *H. pylori* may colonise the antrum of the stomach, where it protects itself from destruction by acid by secreting a urease enzyme, which breaks down urea to ammonia. In this way, it surrounds itself with an alkaline microenvironment. Duodenal mucosa may also be colonised by *H. pylori* at a later stage. *H. pylori* could lead to the formation of duodenal ulcers: firstly, by preventing the feedback loop which normally balances acid and gastrin secretion, so that fasting gastrin and hence acid production is increased; secondly, by production of exotoxins that could directly damage gastric cells (Fig. 39). Duodenal ulcers are probably the result of local damage to the mucosa so that it is no longer able to resist the increased acid levels. The role of *H. pylori* in gastric ulcers is thought to be similar.

Drugs that block acid secretion may allow the ulcer to heal, but *H. pylori* persists and relapse is frequent (about 90% at 12 months). Treatment to eradicate *H. pylori* reduces the recurrence rate dramatically.

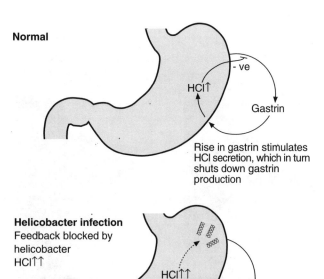

Normal

HCl↑

- ve

Gastrin

Rise in gastrin stimulates HCl secretion, which in turn shuts down gastrin production

Helicobacter infection
Feedback blocked by helicobacter
HCl↑↑

HCl↑↑

Gastrin↑

Duodenal ulcer

Fig. 39
Helicobacter in peptic ulcer disease.

A rare cause of severe peptic ulceration is a gastrin-secreting tumour (usually but not always benign) which stimulates maximal gastric acid secretion (Zollinger–Ellison syndrome).

Regimens for *Helicobacter* eradication
These are still under extensive study and the best regimen is not yet clear. These two are widely used:

1. Bismuth based: usually *chelated bismuth* and two antibiotics (metronidazole or tinidazole, and either amoxycillin or tetracycline, all in high doses).
2. Omeprazole based: usually high-dose omeprazole and one antibiotic (either amoxycillin or clarithro-mycin) or two antibiotics (amoxycillin and metro-nidazole).

NSAIDs

These may cause peptic ulcer (especially gastric) by de-creasing local prostaglandin secretion in the gastric mucosa and hence mucosal blood flow, mucus secre-tion and other protective factors. This may occur regardless of the route of administration of the NSAID. Many NSAIDs may also have a direct irritant effect on the gastric mucosa.

Appropriate treatment is withdrawal of the NSAID if possible and if necessary, antisecretory drugs (see below), or the prostaglandin analogue *misoprostol* may be used.

Control of acid secretion in the stomach

External controls include the vagus nerve secreting acetyl choline, histamine type II receptors and gastrin secreted by the antrum of the stomach: all of these mechanisms act ultimately via the proton pump (Fig. 40). Acid secretion is also stimulated by prostaglandin receptors on the luminal surface of the cell.

Acid-modifying drugs

Antacids

Antacids are weak alkali which simply neutralise the acid secreted by the parietal cells. They are, therefore, effective at relieving symptoms caused by excessive acid secretion.

Aluminium hydroxide or magnesium trisilicate are not absorbed and so cause no systemic effects. They may have local effects within the gastrointestinal tract, e.g. aluminium salts cause constipation, while magnesium salts cause diarrhoea. They may also reduce the absorption of other drugs, such as tetracyclines or digoxin. They are used mainly for symptom relief.

Sodium bicarbonate is sometimes taken as a popular home remedy for dyspepsia. It is not recommended because it is absorbed and if used in large amounts can cause systemic alkalosis.

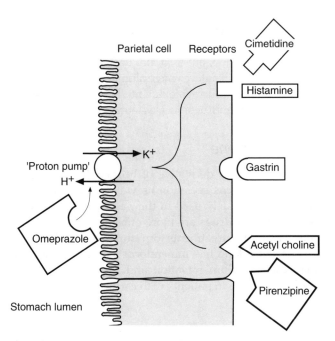

Fig. 40
The pharmacology of acid secretion.

Histamine receptor antagonists

Acid secretion is promoted by histamine receptors (type 2) on the parietal cells. Antagonists at H_2 receptors competitively antagonise the effects of histamine and so decrease acid secretion, especially at night and fasting, and to a lesser extent after food. This is sufficient to allow healing of gastric or duodenal ulcers.

Cimetidine and ranitidine are both well absorbed after oral administration, but both can also be given intravenously. They are excreted unchanged by the kidney.

Therapeutic uses

Antagonists at H_2 receptors are effective at reducing acid secretion and healing almost all duodenal ulcers after 4–8 weeks. Gastric ulcers heal more slowly and may require higher doses for longer. Because of the high relapse rate after such antisecretory therapy, many patients take H_2 receptor antagonists indefinitely, or in repeated courses. These drugs are also effective in reflux oesophagitis (see below), but here long-term therapy is often necessary. They are often used, largely inappropriately, simply for symptom relief in many patients who have dyspepsia without any clear organic lesion.

Adverse effects

Cimetidine has weak antiandrogen effects and occasionally causes gynaecomastia in long-term use. This is less common with ranitidine. Either may cause confusion and drowsiness in the elderly.

Interactions

Cimetidine inhibits drug-metabolising enzymes in the liver and may increase the effects and toxicity of many drugs (see Ch. 17).

Proton pump inhibitors

The H^+/K^+-ATPase proton pump/enzyme is irreversibly inhibited by these drugs, and so acid production ceases. Acid secretion can only resume when new enzyme has been formed.

Omeprazole is metabolised by the liver. Because of the irreversible inhibition of the proton pump, its duration of action is considerably longer than its half-life and omeprazole is usually administered once per day.

Therapeutic uses

Omeprazole is the most effective antisecretory drug, used to treat peptic ulcers that have failed to respond to H_2 receptor antagonists, where its rate of healing is faster but the relapse rate is the same. It is also very effective in treating severe reflux erosive oesophagitis, where prolonged therapy is often necessary. It is used to treat the Zollinger–Ellison syndrome, which is caused by a gastrin-secreting tumour causing excessive acid secretion and severe ulceration.

Adverse effects

- Headache
- Nausea, vomiting and diarrhoea.

Interactions

Omeprazole can inhibit some hepatic drug-metabolising enzymes.

Anticholinergic drugs

Acid secretion is promoted by acetyl choline release from parasympathetic vagal nerve endings. The receptors are muscarinic. Anticholinergic drugs can decrease acid secretion.

Pirenzipine is a muscarinic receptor antagonist, relatively selective for acid secretion. It can be used to decrease acid secretion and heal ulcers. It is slower to act than the H_2 receptor antagonists and has more adverse effects with no improvement in relapse rate; it is relatively little used. Although selective, pirenzipine may still cause some typical anticholinergic adverse effects, such as dry mouth, constipation, urinary retention, etc.

Prostaglandin analogues

Prostaglandin E_1 may exert two separate actions in the stomach; firstly, it decreases acid secretion by an action on a receptor on the surface of the parietal cell; secondly, it may have a cytoprotective effect, which is not well understood but which involves increased mucosal blood flow and increased mucus and duodenal bicarbonate secretion.

Misoprostol is an analogue of PGE_1 with a half-life of 2 hours. It is well absorbed and is metabolised to active metabolites.

Therapeutic uses

The antisecretory effect allows healing of peptic ulcers, but this is no better than H_2 receptor antagonists and misoprostol has more adverse effects. Misoprostol may have a particular role in the treatment and prophylaxis of ulcers caused by NSAIDs, and this is its main use. Prophylactic therapy may be advisable in patients at high risk (e.g. those who require a NSAID despite a previous history of peptic ulcer disease); its routine use in all patients taking NSAIDs is not justified.

Contraindication. In pregnant women it may cause uterine contractions and miscarriages.

Adverse effects

- Crampy abdominal pains
- Diarrhoea.

Drugs with no effect on acid secretion

These drugs are believed to form a protective coating over the ulcer crater and allow healing to occur underneath. They may also have a separate action in stimulating local prostaglandin release.

Chelated bismuth

This drug was used to treat peptic ulcer disease for many years, but was displaced by the H_2 receptor antagonists since they were equally effective and more pleasant to take. Later, its role in treating *H. pylori* in peptic ulcers was appreciated (see above). Chelated bismuth is now known to have antihelicobacter effects, especially when used with antibiotics. Chelated bismuth also has an action in protecting the ulcer crater and allowing healing. It is given orally and a small quantity is absorbed; this is later excreted through the kidney.

Therapeutic uses

Treatment of peptic ulcer disease either alone for 6 weeks to heal the ulcer or for a 2-week course with antibiotics to eradicate helicobacter and reduce the recurrence rate of peptic ulcer disease.

Adverse effects

- Metallic taste
- Blackening of faeces
- Encephalopathy, if used in high doses for prolonged periods; bismuth should not be used repeatedly or for more than 2 months at a time.

Sucralfate

Sucralfate is an aluminium salt of sucrose. It acts locally and is not absorbed systemically. It is used to treat peptic ulcers and has healing rates similar to those for the H_2 receptor antagonists. It is less popular because it has to be taken several times per day. The only adverse effect of note is constipation, but it should be avoided in patients with chronic renal failure where aluminium accumulation can be a problem. Sucralfate can interfere with the absorption of some other drugs, such as tetracyclines.

Carbenoxolone

Carbenoxolone is a derivative of licorice. It may stimulate gastric mucus secretion as well as protecting the ulcer. It was widely used in the past but less so today because newer drugs are more effective and less toxic. It is also used in treatments for reflux oesophagitis.

Carbenoxolone has mineralocorticocoid effects and may cause sodium retention and hypokalaemia; this could be serious in patients with cardiac failure.

11.2 Gastrooesophageal reflux

Gastric contents may regurgitate into the oesophagus in some patients with an incompetent gastro-oesophageal sphincter, causing heartburn or severe pain. In severe cases, complications such as erosions, bleeding and stricture may occur. Management involves general measures (weight loss if obese, avoiding tight clothes around the waist, avoiding stooping, elevating the head of the bed to reduce nocturnal reflux), and often drug therapy.

Antacids: particularly antacids combined with alginate, which coats the oesophagus and reduces the contact with acid.

Antisecretory drugs: high dose H_2 receptor antagonists are used but are generally less successful than in peptic ulcer disease; long-term therapy is usually necessary. *Omeprazole* is highly effective in this condition, and this is its main use. Long-term use may be necessary in some patients.

Prokinetic drugs. *Metoclopramide and domperidone* are discussed under antiemetics (see below) but both increase lower oesophageal sphincter pressure and increase gastric clearance, in addition to their central effects.

Cisapride promotes gastrointestinal motility and increases lower oesophageal pressure by causing acetyl choline release from the nerve endings of the myenteric plexus. It is well absorbed and metabolised in the liver with a short half-life. It may cause diarrhoea.

11.3 Nausea and vomiting

These are common non-specific features of disease or drug toxicity and the cause should be diagnosed and treated where possible. Vomiting is the result of activation of the vomiting centre in the brainstem, mainly via the vagus nerve. The vomiting centre is influenced by the vestibular apparatus, by the cerebral cortex, by afferents from the gastrointestinal tract and by the chemoreceptor trigger zone, through muscarinic and histamine (H_1) receptors. The chemoreceptor trigger zone is another centre within the brainstem, which is activated by afferents (often D_2 dopaminergic) similar to those of the vomiting centre, but in addition by toxins including drugs.

Antiemetics

Antiemetics are drugs used to treat vomiting and nausea symptomatically, and they may act in several ways (Fig. 41).

Anticholinergic drugs. Act on the vomiting centre especially, as well as on the gastrointestinal tract directly, for example *hyoscine*. Adverse effects include dry mouth etc., occasionally confusion and agitation.

Antihistamines. These act on H_1 receptors in the vomiting centre, as well as having weak anticholinergic and sedating effects. They are frequently used to treat motion sickness or vestibular disease (often inappropriately in the elderly). Example: *promethazine.*

Phenothiazines. In addition to anticholinergic sedative and H_1 blocking effects, phenothiazines (Chapter 6) block dopamine receptors in the chemoreceptor trigger zone. Example: *prochlorperazine.* Adverse effects include Parkinsonism (see Ch. 6).

Metoclopramide

This is a dopamine receptor antagonist and acts in the chemoreceptor trigger zone. It has direct effects on the gastrointestinal tract (see above). It is given orally or parenterally for most causes of vomiting, although it is not effective for motion sickness.

Adverse effects include acute extrapyramidal reactions, such as oculogyric crisis, especially in children (treat with parenteral anticholinergic such as benztropine). Increased prolactin concentrations and gynaecomastia occur in prolonged use.

Domperidone is similar but is less likely to cause extrapyramidal reactions; it can, however, cause cardiac arrhythmias when given parenterally in high dose.

5-HT antagonists

Ondansetron is a 5-HT_3 antagonist, which is very effective in treating nausea and vomiting, particularly after anticancer chemotherapy. Its exact mode of action is unclear but is probably both central and peripheral. Its adverse effects include constipation and headache. It is reserved for cases where other drugs are ineffective.

11.4 Constipation and diarrhoea

Disturbances of bowel habit are common and often resolve spontaneously with no treatment. The cause should be identified if possible and treated as necessary. Alteration of bowel motility may be an adverse effect of many drugs.

Laxatives

Laxatives are drugs used to treat constipation (Fig. 42). There are many available, and it is important to adjust the dose to achieve the desired effect. The first line of treatment for constipation should be dietary modification, with increased fibre and fluids, and careful education of the patient. If drug treatment is required, the bulking agents are the first choice, followed by the osmotic laxatives, with the stimulant drugs reserved for intermittent use. The faecal softeners are less often used.

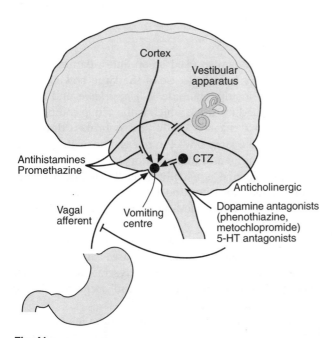

Fig. 41
Central actions of antiemetics.

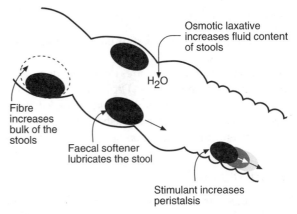

Fig. 42
Laxatives.

Bulking agents

These absorb water, swell and increase the bulk of the stool. This increased bulk stimulates normal peristalsis and hence defaecation. They may take a few days to act fully and may cause flatulence and crampy abdominal pain at first. They are given orally. Examples: *bran, ispaghula.*

Osmotic laxatives

These reduce absorption of water from the bowel. They, therefore, soften the stool and increase its bulk, stimulating peristalsis. *Lactulose* is a disaccharide which is broken down by colonic bacteria to acetic and lactic acid, which cause the osmotic effects. Adverse effects include abdominal pain and flatulence. *Phosphate* or *magnesium* salts are used as enemas.

Stimulants

These stimulate peristalsis and promote defaecation. They are used in cases of severe chronic constipation or where a more rapid effect (within 6–8 hours) is required. The major adverse effects occur in chronic use, where atony of the bowel may occur, creating a vicious cycle of laxative use/constipation/laxative use for the patient. They are usually given orally. Examples: *senna, bisacodyl, castor oil.*

Faecal softeners

These lubricate and soften the stool and are usually given orally. Examples: *dioctyl sodium sulphosuccinate, liquid paraffin.*

Antidiarrhoeals

In treating diarrhoea, especially in children, it is vitally important to replace fluid and electrolyte losses. Since most cases of diarrhoea are self limiting, this is often all that is necessary, and the use of specific antidiarrhoeal drugs is often inappropriate.

Antimotility drugs

These reduce peristalsis by stimulating opioid receptors in the bowel.

Loperamide, diphenoxylate are pethidine derivatives that act only in the bowel. Diphenoxylate is often combined with atropine. *Codeine phosphate* and *morphine* (Ch. 7) are occasionally used also.

Adverse effect is constipation.

Adsorbents

Some of these absorb water without increasing stool bulk, so making the stool firmer and smaller, for example *kaolin.*

Antispasmodics

These are anticholinergic drugs that decrease bowel motility by reducing peristalsis and are used orally to treat painful spasm of the large bowel in the irritable bowel syndrome. Examples: *mebeverine*, which has little systemic anticholinergic effect; *propantheline*, which has more systemic effects and which is also used parenterally to relieve severe pain associated with spasm, e.g. in biliary colic.

11.5 Inflammatory bowel disease

Ulcerative colitis is a chronic inflammatory disease of unknown cause that affects the large bowel. Crohn's disease is also a chronic inflammatory disease of unknown cause, which affects mainly the small bowel but also the large bowel and other parts of the gastrointestinal tract. Both diseases typically undergo exacerbations and remissions, and the aim of treatment is to resolve the acute episodes and prolong remissions. In addition to drug therapy, treatment involves correction of any nutritional deficiencies and sometimes surgery for complications or severe uncontrolled disease.

Anti-inflammatories

Drug treatment is with anti-inflammatory drugs, especially the corticosteroids, which are used systemically in severe acute attacks (e.g. prednisolone or hydrocortisone). They may also be given locally by means of enemas for less severe acute attacks involving the large bowel, or as maintenance therapy. Other anti-inflammatories such as *azathioprine* (see Ch. 9) are also occasionally used.

Sulphasalazine

Sulphasalazine is also used as an anti-inflammatory in inflammatory bowel disease of the large bowel. It is a complex of a sulphonamide, *sulphapyridine*, and 5 *aminosalicylic* acid (5-ASA), which is the active component. The complex is taken orally and is broken down by bacteria in the large bowel to release the 5-ASA, which acts locally as an anti-inflammatory.

Sulphasalazine is usually given to maintain remission but may also be used in acute attacks. It is also used as a disease-modifying drug in rheumatoid arthritis (see Ch. 9).

Adverse effects are mainly because of the sulphapyridine content; headache, nausea and vomiting, rashes and occasionally blood dyscrasias and renal dysfunction; infertility in males can occur because of decreased sperm count.

Other forms: *Olsalazine* is two molecules of 5-ASA combined, and *mesalazine* is a delayed release form of 5-ASA. 5-ASA can also be given as an enema.

11.6 **Gall stones**

Bile acids

In the developed world, gall stones are usually made of cholesterol. Bile acids may be used to gradually dissolve cholesterol gallstones. This is only suitable for small stones, as 3–6 months treatment is required. Recurrence is common. Bile acid treatment for gall stones is generally reserved for patients who are unfit for surgery.

Examples: *chenodeoxycholic acid, ursodeoxycholic acid.*
Adverse effects: diarrhoea.

Self-assessment: questions

Multiple choice questions

1. In duodenal ulcers:
   a. *H. pylori* is present in almost all cases
   b. Relapse after treatment with cimetidine is rare
   c. *H. pylori* secretes a urease enzyme
   d. Basal acid secretion is increased
   e. Attempts to eradicate *H. pylori* are rarely successful

2. In conditions where gastric acid secretion causes symptoms:
   a. Antacids are mainly used for symptomatic relief
   b. H_2 receptor antagonists block all acid secretion
   c. Ranitidine may commonly cause drug interactions
   d. The final common pathway of all stimuli to acid secretion is the proton pump
   e. Omeprazole is very effective in reflux oesophagitis

3. In treating peptic ulcer disease:
   a. Misoprostol is used to treat the gastrointestinal adverse effect of NSAIDs
   b. All patients taking NSAIDs should also take misoprostol
   c. Chelated bismuth can be used to treat acute peptic ulcer
   d. Long-term bismuth is used to maintain remission in peptic ulcer disease
   e. Sucralfate may cause diarrhoea

4. In the treatment of gastrooesophageal reflux:
   a. Metoclopramide may enhance drug absorption
   b. Metoclopramide may cause severe dystonic reactions
   c. Hyperprolactinaemia is a result of antidopaminergic drugs
   d. Domperidone increases large bowel motility
   e. Cisapride may cause anticholinergic adverse effects

5. Drugs used to treat nausea include:
   a. Ondansetron
   b. Prochlorperazine
   c. Bromocriptine
   d. Atropine
   e. Dexamethasone

6. Bowel disturbance may arise as a result of treatment with:
   a. Disopyramide
   b. Omeprazole
   c. Erythromycin
   d. Iron salts
   e. Morphine

7. In treating disturbances of bowel motility:
   a. Rehydration is more important than using antidiarrhoeal drugs

   b. Sulphasalazine is used to treat irritable bowel syndrome
   c. Corticosteroids are the main anti-inflammatories used to treat acute ulcerative colitis
   d. Steroids are always used topically in inflammatory bowel disease
   e. Overdose of diphenoxylate may be treated with naloxone

Case histories

History 1

A patient complaining of upper abdominal pain is endoscoped and found to have a duodenal ulcer. Antral biopsies show *H. pylori*.

1. Should this patient receive treatment to eradicate the *Helicobacter* on first presentation?
2. If so, what treatment should be given to eradicate *Helicobacter*?
3. What treatment might be given to heal the peptic ulcer?
4. If anti-helicobacter therapy is not given, what are the risks of recurrence?
5. The patient later develops osteoarthritis of the knee; should he be given a non-steroidal anti-inflammatory drug?

History 2

A patient has gastrooesophageal reflux proven on endoscopy.

1. Apart from non-pharmacological treatments, what drugs might be considered?
2. How might metoclopramide be helpful?
3. What drugs might aggravate this condition?
4. How should severe cases be treated?
5. What are the adverse effects of omeprazole?

History 3

An elderly patient resident in a nursing home is constipated, i.e. no bowel motion passed for 5 days.

1. What drugs might exacerbate constipation?
2. What other causative factors should be considered in this patient's constipation?
3. If dietary treatment is unsuccessful in this patient, what drug treatment should be considered?
4. What are the harmful effects of long-term use of senna or other stimulant laxatives?
5. What drug therapies might be useful in acute severe constipation?

Self-assessment: answers

Multiple choice answers

1. a. **True.** Its association with gastric ulcers is less certain.
   b. **False.** Relapse is frequent since the cause of the peptic ulcer, the *H. pylori* infection, persists.
   c. **True.** This is how it protects itself from stomach acid.
   d. **True.** As a result of blockage of negative feedback on gastrin.
   e. **False.** Triple therapy with bismuth and antibiotics is successful in about 90% of cases.

2. a. **True.** Very high but unpalatable doses can be used to heal ulcers also.
   b. **False.** Acid production is reduced by about 70–80%.
   c. **False.** Cimetidine, however, does, because of its effects on liver enzymes.
   d. **True.** Hence omeprazole is the most effective of all antisecretory drugs.
   e. **True.** Again, omeprazole is the most effective treatment.

3. a. **True.** By replacing the decreased mucosal prostaglandins.
   b. **False.** It is unnecessary in many patients, has adverse effects of its own and adds considerably to the costs.
   c. **True.** Less widely used today because it has to be taken four times per day compared to once per day for the H_2 receptor antagonists.
   d. **False.** There would be a serious risk of bismuth encephalopathy.
   e. **False.** Sucralfate tends to cause constipation.

4. a. **True.** For instance, used with paracetamol in patients with migraine.
   b. **True.** Especially in children or young women.
   c. **True.** Because dopamine inhibits prolactin release from the pituitary.
   d. **False.** Domperidone may stimulate upper gastrointestinal motility, but not lower.
   e. **False.** Cisapride is procholinergic, not anticholinergic.

5. a. **True.** A $5-HT_3$ antagonist.
   b. **True.** Widely and perhaps excessively used.
   c. **False.** Bromocriptine is a dopamine agonist, and its adverse effects include nausea.
   d. **False.** Although the anticholinergic hyoscine is used.
   e. **True.** Especially after anticancer chemotherapy.

6. a. **True.** Anticholinergic, so may cause constipation.
   b. **True.** Diarrhoea.
   c. **True.** Diarrhoea, and so may many other antibiotics.
   d. **True.** Constipation.
   e. **True.** Constipation.

7. a. **True.** Often forgotten.
   b. **False.** Sulphasalazine is used to treat inflammatory bowel disease of the colon.
   c. **True.** Topically or systemically.
   d. **False.** Systemic steroids are used in severe cases.
   e. **True.** Diphenoxylate is an opioid.

Case history answers

History 1

1. In general, current opinion is that he should not. The argument against treating all patients on first presentation is that the regimens used for eradicating *Helicobacter* at present have a high incidence of adverse effects, and that eradication should be reserved for recurrent or complicated cases. The case for early treatment is becoming more widely accepted.
2. Triple therapy with bismuth, metronidazole, and amoxycillin or tetracycline is the standard therapy at present: many other, perhaps more acceptable, regimens are under study.
3. Eradicating the *Helicobacter* is in addition to healing the ulcer, for which a wide range of drugs is available including H_2 receptor antagonists, chelated bismuth, omeprazole or sucralfate.
4. The recurrence rate at 1 year is 80–90%.
5. NSAIDs should be avoided wherever possible in patients with peptic ulcer disease. Patients with osteoarthritis often need only analgesia and not an anti-inflammatory, so paracetamol used regularly might be sufficent. If the patient had a true inflammatory arthropathy, a NSAID might be necessary and prophylactic therapy with misoprostol or ranitidine should be considered.

History 2

1. Drug treatment would normally be an antacid with alginate, drugs to suppress acid secretion, or prokinetic agents — or combinations of these.
2. Metoclopramide increases the tone of the lower oesophageal sphincter and increases gastric emptying.
3. Drugs with an anticholinergic adverse effect decrease lower oesophageal tone, as do smooth muscle relaxants (e.g. calcium-channel blockers).

4. The drug of choice in severe cases is omeprazole which is exceedingly effective and may be needed for long-term maintenance in some patients.
5. Omeprazole may cause headache, diarrhoea and drug interactions. There are some theoretical concerns about the long-term safety of drugs which suppress acid secretion so profoundly, e.g. risk of gastric carcinoma because of failure to detoxify nitrosamines, but these remain unproved.

History 3

1. Drugs with anticholinergic adverse effects, such as tricyclic anticonvulsants or phenothiazines, also opiate analgesics.
2. Hypothryoidism and depression should be excluded. Other factors include poor diet (deficient in fibre), immobility and dehydration.
3. The first line of drug treatment is usually supplementation of fibre intake, either by diet or by use of a bulking agent, followed by an osmotic laxative and finally intermittent use of a stimulant laxative.
4. Atony of the bowel and laxative dependency.
5. Local treatment with suppositories (e.g. glycerin or bisacodyl) or by enema (e.g. phosphate enema) may be useful in acute severe cases: serious pathology, e.g. intestinal obstruction, should be excluded first.

Drugs acting on the endocrine system

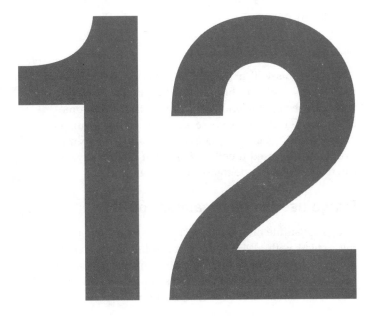

12.1 Diabetes mellitus

Diabetes mellitus (DM) is common, affecting about 1% of the population. In DM, the body becomes unable to regulate the blood glucose, which rises, and the characteristic symptoms of polyuria, polydipsia and weight loss occur. DM is really two distinct disorders. DM of either type is associated with serious long-term complications, including neuropathy, retinopathy, nephropathy and arterial disease. Treatment of DM aims to control the blood glucose, relieve symptoms, and reduce the severity and frequency of the complications.

Non-insulin-dependent DM (NIDDM)

NIDDM is the more common and occurs in middle-aged or elderly patients. There is often a family history. There is resistance at the cellular level to the effects of insulin, and the circulating insulin level is high (this concept is challenged by some recent work that suggests that true insulin is actually low, and that old assays of insulin were flawed). NIDDM is associated with obesity and hypertension.

Treatment of NIDDM involves careful attention to diet, weight loss if obese and, in some patients, the use of oral hypoglycaemic drugs (see below). In some patients with NIDDM, it may be necesssary to use insulin; however, they are not insulin dependent in that if they discontinue their insulin, they are not at risk of ketosis.

Insulin-dependent diabetes

Insulin-dependent diabetes tends to occcur in younger patients and is caused by the autoimmune destruction of the β cells in the islets of the pancreas, which produce insulin. There is, therefore, an insulin deficiency, which prevents most cells from taking up glucose and forces them to metabolise lipids; this leads to ketosis and acidosis. Insulin is needed in addition to diet for treatment; without insulin, the patient will rapidly fall ill and may die.

Management of NIDDM

Many patients will manage on diet alone. If not, then diet is used with sulphonylureas. Sulphonylureas may increase the appetite and, therefore, metformin is sometimes used instead in obese patients. If one drug is unsuccessful, then sulphonylureas and metformin drugs may be used together. Finally, if still unsuccessful, the patient may be treated with insulin.

Drugs used in the treatment of DM

Drugs constitute only one aspect of the management of the patient with DM. Diet and control of body weight are very important, as are education of the patient in the nature and management of his condition and prevention or limitation of the complications.

Insulin

Insulin is a peptide produced normally by the islet cells of the pancreas. It has a range of actions which depend on the type of cell (Fig. 43):

Insulin
- allows the active uptake of glucose and its utilisation in muscle and fat cells
- stimulates synthesis of glycogen in the liver
- inhibits formation of glucose (gluconeogenesis) in the liver
- inhibits breakdown of lipids
- stimulates protein synthesis
- stimulates some cell ion transport mechanisms (e.g. Na^+/K^+-ATPase).

Clinical pharmacokinetics

Insulin must be administered parenterally, usually by subcutaneous injection. It is metabolised by the liver and the kidney, and has a half-life of 9–10 minutes. Slow release preparations have, therefore, been developed.

Formulations of insulin

Pharmaceutical insulin was orginally derived from pigs (porcine insulin) or from cattle (beef insulin). These differed slightly from human insulin, and antibodies sometimes developed. This was avoided by the development of highly purified porcine insulin. Now, however, most patients receive human insulin, produced either by biosynthesis (using genetic engineering to express the gene for human insulin in bacteria) or by chemical modification of porcine insulin. Human insulin is theoretically less immunogenic than porcine insulin but has no real advantage over the highly purified porcine insulins. Human insulins generally are shorter acting than porcine equivalents.

Concerns that human insulin might cause hypoglycaemia more readily than earlier insulins seem unfounded now.

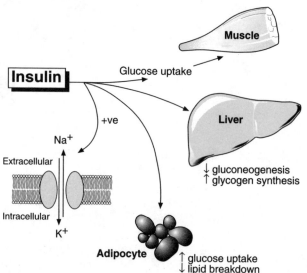

Fig. 43
Action of insulin.

Insulins may be classified according to their duration of action as short, intermediate or long acting.

Short acting: e.g. soluble insulin. Because of its short half-life, its peak effect is at about 1–2 hours when given subcutaneously, and its duration of action is about 4–8 hours. Soluble insulin may also be given intravenously.

Intermediate acting: e.g. insulin zinc suspension (amorphous). The duration of action is prolonged by complexing the insulin with a zinc salt, so that particles form. Insulin is then slowly released from these particles. The peak action is at about 3–6 hours and the duration is about 12–24 hours.

Long acting: e.g. insulin zinc suspension (crystalline). Here crystals of the insulin zinc complex are formed, which break down more slowly still. Peak action is at 5–12 hours and duration of effect is 16–30 hours.

Mixtures of these insulins are also available.

Insulin regimens

Dose and choice of preparations must be determined for each patient individually. Most patients use a short acting and an intermediate or long acting preparation twice a day (before breakfast and the evening meal). Another popular regimen is a long-acting insulin once a day, supplemented around meal times with injections of soluble insulin, three times per day. Many patients will monitor their blood glucose at home and make minor adjustments in dose accordingly.

Adverse effects

Hypoglycaemia is the most common and serious: it is the result of an imbalance between glucose intake (e.g. missing a meal), glucose utilisation (e.g. unusual exercise) and insulin dose. The result is sympathetic activation (palpitations, anxiety and sweating) and neuroglycopenia (visual disturbance, drowsiness or aggression, coma). Treatment is by administration of carbohydrate orally to a conscious patient, or i.v. glucose or i.m. *glucagon* (a peptide hormone and physiological antagonist of insulin). The patient and his family should be trained to spot the warning signs and how to treat hypoglycaemia, including possibly administration of glucagon if the patient goes unconscious.

Lipodystrophy is the atrophy or hypertrophy of fat at the site of injection, less common with the newer insulin preparations.

Antibody formation may arise because of impurities in the preparation and is less common with the highly purified or human insulins. Antibodies could prolong the action of the insulin (often beneficial) but reduce its effects (usually harmful).

Acute diabetic ketoacidosis

This may occur in newly diagnosed IDDM or may arise in IDDM if the insulin dose is inadequate for needs, e.g. during infection or other physiological stress. The patient will become seriously dehydrated, hyperglycaemic and acidotic.

Treatment involves careful monitoring of the clinical state and serum biochemistry, consideration of why the ketoacidosis might have occurred (e.g. infection, myocardial infarction, etc.), rehydration, the fluid deficit may be as much as 5–12 litres) and insulin given as a slow i.v. infusion. It is not usually necessary to treat the acidosis separately.

Oral hypoglycaemic drugs

Sulphonylureas

These act by stimulating release of endogenous insulin from the pancreas. They may also have an extra-pancreatic effect in decreasing breakdown of insulin and increasing the density of insulin receptors on the cell, improving insulin sensitivity.

Glibenclamide is long acting (up to 24 hours) and is metabolised by the liver. *Gliclazide* (6–12 hours) and *tolbutamide* (3–6 hours) are shorter acting and are more suitable for use in elderly patients for this reason. All are metabolised by the liver. *Chlorpropamide* is very long acting (24–48 hours or longer) and should not be used any longer.

Adverse effects:

- Hypoglycaemia
- Gastrointestinal upsets
- Hypersensitivity: rashes etc.

Drug interactions. Sulphonylureas are heavily protein bound and their actions may be increased, e.g. if the patient is given sulphonamides, as a result of displacement from the binding sites.

Biguanides

Metformin is the only biguanide used. It acts by increasing peripheral utilisation of glucose and decreasing absorption of glucose from the gastrointestinal tract and gluconeogenesis. Metformin does not cause hypoglycaemia. It is excreted unchanged by the kidney.

Adverse effects:

- Gastrointestinal upsets are common; nausea, vomiting and anorexia
- Liver or renal disease or congestive cardiac failure: metformin may cause lactic acidosis.

12.2 Corticosteroids

Corticosteroids are hormones produced in the cortex of the adrenal gland: they may be broadly defined as glucocorticoids or mineralocorticoids. Corticosteroid drugs aften show a mixture of both types of activity and the proportion of each varies with dosage levels.

Glucocorticoids: the natural glucocorticoid is hydrocortisone (cortisol), produced under the control of the hypothalamus, which secretes corticotrophin-releasing factor to stimulate the pituitary to secrete adrenocorti-

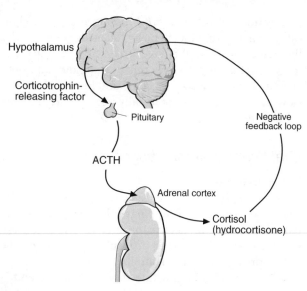

Fig. 44
Hypothalamic–pituitary–adrenal axis.

cotrophic hormone (ACTH). This is termed the hypothalamic–pituitary–adrenal (HPA) axis (Fig. 44).

Mineralocorticoids: although hydrocortisone has some mineralocorticoid effects, the major natural mineralocorticoid is aldosterone, produced in response to the renin–angiotensin–aldosterone (RAA) axis (see Ch. 3)

These hormones or synthetic derivatives can be given as drugs. These are powerful drugs with serious adverse effects and should be reserved for conditions where replacement is necessary, where other drugs have failed or where the illness is so severe that the benefits of treatment outweigh the risks.

Glucocorticoids

The mode of action is uncertain; they bind to receptors in the cytoplasm and the complex is transported into the cell nucleus, where it binds to steroid responsive elements on DNA to encourage new protein synthesis. The protein produced may have several effects; the best described is lipocortin, which in turn inhibits phospholipase A_2 and hence the release of arachidonic acid. This decreases activity in the cyclooxygenase and lipooxygenase pathways of production of inflammatory mediators. Corticosteroids do not appear to act for 12–18 hours and their action lasts for 24–48 hours after they are stopped.

Glucocorticoids are released in times of physiological stress. If absent, the patient may experience an Addisonian crisis, with hypotension, shock and death, when faced with physiological stress such as infection, etc.

Glucocorticoids are also important in carbohydrate and protein metabolism; they promote the formation of glycogen and gluconeogenesis in the liver. Peripheral utilisation of glucose is decreased and the blood glucose may increase. Protein catabolism is increased, breaking down muscle and the matrix of bone.

Clinical pharmacokinetics
Because of the time to achieve any clinical effect, the use of intravenous rather than oral glucocorticoids is often unnecessary. They are well absorbed after oral administration and broken down by liver metabolism.

Therapeutic uses
Replacement therapy: in patients with adrenocortical insufficiency either caused by disease of the adrenal gland (autoimmune, Addison's disease), destruction or removal of the gland or pituitary failure.

Anti-inflammatory effect: glucocorticoids may be used (systemically or topically) to reduce inflammation in a wide variety of conditions (e.g. asthma, inflammatory bowel disease, eczema and other skin conditions, glomerulonephritis, treatment of hypersensitivity, arteritis, amongst others). They are usually started at high doses and then reduced to the lowest level at which disease activity is suppressed, or withdrawn altogether if possible. Wherever possible, topical treatment is preferable to systemic so that adverse effects are minimised.

Chemotherapy: glucocorticoids are also used as part of chemotherapy for acute leukaemias and Hodgkin's lymphoma (see Ch. 15).

Glucocorticoid drugs
Hydrocortisone is used orally in low doses (20–30 mg/day) for replacement therapy in adrenal insufficiency. It is used in high doses (400–1200 mg/day) parenterally to treat severe acute allergy or asthma or inflammatory bowel disease. It is used topically as enemas in inflammatory bowel disease and as creams in skin conditions such as eczema.

Prednisolone is about five times more potent as a glucocorticoid but has less mineralocorticoid action. It is used orally for acute asthma or hypersensitivity or other serious systemic inflammatory conditions (40–60 mg/day initially, reducing to 5–10 mg/day for maintenance).

Methylprednisolone is a derivative of prednisolone which can also be given parenterally and is used especially in treating transplant rejection.

Dexamethasone is about 20 times more potent than hydrocortisone but with almost no mineralocorticoid effect. It is given orally or parenterally for its anti-inflammatory effects, particularly in the treatment of cerebral oedema.

Beclomethasone and budesonide are very potent glucocorticoids used topically, by inhalation to treat asthma (Ch. 10). Many other potent fluorinated glucocorticoids are used in skin conditions.

Tetracosactrin, a synthetic analogue of ACTH, was used by injection in the hope that the adrenals would not be suppressed: in practice, this advantage was slight and the clinical response to tetracosactrin was so variable that this has been largely abandoned. It is used in tests of pituitary–adrenal function.

Mineralocorticoids

These affect sodium balance and cause sodium and water retention and increase Na⁺ reuptake in the distal tubule in exchange for K⁺.

Aldosterone is not used therapeutically. An analogue, *fludrocortisone* is used in replacement therapy for patients with adrenal insufficiency. It has effectively no glucocorticoid activity.

Adverse effects of corticosteroids

The adverse effects of corticosteroids should prompt particular care in the use of these drugs. The frequency of adverse effects is related to their dosage, duration of use and relative glucocorticoid/mineralocorticoid effects, e.g. hydrocortisone will have few adverse effects when used in low doses for replacement therapy, but will have both glucocorticoid and mineralocorticoid adverse effects when used in high doses: dexamethasone, however, will have mostly glucocorticoid adverse effects. Glucocorticoids should be used topically whenever possible to avoid systemic adverse effects (Fig. 45).

Glucocorticoid adverse effects

- Impaired glucose tolerance or sometimes diabetes mellitus
- Osteoporosis, especially of the vertebrae and in the elderly
- Avascular necrosis of the hip

- Cushing's syndrome, with characteristic appearance of moon face, buffalo hump, striae, as well as muscle wasting and thinning of the skin and poor healing
- Immune suppression: there may be reduced resistance to infections such as tuberculosis
- Growth suppression in children: the original disease state is usually more relevant in causing growth suppression than the glucocorticoid
- Mental disturbances: euphoria, agitation or depression
- Cataract
- Striae and thinning of the skin: this may be a particular problem with topical use of potent glucocorticoids
- Dyspepsia: common; peptic ulceration may occur but whether this is caused by glucocorticoids is not certain.

Adrenal suppression. Administering glucocorticoids suppresses the hypothalamus–pituitary–adrenal (HPA) axis; if used in high doses for prolonged periods, the adrenal glands may atrophy. This is also possible but less likely after topical use. To avoid this, it is important to use low doses for as short a time as possible. Withdrawal of treatment after long-term use must be gradual (perhaps over several months) to allow the HPA to recover. Otherwise the patient may experience an Addisonian crisis. Similarly, in patients who have received glucocorticoids for prolonged periods, adrenal insufficiency may occur during physiological stress, e.g. during surgery or after an accident. If such a reaction is suspected, an increased dose of

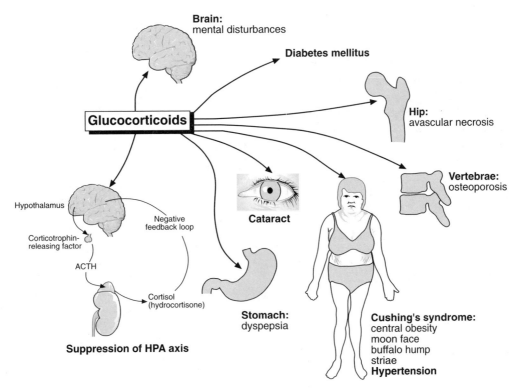

Fig. 45
Adverse effects of glucocorticoids.

hydrocortisone should be administered. All patients prescribed glucocorticoids should be warned of these dangers and should be issued with a 'steroid card', giving details of dosage and possible complications.

Mineralocorticoid adverse effects

- Sodium and water retention, leading to hypertension
- Hypokalaemia.

12.3 The reproductive system

The steroid hormones of the reproductive system are of three broad types:

- oestrogens, produced by the ovary and also in adipose tissue
- progesterone, also produced by the ovary
- testosterone, produced by the testis.

Contraception

The most common therapeutic use of the sex hormones is in oral contraceptives. These are of two types:

- Oestrogen progestogen combinations (the combined pill)
- Progestogen-only pill (minipill).

Oestrogen progestogen combinations

These act by inhibiting ovulation. The oestrogen inhibits release of follicle stimulating hormone (FSH) from the pituitary, while the progestogen blocks luteinising hormone (LH) release. Both are taken for 21 days and then stopped for 7 days before resuming the cycle. During the withdrawal period, there is uterine bleeding similar to menstruation. The tablet should be taken at the same time every day; if missed for more than 12 hours, the contraceptive effect may be lost. Therapy should be started on the first day of a cycle so as to provide contraceptive cover for that cycle; if started later, barrier contraceptives should also be used for that cycle. The failure rate is about 1 per 100 woman years or less.

Clinical pharmacokinetics

The oestrogen most commonly used is the synthetic *ethinyloestradiol* in doses between 50 and 20 µg (the natural oestrogens undergo extensive first-pass metabolism and are unsuitable). Lower dose pills are now recognised as being as effective and have fewer adverse effects. The progestogen is usually *norethisterone* or *levonorgestrel*. These are derivatives of nortestosterone and may have androgenic effects. Other progestogenes without androgenic effects are also used including gestodeen and desogestril.

These synthetic steroids are all absorbed well and are eliminated by conjugation with glucuronide and

Action

Other effects

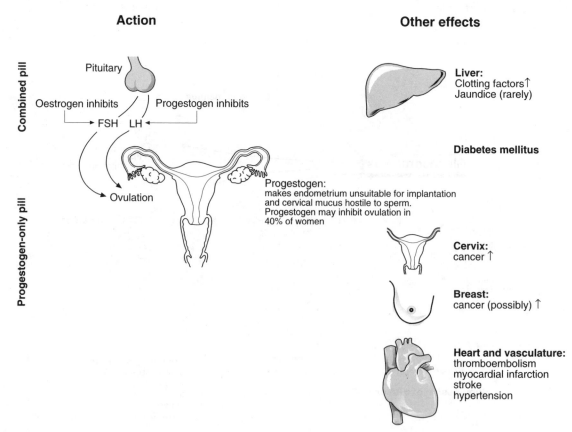

Fig. 46
Action of the combined oral contraceptive.

excreted in bile. There is enterohepatic circulation, i.e. the conjugated oestrogen is broken down in the gut by bacteria and the free oestrogen is reabsorbed. There are a wide variety of preparations available.

Other uses. High doses of the combined pill can be given for two doses as a contraceptive for up to 72 hours after unprotected intercourse. The combined pill is sometimes used for cycle regulation in women with dysmenorrhoea or dysfunctional uterine bleeding.

Adverse effects

- The most serious involve the cardiovascular system and are related to the oestrogen dose
  - Venous thromboembolic disease, i.e. deep venous thrombosis or pulmonary embolism. This was more common with higher oestrogen dose pills initially used and is caused by a decrease in antithrombin III production and increase in fibrinogen production by the liver. This may be a particular risk around the time of surgery, and women having elective operations should discontinue the combined pill for 4 weeks before the operation and for 2 weeks after
  - Myocardial infarction and stroke: these are more common with higher oestrogen dose pills, in older women (>35 years), and smokers, probably because of the alteration of clotting factors and increased platelet aggregation
  - Hypertension; many women will experience a slight rise in blood pressure of little significance. In about 5–10%, the rise is greater and withdrawal of the combined pill may be necessary
- Malignant disease: the combined pill protects against endometrial and ovarian malignancy but is associated with an increased risk of cervical carcinoma and possibly breast carcinoma
- Glucose intolerance and diabetes
- Headache
- Menstrual irregularity in the first months of treatment
- Chloasma
- Rarely; cholestatic jaundice, hepatic tumours.

Contraindications to the combined pill

- History of thromboembolic disease
- Liver disease
- Undiagnosed vaginal bleeding
- Hyperlipidaemia
- Breast, endometrial or hepatic carcinoma.

Use with caution in:

- Diabetes mellitus
- Smokers
- Older patients (aged over 35 years)
- Hypertensives
- Migraine.

The progestogen-only pill

This works by altering the cervical mucus and the endometrium so that fertilisation or subsequent implantation is unlikely. In about 40% of women, ovulation is also inhibited. Although the failure rate is higher than the combined pill (about 2/100 woman years), it may be more suitable for patients with contraindications to oestrogens. The tablet is taken constantly with no breaks. It should be taken at the same time every day: if it is delayed for more than 3 hours, the contraceptive effect may be lost.

The progestogens used are the same as in the combined pill, but in a lower dose, e.g. in the combined pill, norethisterone may be given in doses of 250 µg/day while in progestogen-only pills, the dose is 30 µg/day.

Medroxyprogesterone is a depot progestogen given by injection: a single dose may provide contraception for 3 months.

Adverse effects of progestogens

- Menstrual irregularities
- Nausea and vomiting
- Breast discomfort.

Drug interactions

These may be very important for both the combined and the progestogen-only pills as an unwanted pregnancy may occur. Enzyme inducers (see Ch. 1) decrease the action of the combined pill, as do some broad-spectrum antibiotics that interfere with enterohepatic circulation, e.g. amoxycillin.

Hormone replacement therapy

Around the menopause, many women will experience distressing vasomotor symptoms — hot flushes, as well as vaginitis — caused largely by the fall in serum oestrogen levels. Other effects of the menopause include a hastening of osteoporosis and an increased risk of cardiovascular disease. Many of these symptoms and problems can be avoided by administering low doses of oestrogens (hormone replacement therapy, HRT). These are given as once daily oral doses, e.g. *conjugated equine oestrogens*, or *oestradiol*.

For the treatment of the vasomotor symptoms, HRT should be given for 6–12 months. The optimum duration of therapy for protection against osteoporosis and cardiac disease is not certain but is probably about 5–10 years.

Adverse effects

Adverse effects are similar to those for the other oestrogen uses, although, because of the lower doses used, the adverse cardiovascular effects are not seen. Overall, problems with cardiac disease are reduced compared with women not taking HRT.

However, other problems may be important;

- Increase in the risk of endometrial carcinoma: this can be avoided by giving progestogens in addition to the oestrogen for 10–12 days in every 28. (This is of course unnecessary in women who have had a hysterectomy.) This will cause a withdrawal bleed which some women dislike
- A possible increase in the risk of breast cancer in women who use long-term HRT (by 10–30%).

In women whose major problem is vaginal dryness, an oestrogen cream applied to the affected area intermittently may be more appropriate than systemic therapy.

Contraindications to HRT are fewer than to the use of higher-dose oestrogens as contraceptives.

Other uses

Cancer treatment

Antioestrogen therapy

Breast cancer cells may have oestrogen receptors. Reducing oestrogen levels (by oophorectomy) is beneficial in about 60% of such cases, as well as in about 10% where oestrogen receptors are not identified.

Tamoxifen is an oestrogen receptor antagonist used to treat breast cancer. It may cause a response in about 30–40% of women. Adverse effects include hot flushes and gastrointestinal upsets.

Aminoglutethimide is a second-line therapy, which prevents the formation of oestrogens. It also prevents the formation of hydrocortisone, which must be given with it to prevent an Addisonian crisis.

LHRH and its analogues

Luteinising hormone-releasing hormone (LHRH) is a peptide released in a pulsatile fashion by the hypothalamus, which stimulates LH release and hence oestrogen production in females or testosterone in males.

Analogues of LHRH (e.g. goserelin) can be given in slow release depot injections to provide constant stimulation; this downregulates the LHRH receptors so that LH release falls off and oestrogen or testosterone fall to very low levels. They are used to treat prostatic carcinoma and, increasingly, in the treatment of breast cancer or endometriosis.

Infertility

Clomiphene is used in the treatment of infertility. It is an oestrogen antagonist at central receptors in the hypothalamus. By blocking these receptors, the normal negative feedback control on FSH and LH release is prevented. The result is increased ovulation increasing the possibilities for fertilisation. The main adverse effect is the risk of overstimulation and multiple pregnancy.

Synthetic LHRH (*gonadorelin*) is given by intermittent injection to simulate pulsatile secretion to cause LH release in the treatment of infertility.

Termination of pregnancy

Mifepristone is a semi-synthetic steroid, used with prostaglandins to cause termination of pregnancy up to 9 weeks. It acts as a progestogen antagonist, preventing endometrial maturation and increasing activity of the myometrium. The combination is effective in 95% of patients but may cause severe uterine pain and hypotension. The use of mifepristone is currently closely regulated and is confined to approved clinics.

Androgen deficiency

Testosterone is normally produced by the testis. Synthetic testosterone can be given in cases of deficiency, after orchidectomy, or in primary deficiency states. In these patients, it will prevent osteoporosis and increase the libido.

Dysfunctional bleeding

The combined pill is sometimes used for cycle regulation in women with dysmenorrhoea or dysfunctional uterine bleeding.

Danazol inhibits the release of pituitary gonadotrophins and is antioestrogen, antiandrogen and antiprogestogen. It is used to treat endometriosis and menorrhagia. Adverse effects include gastrointestinal upsets and virilisation.

12.4 Thyroid disease

Hyperthyroidism

Hyperthyroidism most often results from an autoimmune condition, Graves' disease, in which autoantibodies stimulate the thyroid cells. The resulting high circulating concentrations of thyroxine suppress the release of thyroid-stimulating hormone (TSH) from the pituitary. Graves' disease tends to undergo spontaneous remission in time, and treatment does not cure the condition but rather suppresses the hyperthyroidism until a remission occurs. Some patients will experience only one episode: about half will experience repeated episodes and may need a more definitive procedure such as radioactive iodine or surgery (Fig. 47).

Hyperthyroidism may also arise from a single toxic adenoma, or from a toxic multinodular goitre. In these cases, remission is less likely and long-term therapy or definitive procedure will probably be needed.

In hyperthyroidism, the patient experiences increased metabolism and so may suffer classical symptoms including weight loss, anxiety, tremor, palpitations and diarrhoea. In the elderly, these symptoms may be less clear and hyperthyroidism more difficult to diagnose.

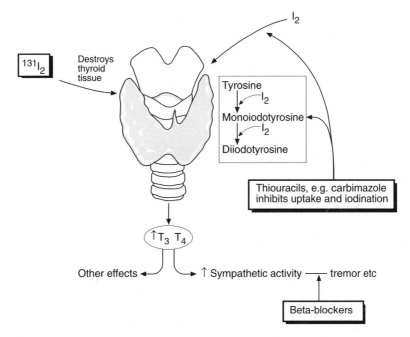

Fig. 47
Hyperthyroidism.

Drugs used to treat hyperthyroidism

Thiouracils

Mode of action. These drugs inhibit the formation of thyroxine by inhibiting the uptake of iodine by the thyroid, the iodination of tyrosine and the coupling of iodinated tyrosine to form thyroxine. Carbimazole may have additional properties, influencing the immunological disorders in Graves' disease and increasing the likelihood of remisssion.

Clinical pharmacokinetics and examples. Carbimazole is metabolised to methimazole (which is itself used widely in the USA and Europe, while carbimazole is favoured in the UK) which accumulates in the thyroid. If given to pregnant women, carbimazole can cross the placenta and can result in fetal hyperthyroidism or goitre. *Propylthiouracil* is similar.

Therapeutic use. Carbimazole is given in high doses initially until the patient becomes euthyroid (usually 4–8 weeks) and is then gradually reduced over 12 months, while monitoring symptoms and thyroid function tests. Repeated courses or continuous therapy will be necessary in some patients. Some endocrinologists combine thyroxine with carbimazole once the patient is euthyroid (blocking replacement regimen) and may achieve better results than with carbimazole alone. Non-specific beta-blockers, such as propranolol (Ch. 3) are usually given (if there are no contraindications) to improve many of the sympathetically mediated symptoms at the start of treatment before the thiouracils have reached their full effect.

Adverse effects. Allergy with rash and fever can occur. Carbimazole may cause neutropenia which, if treatment is not stopped, may develop into full agranulocytosis. This may arise suddenly, and patients must be carefully warned to report any evidence of infection, such as a sore throat, immediately. A full blood count should then be checked straightaway and if there is any evidence of neutropenia, the carbimazole should be withdrawn.

Hepatitis and arthralgia may rarely occur.

Propylthiouracil is less likely to cause agranulocytosis.

Potassium iodide or iodine solution

Paradoxically, this causes an immediate reduction in the plasma thyroid hormone concentrations, as well as inhibiting thyroxine formation. The vascularity of the gland is also decreased. The effect is transient, lasting only 3–4 weeks, but is valuable in managing patients awaiting thyroid surgery or in thyroid crisis (see below).

Radioactive iodine

Isotopic ^{131}I is well absorbed and concentrated in the thyroid where it causes permanent damage to the hormone-producing tissue. A single oral dose is usually effective. Standard antithyroid therapy is used before and after ^{131}I administration since ^{131}I takes 4–6 weeks to work. There is a very high incidence of hypothyroidism subsequently, but treating hypothyroidism is easier than treating hyperthyroidism. There is no evidence of any risk of later malignancy or of genetic damage. It is used in patients who have failed to respond to medical therapy or who have relapsed, or increasingly as first-line therapy for hyperthyroidism, especially in the elderly.

Thyroid crisis

This is severe sudden hyperthyroidism perhaps precipitated by physiological stress, surgery, etc. The patient develops fever, tachycardia, dehydration and encephalopathy. Treatment is by intravenous fluids, beta-blockers, iodine solution, corticosteroids and carbimazole or propylthiouracil.

Hypothyroidism

Hypothyroidism may result from autoimmune thyroiditis (Hashimoto's), thyroidectomy, radioiodine, or, in some parts of the world, from iodine deficiency. Rarely, it may be part of hypopituitarism. The patient is most often elderly and female and may complain of tiredness and lethargy. Other features include coarsening of the skin and hair, bradycardia, constipation, menorrhagia and slowing of the tendon reflexes. The concentration of free thyroxine in the blood is reduced, while that of thyroid-stimulating hormone from the pituitary is usually greatly increased.

Treatment is by L-thyroxine, given orally. The dose is adjusted according to patient symptoms and in response to the concentration of thyroid-stimulating hormone which should be maintained within the normal range.

Adverse effects of L-thyroxine are mainly those of overdose, mimicking hyperthyroidism. In patients with ischaemic heart disease, L-thyroxine should be started in a low dose and should be increased very slowly; otherwise, an attack of angina or a myocardial infarction may be precipitated.

12.5 Calcium metabolism

Vitamin D_2 (*calciferol*) is a fat-soluble vitamin that is formed in the skin on exposure to UV light or may be derived from the diet. Calciferol is then activated first in the liver and then in the kidney to 1.25-dihydroxycholecalciferol. This increases the serum Ca^{2+} by enhancing the absorption of Ca^{2+} from the gastrointestinal tract and the reabsorption of Ca^{2+} and phosphate from the renal tubule. It also stimulates osteoclasts to increase bone turnover and further increase serum Ca^{2+}. Deficiencies of vitamin D may be dietary (especially in vegetarians and the elderly) or be the result of malabsorption, liver disease or renal disease. The clinical result is osteomalacia (known in children as rickets).

Calciferol

Calciferol is used in vitamin D-deficiency states, malabsorption, liver and renal disease (in which very high doses may be required) and hypoparathyroidism. Its use in osteoporosis is controversial. Calciferol may be administered orally. *1-α-hydroxycholecalciferol* is a more potent analogue.

Adverse effects. Hypercalcaemia may occur and careful monitoring of serum Ca^{2+} is necessary.

Biphosphonates

These bind to hydroxyapatite crystals in bone and reduce the breakdown of bone. They can be used to treat Paget's disease of the bones and hypercalcaemia of malignancy. Intermittent treatment with biphosphonates may also be useful in patients with severe osteoporosis complicated by vertebral fractures.

Examples: *etidronate* (oral or i.v.), *pamidronate* (i.v. only).

Adverse effects. Gastrointestinal upsets, hypocalcaemia. Excessive dose may inhibit osteoblasts as well as osteoclasts: this may cause fractures in patients with Paget's disease.

Calcitonin

This is a peptide secreted by the C cells of the thyroid, which lowers serum calcium by decreasing bone turnover and increasing excretion of calcium through the kidneys. It is used to treat Paget's disease. Its adverse effects include flushing of the face and nausea.

12.6 Other pituitary hormones

Antidiuretic hormone

Cranial diabetes insipidus (DI) is caused by a deficiency of antidiuretic hormone (ADH, also known as vasopressin) a peptide which is secreted from the posterior pituitary (cranial DI). This reduces the resorption of water in the renal collecting tubules. Its absence leads to polyuria, and polydipsia or dehydration with hypernatraemia. Treatment is by synthetic analogues, e.g. *desmopressin*, which is given as a nasal spray. The dose is adjusted according to effect. The major adverse effect is water intoxication if too much is used. *Arginine vasopressin* may be used parenterally. It may cause severe vasoconstriction and is used for this purpose in the treatment of bleeding from oesophageal varices.

Somatropin

This is an analogue of human growth hormone and is used in the treatment of short stature in growth hormone-deficient children.

Self-assessment: questions

Multiple choice questions

1. Drugs which may impair glucose tolerance include:
   a. Bendrofluazide
   b. Prednisolone
   c. Oral contraceptives
   d. Enalapril
   e. Benzylpenicillin

2. Carbimazole:
   a. Is a prodrug
   b. May cause hypothyroidism
   c. May cause thrombocytopenia
   d. Blocks iodine uptake in the gastrointestinal tract
   e. Treatment is rarely followed by relapse

3. In treating hyperthyroidism:
   a. High-dose potassium iodide is useful in the long-term treatment of hyperthyroidism
   b. Patients may be treated with ^{131}I while still taking carbimazole
   c. There is a high risk of hypothyroidism in patients treated with ^{131}I
   d. Hypothyroidism may be treated with dietary iodine supplements
   e. Treatment of hypothyroidism is best monitored by measuring serum thyroxine

4. Insulin
   a. Is formed in the liver
   b. Insulin tends to increase body weight
   c. In patients treated with insulin, diet is unimportant
   d. Human insulin is more likely to cause hypoglycaemia than porcine insulin
   e. Good control of IDDM results in a decreased risk of serious complications

5. The following statements are correct:
   a. IDDM is more common than NIDDM
   b. Patients with IDDM should change their treatment only on the advice of their doctor
   c. Hypoglycaemia is the most common adverse effect of insulin
   d. Soluble insulin may be given i.v.
   e. In hypoglycaemia, high-dose i.m. glucose should be given

6. The following statements are correct:
   a. In diabetic ketoacidosis, dehydration may be life theatening
   b. Acidosis requires urgent treatment with i.v. sodium bicarbonate
   c. Crystalline insulin is used for its long duration of action

   d. Patients treated with insulin can monitor their own blood glucose
   e. Antibodies to insulin are more common with porcine than human insulin

7. Concerning oral hypoglycaemics in NIDDM:
   a. Sulphonylureas can be used to treat a patient who has developed DM because of pancreatitis.
   b. Chlorpropamide is appropriate for elderly patients
   c. Sulphonylureas are not the drug of choice in obese patients with NIDDM
   d. Metformin may cause lactic acidosis in some patients
   e. Hypoglycaemia is a common adverse effect of oral hypoglycaemic drugs

8. Concerning calcium metabolism:
   a. Vitamin D causes calcium resorption from the kidney
   b. Vitamin D can be manufactured in the body
   c. Vitamin D is found in fresh fruit and vegetables
   d. Vitamin D and Ca^{2+} are used to treat hypoparathyroidism
   e. Vitamin D etidronate stabilises bone and reduces hypocalcaemia in malignant disease

9. Systemic glucocorticoids may cause:
   a. Psychosis
   b. Opportunistic infections
   c. Osteomalacia
   d. Suppression of the renin–angiotensin–aldosterone axis
   e. Skin changes

10. Corticosteroids:
    a. Hydrocortisone has no mineralocorticoid effects
    b. Glucocorticoids are potent anti-inflammatory drugs
    c. Hydrocortisone is a naturally occurring hormone
    d. ACTH is often used to treat inflammatory disease
    e. Aldosterone can be given to treat adrenal insufficiency

11. Diseases in which corticosteroids are used include:
    a. Addison's   d. Cellulitis
    b. Conn's   e. Lymphoma
    c. Asthma

12. In contraception:
    a. The combined oral contraceptive (COC) may cause ischaemic heart disease
    b. The failure rate for the progestogen-only pill is lower than for the COC

c. The progestogens used in the COC may have androgenic effects

d. Enterohepatic circulation of oestrogen occurs

e. COC may be involved in a variety of drug interactions

13. In contraception:
    a. Low-dose oestrogen COCs are less likely to cause thromboembolic disease than older high-dose preparations
    b. COC should never be used in women over the age of 35
    c. COC decreases the risk of uterine carcinoma
    d. COC should not be used in women who smoke
    e. The progestogen-only pill is safe in women with a history of thromboembolic disease

14. Postmenopausal hormone replacement therapy:
    a. Is contraindicated in women with ischaemic heart disease
    b. If given to patients with a uterus, should include a progestogen as well as an oestrogen
    c. If given long term, may decrease the risks of osteoporosis
    d. Decreases the risks of breast cancer
    e. Should not be started for at least a year after the last period

Case histories

History 1

A 28-year-old woman presents with hyperthyroidism caused by Graves' disease.

1. What treatment or treatments would be appropriate as first line?
2. What possible adverse effects of treatment must she be warned about?
3. While being treated for hyperthyroidism, she becomes pregnant: what are the risks to the fetus?
4. She is treated for 12 months, but on stopping therapy, she quickly relapses: what treatment options should be considered now?
5. What drugs may interfere with the interpretation of thyroid function tests?

History 2

An obese 68-year-old woman with hypertension complains of thirst and polyuria and is noted to have glycosuria. Blood sugar analysis confirms that she is diabetic.

1. What are the main lines of treatment to recommend to this woman?
2. What maintenance drug treatment should be considered first line?

3. If this fails, what should be second line?
4. What drugs may have precipitated her diabetes?
5. When might insulin therapy be considered in such a patient?

History 3

A 25-year-old man presents with 3-day history of vomiting, polyuria and thirst. There is no previous history. Urinalysis shows glycosuria and ketonuria, and blood glucose is high.

1. What is the diagnosis?
2. What treatment should he be given?
3. How are insulins administered?
4. He is treated for diabetes mellitus over the next 3 years. However, one day he is found unconscious. What diagnosis should be considered first?
5. How should he now be treated?

History 4

A 58-year-old woman is given high-dose prednisolone for several months because of giant cell arteritis, an inflammatory disease. Her condition responds well to this.

1. What problems may arise if her prednisolone is suddenly stopped?
2. She complains of swollen ankles: why might this be?
3. What musculoskeletal changes might she experience?
4. What other adverse effects might she experience?
5. She fractures her hip in a fall and requires surgery. What complications might she suffer because of her therapy around the time of operation?

History 5

A 19-year-old woman wishes to go on oral contraceptive.

1. She is worried because she has heard that the combined oral contraceptive (COC) pill can cause cancer: what can you tell her?
2. She smokes: is this a particular problem?
3. She is started on a combined oestrogen progestogen pill: she telephones you 6 months later to say that she forgot to take her pill yesterday and to ask what she should do.
4. She complains of pleuritic chest pain 6 months later again; what drug-related diagnosis should be considered?
5. She later develops epilepsy and is treated with carbamazepine; she wishes to continue the oral contraceptive: are there any problems with this?

History 6

A 50-year-old woman develops irregular periods. She complains of hot flushes, about 3 months after her last period, as well as feeling tired and irritable. She asks whether she should have hormone replacement therapy.

1. What are the likely benefits to this patient of short-term (6 months) treatment with HRT?

2. She asks about osteoporosis, since there is a family history of fractured hips: what should you tell her about this and HRT?

3. There is also a strong family history of ischaemic heart disease. Would you expect HRT to increase or decrease the risks of this?

4. Are doses of oestrogen in HRT higher than in combined oral contraceptives?

5. She is concerned particularly about vaginal dryness. Will HRT help this?

Self-assessment: answers

Multiple choice answers

1. a. **True.** This is a thiazide diuretic.
   b. **True.** Glucocorticoids cause a rise in blood glucose by several mechanisms.
   c. **True.** But not usually clinically significant.
   d. **False.** ACE inhibitors may even increase insulin sensitivity.
   e. **False.** No effect on the pancreas or peripheral cells.

2. a. **True.** Converted to methimazole.
   b. **True.** If used in high doses for prolonged periods.
   c. **False.** May cause agranulocytosis.
   d. **False.** Blocks iodine uptake by the thyroid gland.
   e. **False.** Carbimazole does not reverse the underlying cause and relapse is common.

3. a. **False.** Short-term use only.
   b. **False.** Carbimazole would impede uptake of ^{131}I into the thyroid. The patient should be off carbimazole for several days beforehand.
   c. **True.** Whether caused by the ^{131}I or to the natural history of the condition.
   d. **False.** Thyroxine is needed.
   e. **False.** TSH is the best measure.

4. a. **False.** Insulin is formed in the pancreas.
   b. **True.** Insulin tends to stimulate appetite.
   c. **False.** Diet is exceedingly important in all diabetics.
   d. **False.** There is no evidence of this.
   e. **True.** Although many patients even with poor control do not develop complications: there is still much to be understood about the cause of diabetic complications.

5. a. **False.** NIDDM is far more common.
   b. **False.** Patients should be sufficiently knowledgeable about their condition to adjust their dose of insulin by themselves.
   c. **True.** This may be life threatening.
   d. **True.** This is the only insulin that may be given in any way other than subcutaneously.
   e. **False.** High concentrations of insulin are very hyperosmolar and severe tissue necrosis would be likely. Glucose should be given either orally or, if the patient is unconscious, intravenously.

6. a. **True.** The extent of the dehydration is commonly underestimated.
   b. **False.** Acidosis usually corrects itself when dehydration and hyperglycaemia are treated.
   c. **True.** Often in combination with a short-acting insulin.

d. **True.** And may adjust their dose of insulin accordingly.
   e. **True.** But with purified porcine insulins, this is of little clinical importance.

7. a. **False.** Because sulphonylureas depend mainly for their action on stimulating release of endogenous insulin.
   b. **False.** Its half-life is so long that it may accumulate and cause dangerous hypoglycaemia in the elderly.
   c. **True.** Because by stimulating insulin release they may increase the appetite.
   d. **True.** In patients with liver or renal disease.
   e. **True.** For the sulphonylureas.

8. a. **True.** One of its major actions.
   b. **True.** In the skin, vitamin D can be formed from cholesterol by the action of UV light.
   c. **False.** Milk and other dairy products are the best sources.
   d. **True.** Since the effect of hypoparathyroidism is hypocalcaemia.
   e. **True.** Its major use.

9. a. **True.** Usually depression, occasionally mania.
   b. **True.** Because of immune suppression.
   c. **False.** Osteoporosis, not osteomalacia.
   d. **False.** This axis is not dependent on CRF or ACTH.
   e. **True.** Striae and easy bruising.

10. a. **False.** Fluid retention is a common adverse effect of hydrocortisone.
    b. **True.** Their major use.
    c. **True.** Usually known as cortisol, for some reason.
    d. **False.** In the past yes but rarely used today.
    e. **False.** If mineralocorticoid replacement is needed, fludrocortisone is used.

11. a. **True.** This is adrenocortical insufficiency.
    b. **False.** This is primary hyperaldosteronism caused by tumour-secreting aldosterone.
    c. **True.** Usually by inhalation.
    d. **False.** Might even exacerbate this by causing immune suppression.
    e. **True.** For Hodgkin's and some other types.

12. a. **True.** But less likely with low-dose oestrogen types used today.
    b. **False.** About 2/100 as opposed to 1/100 for the COC.
    c. **True.** Since they are testosterone derivatives such as norethisterone or levonorgestril.
    d. **True.** Important for its action.
    e. **True.** With enzyme inducers and broad-spectrum antibiotics for instance.

13. a. **True.** Hence their widespread use today, while the high-dose pills are reserved for special circumstances.
    b. **False.** However, the risks are undoubtedly increased, and other risk factors should be considered before using them in older women.
    c. **True.** But may increase the risk of cervical and possibly breast cancer.
    d. **False.** Although again the risk is increased and women should be warned against smoking, particularly in combination with other risk factors.
    e. **True.** Although this is still mentioned as a contraindication in the data sheets of most of these drugs.

14. a. **False.** Probably even decreases risk of progression of IHD.
    b. **True.** Otherwise there is a risk of endometrial carcinoma.
    c. **True.** But therapy for 5–10 years is needed.
    d. **False.** May increase the risks of breast cancer (controversial).
    e. **False.** Vasomotor symptoms may start even before the last period and may be treated.

Case history answers

History 1

1. Carbimazole (perhaps with thyroxine added at a later stage when euthyroid again) and a non-specific beta-blocker (if not contraindicated).
2. The risks of agranulocytosis on carbimazole: she must be warned to return immediately if she develops any signs of infection, such as a sore throat, so that her white cell count can be checked.
3. The antibodies which cause hyperthyroidism in Graves' can cross the placenta and cause neonatal hyperthyroidism: carbimazole may cause a goitre in a fetus and this may lead to complications in the delivery.
4. The options are long-term carbimazole, surgery or radioiodine (even in someone so young, this is a safe treatment).
5. Oral contraceptives increase production of thyroid-binding globulin, giving rise to increased serum total thyroxine concentrations (but not free thyroxine or TSH which remain normal). Some heavily protein-bound drugs (such as phenytoin) can cause displacement of thyroxine from protein-binding sites and lower total (but not free thyroxine).

History 2

1. Weight loss, diet and perhaps oral hypoglycaemics. She should be educated about life style, smoking, etc.

2. Metformin is most appropriate in an obese patient.
3. Sulphonylureas might be considered second line, in addition to metformin. They should probably not be used alone, if avoidable, in an obese patient since they tend to stimulate the appetite.
4. Since she is hypertensive, thiazide diuretics might have been a precipitant: many other drugs, e.g. corticosteroids, are also possible. However, hypertension and diabetes are associated even in the absence of drug therapy.
5. Insulin should be considered if oral drugs fail to control her blood sugar, or during periods of intercurrent illness (e.g. infections etc.) or surgery, when her diabetes is likely to go out of control.

History 3

1. Diabetic ketoacidosis.
2. Intravenous fluids to rehydrate, intravenous insulin to lower the blood sugar and K^+ supplements as appropriate, depending on the serum K^+. The precipitating cause should be identified and treated where possible.
3. Soluble insulin may be given i.v., i.m., or s.c.; all others are given s.c. only.
4. Hypoglycaemia.
5. He should be treated without delay, even if the diagnosis cannot be immediately confirmed: intravenous glucose can be given by trained staff, but in the absence of these, intramuscular glucagon can be given by someone with very little training.

History 4

1. She might experience an Addisonian crisis with hypotension, collapse and death, since her hypothalamic pituitary adrenal axis is almost certainly suppressed and will need some time to recover. She might also experience a flare up of disease activity.
2. Prednisolone has some mineralocorticoid effects and will cause Na^+ and fluid retention.
3. She is at risk of osteoporosis and muscle wasting.
4. Impaired glucose tolerance, Cushingoid appearance, immune suppression are the most common.
5. Risk of an Addisonian crisis unless given additional parenteral steroids before operation, poor healing of wounds which may delay recovery afterwards.

History 5

1. The combined oral contraceptive protects against endometrial and ovarian carcinoma, but is associated with an increased incidence of cervical carcinoma. This may be due to lifestyle rather than a direct drug effect. There may also be an increase in the incidence of breast carcinoma, although this is controversial.

2. She is at higher risk of myocardial infarction or cerebrovascular accident while taking a COC and smoking: she should be advised to stop smoking. However, in a young woman this would not be a contraindication to the COC.
3. If she is less than 12 hours late, she should take the pill as soon as possible and the next at the usual time. If more than 12 hours late, the pill may be ineffective: she should continue taking the pill as usual, but use additional barrier contraceptive methods for the next 7 days. If there were less than seven tablets left in the pack, she should begin the next pack without the usual 7-day break .
4. Pulmonary embolism.
5. Carbamazepine may induce liver enzymes and reduce the efficacy of the COC. She may need a high-oestrogen dose pill.

History 6

1. Improvement in vasomotor and other symptoms of the menopause: no prophylactic effects can be anticipated in such short-term therapy.
2. Osteoporosis is common in women as there is increased bone loss after the menopause. HRT given for periods of 5–10 years reduces this — but there are concerns that there may be an increased bone loss when HRT is stopped.
3. HRT probably decreases the risks of ischaemic heart disease.
4. The doses of oestrogen used in HRT are lower than in COC and, therefore, fewer adverse effects are to be expected.
5. Systemic HRT will improve vaginal dryness, but if this the predominant symptom, the patient may prefer to use just a local vaginal oestrogen ointment.

Antibiotics (antimicrobials)

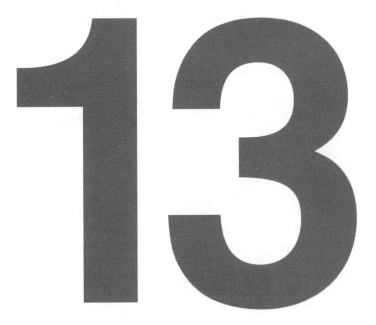

13.1 Action of antibiotics

Antimicrobials are drugs used to treat infection. They may be antibacterial (often called antibiotics, since many are derivatives of naturally produced chemicals), antiviral, antifungal, antiprotozoal or anthelminthic (see Ch. 14). Antibiotics may either kill the microorganism (bactericidal) or may retard their growth (bacteriostatic) so that the body's own immune system can overcome the infection. In clinical use, this distinction is usually not important, but bacteriostatic drugs should not be used in immunosuppressed patients, nor in life-threatening diseases like endocarditis or meningitis.

Spectrum

Antibiotics may affect a narrow or broad range or spectrum of bacteria. Broad-spectrum antibiotics are popular because doctors often fail to take adequate cultures or to consider the use of a narrow-spectrum drug, but in general they are more expensive and are particularly likely to encourage the development of antibiotic resistance. They are also associated with more adverse effects. These include the development of superinfection, in which an antibiotic, usually broad spectrum, eliminates normal bacterial flora and allows organisms which are normally not pathogenic (e.g. fungi or resistant bacteria) to flourish.

Principles for prescribing antibiotics

Antibiotics are often abused, i.e. used excessively or inappropriately, for example to treat minor viral infections (especially in childhood). Broad principles for the use of antibiotics, therefore include:

1. Make a diagnosis of bacterial infection (fever alone does not always imply bacterial infection) and its site and consider the likely organisms, e.g. in lobar pneumonia, the likely organism is *Streptococcus pneumoniae.*
2. Wherever possible, and particularly in all serious infections, take appropriate specimens (blood, sputum, pus, urine, swabs) for culture and antibiotic sensitivity testing, and perhaps for microscopy and Gram staining. It is not always practical to do this.
3. Consider the need for antibiotic therapy at all, e.g. antibiotics are usually inappropriate in gastroenteritis or many skin infections.
4. If cultures have been taken, is there a need for urgent therapy before results are available. Empirical antibiotic therapy may be necessary in seriously ill patients but may prevent the confirmation of the diagnosis of infection later or the identification of the infecting organism. This may be particularly important when there is a subsequent failure to respond or only partial response to the chosen antibiotic.

5. Select the most appropriate drug, its dose and route of administration. Consider:
    a. the organism: what antibiotics is it sensitive to? This would ideally be based on microbiological sensitivity testing but may have to be a 'best guess' if the organism or its sensitivities are not known.
    b. the patient: age, allergy, renal or hepatic function, diminished resistance to infection (malnutrition, malignant disease, immunosuppression, including by drugs such as corticosteroids), pregnancy or genetic factors (may all influence choice of or response to antibiotics).
    c. the severity of the infection: this will influence the choice of drug and route of administration. Some antibiotics are not absorbed when given orally (e.g. aminoglycosides). In seriously ill patients, parenteral administration is more reliable.
    d. the site of infection: antibiotics often do not penetrate abscess cavities well, and abscesses in general require drainage in addition. Some antibiotics may not penetrate to the site of infection (e.g. aminoglycosides are inappropriate for meningitis).
    e. the presence of foreign bodies: such as a prosthetic heart valve or a piece of glass in a skin wound, again likely to diminish or prevent response to antibiotics.
6. Monitor success of therapy clinically, or microbiologically by repeated cultures as appropriate. Some antibiotics with serious concentration-related toxicity also require monitoring of plasma concentrations (e.g. gentamicin).
7. Combinations of antibiotics are occasionally used:
    a. where there is a mixed infection, e.g. in peritonitis
    b. where the two antibiotics can produce a greater effect than one alone (synergism), e.g. penicillin and gentamicin in treating infective endocarditis
    c. where the infecting organism is not known and broad-spectrum cover is required urgently, e.g. septicaemia
    d. to prevent the development of resistance to one antibiotic, e.g. in tuberculosis.
8. Antibiotics may also be used occasionally for prophylaxis, i.e. to prevent the development of infection rather than to treat established infection. Examples are in some abdominal or orthopaedic surgery, in dental procedures for patients at risk of infective endocarditis, or in the close contacts of patients who have meningococcal meningitis. The duration of prophylactic use is brief (usually 24 hours or less), and the choice of drug is based on previous experience of what organisms are likely.

Sites of action

Antibiotics may act at different sites (Fig. 48):

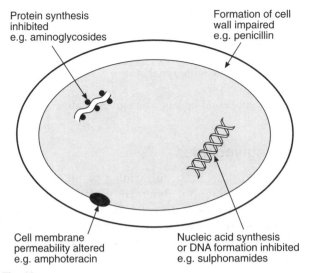

Fig. 48
Modes of action of antibiotics.

- by inhibiting formation of the bacterial cell wall, e.g. penicillin and cephalosporins
- by inhibiting bacterial protein synthesis, e.g. tetracyclines, aminoglycosides, erythromycin, chloramphenicol
- by inhibiting nucleic acid synthesis, either at an early stage, e.g. sulphonamides, trimethoprim, or later, e.g. ciprofloxacin, rifampicin
- by altering the permeability of cytoplasmic membranes, e.g. amphotericin (an antifungal, see Ch. 14).

Antimicrobial resistance

The increased use of an antibiotic encourages the emergence of resistant strains of bacteria. There are geographic variations in antibiotic resistance depending on local prescribing trends. For safe empirical therapy, it is important to know the local patterns of resistance and help should be sought from a microbiologist. The reasons for resistance vary. Some antibiotics would never affect an organism because of its structure and their site of action. For example, Gram-negative bacilli are resistant to benzylpenicillin.

Some bacteria acquire resistance. These traits may arise as new mutations or may be transferred from organism to organism by plasmids (DNA packages) either by conjugation or transduction, or by bacteriophage viruses.

Resistance can occur through a number of mechanisms:

- the production of an enzyme which breaks down the antibiotic, e.g. β-lactamase and many penicillins
- the cell membrane becomes impermeable to a drug, e.g. tetracyclines
- structural or biochemical alteration within the organism which makes it less susceptible, e.g. alteration of ribosomal structure may lead to erythromycin resistance.

13.2 Major antibiotics

Penicillins

Penicillins contain a β-lactam ring which inhibits the formation of peptidoglycan crosslinks in bacterial cell walls (especially in Gram-positive organisms). The wall is weakened and water enters the cell by osmosis and causes cells to burst. Penicillins are bactericidal but can act only on dividing cells. They are not toxic to animal cells which have no cell wall.

Clinical pharmacokinetics
The penicillins are poorly lipid soluble and do not cross the blood–brain barrier in appreciable concentrations unless it is inflamed (so they are effective in meningitis). They are actively excreted unchanged by the kidney, but the dose should be reduced in severe renal failure. This tubular secretion can be blocked by probenecid to potentiate penicillin's action.

Resistance
This is usually the result of production of β-lactamase in the bacteria which destroys the β-lactam ring. It occurs in organisms such as *Staphylococcus aureus* (90% of strains), *Haemophilus influenzae* and *Neisseria gonorrhoea* (about 5–10%).

Examples
There are now a wide variety of penicillins, which may be acid labile (i.e. broken down by the stomach acid and so inactive when given orally) or acid stable, or may be narrow or broad spectrum in action.

Benzylpenicillin (penicillin G) is acid labile and β-lactamase sensitive and is only given parenterally. It is the most potent penicillin but has a relatively narrow spectrum covering *Streptococcus pyogenes*, *S. pneumoniae*, *Neisseria meningitidis* or *N. gonorrhoeae*, treponemes, *Listeria*, *Actinomyces* and many anaerobic organisms, e.g. *Clostridia*.

Phenoxymethylpenicillin (penicillin V) is acid stable and is given orally for minor infections; it is otherwise similar to benzylpenicillin.

Ampicillin is less active than benzylpenicillin against Gram-positive bacteria but has a wider spectrum including (in addition to those above) *Streptococcus faecalis*, *Haemophilus influenza*, and some *Escherichia coli*, *Klebsiella* and *Proteus* strains. It is acid stable and is given orally or parenterally, but is β-lactamase sensitive.

Amoxycillin is similar but better absorbed orally. Amoxycillin is sometimes combined with *clavulanic acid*, which is a β-lactam with little antibacterial effect but which binds strongly to β-lactamase. It, therefore, blocks the action of β-lactamase and extends the spectrum of amoxycillin.

Flucloxacillin is acid stable and is given orally or parenterally. It is β-lactamase resistant and is used as a narrow spectrum drug for *Staphylococcus aureus* infections.

Azlocillin is not acid stable and is only used parenterally. It is β-lactamase sensitive and has a broad spectrum, which includes *Pseudomonas aeruginosa* and *Proteus* species. It is used intravenously for life-threatening infections, especially in immunocompromised patients, in combination with an aminoglycoside.

Adverse effects

These are relatively unusual.

- Allergy occurs in 0.7% to 10% of patients, ranging from urticaria to potentially fatal anaphylaxis; patients should always be asked about a history of previous exposure and adverse effects. Rashes are common with ampicillin or amoxycillin (almost invariable if they are given in error to patients with infectious mononucleosis) and do not represent a true allergy
- Superinfections (e.g. oral thrush caused by *Candida*)
- Diarrhoea: especially with ampicillin (20%), less common with amoxycillin, as it is better absorbed
- Rare: blood dyscrasia or haemolysis; nephritis (ampicillin).

Drug interactions

The use for ampicillin (or other broad-spectrum antibiotics) may decrease the effectiveness of oral contraceptives by diminishing enterohepatic circulation.

Cephalosporins

Cephalosporins also owe their activity to a β-lactam ring and are bactericidal. They are broad-spectrum antibiotics. There are many different cephalosporins with varying side chains; these alter pharmacokinetics, spectrum of activity and β-lactamase resistance. Cephalosporins are relatively expensive and, although good alternatives to penicillins when a broad-spectrum drug is required, should not be used as first choice unless the organism is known to be sensitive. Some cephalosporins (e.g. cefotaxime) may be indicated for empirical use to treat life-threatening infections where the organism is probably sensitive.

Examples and clinical pharmacokinetics

Cephradine and *cephalexin* are well absorbed orally; cephradine can also be given parenterally. They cover mostly Gram-positive organisms, such as *Streptococcus pyogenes*, *S. pneumoniae* and *Staphylococcus aureus*, as well as some Gram-negative bacteria, although they are less effective in this than later cephalosporins. They are excreted by the kidney (reduce dose in renal failure).

Cefuroxime can be given parenterally or as an oral prodrug. It has a broader spectrum, including many Gram-negative bacilli.

Cefotaxime is given parenterally. It has an even broader spectrum, including many *Enterobacter*, *E. coli* and *Proteus* strains.

Adverse effects

- Allergy (10–20% of patients with penicillin allergy are also allergic to cephalosporins)
- Nephritis and acute renal failure
- Superinfections
- Gastrointestinal upsets when given orally.

Aminoglycosides

Aminoglycosides cause misreading of mRNA by the ribosome, leading to abnormal protein production. They are bactericidal. To enter the bacterium, aminoglycosides need to be actively transported across the cell membrane: this does not occur in anaerobic organisms, which are, therefore, resistant.

Clinical pharmacokinetics

These are poorly lipid soluble and, therefore, not absorbed orally: parenteral administration is required for systemic effect. They do not enter the CNS even when the meninges are inflamed. They are not metabolised and are excreted unchanged by the kidney (where very high concentrations may occur, perhaps causing toxic tubular damage) by glomerular filtration (no active secretion). Their clearance is markedly reduced in renal impairment and toxic concentrations are more likely.

Resistance results from bacterial enzymes which break down aminoglycosides or to their decreased transport into the cells.

Examples

Gentamicin is the most commonly used, covering Gram-negative aerobes, e.g. enteric organisms (*E. coli*, *Klebsiella*, *S. faecalis*, *Pseudomonas* and *Proteus spp.*), and is also used in antibiotic combinations against *Staphylococcus aureus*. They are not active against aerobic *Streptococci*. In addition to treating known sensitive organisms, it is used often blindly with other antibiotics in severe infections of unknown cause.

Streptomycin was formerly the mainstay of antituberculous therapy but is now rarely used in the developed world.

Tobramycin: used for pseudomonas and for some gentamicin-resistant organisms.

Some aminoglycosides, e.g. gentamicin, may also be applied topically for local effect, for example in ear and eye ointments. *Neomycin* is used orally for decontamination of the gastrointestinal tract (e.g. in hepatic encephalopathy).

Adverse effects

Although effective, the aminoglycosides are toxic, and this is plasma concentration related. It is essential to *monitor plasma concentrations* (usually trough and peak, i.e. shortly before and after administration of a dose) to ensure adequate concentrations for bactericidal effect, while minimising adverse effects, every 2–3 days during treatment. The main adverse effects are:

- Nephrotoxicity
- Toxic to the 8th cranial nerve (ototoxic), especially the vestibular division

Other adverse effects are not dose related, and are relatively rare, e.g. allergies, eosinophilia.

Macrolides

These are broad-spectrum antibiotics which are relatively non-toxic but to which resistance develops rapidly. They inhibit protein synthesis by binding to the ribosome and are bacteriostatic at usual doses but bactericidal in high doses.

Examples and clinical pharmacokinetics

Erythromycin is acid labile but is given as an enterically coated tablet; however, absorption is erratic and poor. It is excreted unchanged in bile and is reabsorbed lower down the gastrointestinal tract (enterohepatic circulation). It may be given orally or parenterally. Erythromycin is widely distributed in the body except to the brain and cerebrospinal fluid, and the spectrum includes *Staphylococcus aureus*, *Streptococcus pyogenes*, *Streptococcus pneumoniae*. It is especially useful in these infections as an alternative to penicillins in allergic patients. In addition, it is specifically indicated in *Legionella pneumoniae*, *Mycoplasma pneumoniae* and *Chlamydia* infections.

Newer macrolides such as *clarithromycin*, or *azithromycin* may have fewer adverse effects.

Adverse effects

- Gastrointestinal upsets (common)
- Rarely hypersensitivity, or cholestatic jaundice.

Clindamycin

Clindamycin, although chemically distinct, is similar to erythromycin in mode of action and spectrum. It is rapidly absorbed and penetrates most tissues well, except the CNS. It is particularly useful systemically for *S. aureus* (especially osteomyelitis as it penetrates bone well) and anaerobic infections.

Adverse effects

Diarrhoea is common. *Pseudomembranous colitis* is a serious inflammation of the large bowel caused by a superinfection with a strain of *Clostridium difficile* which secretes a toxin that damages the mucosal lining; this may occur after any antibiotic but is especially common after clindamycin, which severely limits its use.

Sulphonamides and trimethoprim

Sulphonamides are rarely used alone today. Trimethoprim is not chemically related but is considered here because their modes of action are complementary.

Mode of action

Sulphonamides are competitive antagonists of para-aminobenzoic acid (PABA), a precursor of folic acid that is essential for the synthesis of purine nucleotides for DNA and RNA. Animals do not manufacture folate, depending on absorbed folate and so are unaffected. Folate is metabolised by the enzyme dihydrofolate reductase to the active tetrahydrofolic acid. *Trimethoprim* inhibits this enzyme in bacteria and to a lesser degree in animals, as the animal enzyme is far less sensitive than that in bacteria. Individually, these drugs are bacteriostatic; but a combination, *cotrimoxazole*, of a sulphonamide (*sulphamethoxazole*) and trimethoprim is bactericidal.

Clinical pharmacokinetics

Most sulphonamides are well absorbed orally and they are widely distributed including to the CNS. Most are excreted by the kidney unchanged.

They are effective against Gram-positive and many Gram-negative organisms but are rarely used alone now. Trimethoprim is also well absorbed and excreted by the kidneys, with a similar spectrum. Cotrimoxazole is widely used for urinary and upper respiratory tract infections but should not be the drug of choice because of its adverse effects. It is the drug of choice for the treatment and prevention of pneumonia caused by *Pneumocystis carinii* in immunosuppressed patients. Trimethoprim is increasingly used alone for urinary tract and upper respiratory tract infections, as it is less toxic than the combination and equally effective.

Adverse effects

- Gastrointestinal upsets
- Less common but more serious:
  — sulphonamides: allergy, rash, fever agranulocytosis Stevens–Johnson syndrome (a severe skin reaction) haemolysis in patients with glucose 6-phosphatase deficiency renal toxicity: sulphonamides may form crystals in an acid urine leading to tubular damage and severe renal impairment
  — trimethoprim: macrocytic anaemia thrombocytopenia
  — cotrimoxazole: aplastic anaemia (especially in the elderly).

Drug interactions

Sulphonamides can decrease metabolism of phenytoin, warfarin and some oral hypoglycaemics, increasing their effects.

Quinolones

The quinolones are effective but expensive antibiotics; less expensive drugs are often equally effective, especially for minor infections. With increased use, resistance to these drugs is becoming more common. The quinolones should in general be reserve drugs and not first-line treatment.

Quinolones inhibit DNA gyrase and prevent recoiling of DNA after replication. This is bactericidal to dividing cells.

Examples and clinical pharmacokinetics

Nalidixic acid, the first quinolone, is used as a urinary antiseptic and for lower urinary tract infections, as it has no systemic antibacterial effect.

Ciprofloxacin is a fluoroquinolone with a broad spectrum against Gram-negative bacilli and *Pseudomonas*, it can be given orally or i.v. to treat a wide range of infections, including respiratory and urinary tract infections as well as more serious infections, such as peritonitis and *Salmonella*. Activity against anaerobic organisms or *Streptococcus pneumoniae* is poor and it should not be first choice for respiratory tract infections.

Adverse effects

- Gastrointestinal upsets
- Fluorouinolones may block the inhibitory neurotransmitter GABA, and this may cause confusion in the elderly and lower the fitting threshold. They are also contraindicated in epileptics
- Allergy and anaphylaxis
- Possibly damage to growing cartilage: not recommended for pregnant women or children.

Drug interactions

Ciprofloxacin is a liver enzyme inhibitor and may cause life-threatening interactions with theophylline.

Tetracyclines

These bind to the ribosome and interfere with protein synthesis. They are bacteriostatic.

Examples and clinical pharmacokinetics

Tetracycline, oxytetracycline have short half-lives, while *doxycycline* has a longer half-life and can be given once per day. These drugs are only partly absorbed. They bind avidly to heavy metal ions and so absorption is greatly reduced if taken with food, milk, antacids or iron tablets. They should be taken at least half an hour before food.

Tetracyclines concentrate in bones and teeth. They are excreted mostly in urine, partly in bile. They are broad-spectrum antibiotics, active against most bacteria except *Proteus* or *Pseudomonas*. Resistance is frequent. Tetracyclines are specifically indicated for *Mycoplasma*, *Rickettsia*, *Chlamydia* and *Brucella* infections. Their most common use today is for acne, given either orally or topically.

Adverse effects

- Gastrointestinal upset

- Superinfection
- Discolouration and deformity in growing teeth and bones (contraindicated in pregnancy and in children <12 years)
- Renal impairment (should also be avoided in renal disease).

Metronidazole

Metronidazole binds to DNA and blocks replication.

Pharmacokinetics. It is well absorbed after oral or rectal administration and can also be given intravenously. It is widely distributed in the body (including into abscess cavities) and is metabolised by the liver.

Uses. Metronidazole is active against anaerobic organisms (e.g. *Bacteroides, Clostridia*), which are encountered particularly in abdominal surgery. It is also used against *Trichomonas, Giardia* and *Entamoeba* infections and can be used to treat pseudomembranous colitis. Increasingly, it is used as part of the treatment of *Helicobacter pyloris* infection of the stomach and duodenum associated with peptic ulcer disease. It is used also to treat a variety of dental infections, particularly dental abscess.

Adverse effects

- Nausea, anorexia and a metallic taste
- Ataxia, caused by peripheral neuropathy
- Disulfiram-like reaction (Ch. 18): metronidazole inhibits alcohol dehydrogenase, and patients receiving it who drink alcohol may experience unpleasant reactions (flushing, abdominal pain, hypotension) as alcohol is metabolised to toxins such as acetaldehyde. Patients taking metronidazole should be advised not to drink alcohol
- Possibly teratogenic if taken in the first trimester of pregnancy.

Drug interactions

Metronidazole may inhibit the metabolism of warfarin.

Nitrofurantoin

This is used as a urinary antiseptic and to treat Gram-negative infections in the lower urinary tract. It is taken orally and is well absorbed and is excreted unchanged in the urine. It only exerts its antimicrobial effect when it is concentrated in the urine and so has no systemic antibacterial effect. It is ineffective in renal failure because of failure to concentrate. Resistance develops relatively quickly.

Adverse effects

- Gastrointestinal upsets
- Allergy (including pulmonary fibrosis)
- Polyneuritis.

Fucidin

Fucidin is active only against *Staphylococcus aureus* (by inhibiting bacterial protein synthesis) and is not affected by β-lactamase. It is usually only used with flucloxacillin to reduce the development of resistance. It is well absorbed and widely distributed, including to bone (useful in osteomyelitis). It can be given orally or parenterally. It is metabolised in the liver.

Adverse effects

- Gastrointestinal upsets
- Hepatitis and jaundice.

Vancomycin

This interferes with bacterial cell wall formation and is only effective against Gram-positive organisms. It is not absorbed after oral administration and must be given parenterally. It is excreted by the kidney. It is used intravenously to treat serious or resistant *Staphylococcus aureus* infections and for prophylaxis of endocarditis in penicillin-allergic patients. It is given orally to treat pseudomembranous colitis (see above).

Teicoplanin is similar but less toxic.

Adverse effects

Although not an aminoglycoside, vancomycin's toxicity is similar and likewise *monitoring of plasma concentrations* is essential.

- Nephrotoxicity
- Ototoxicity
- Allergy.

Chloramphenicol

This inhibits bacterial protein synthesis. It is well absorbed and widely distributed, including to the CNS. It is metabolised by glucuronidation in the liver.

Although an effective broad-spectrum antibiotic, its uses are limited by its serious toxicity. The major indication is to treat bacterial meningitis caused by *Haemophilus influenza*, or to *Neisseria meningitidis* (initially in addition to benzylpenicillin or alone if patient is penicillin allergic) or if organism is unknown. It is also specifically used for *Rickettsia* (typhus).

Adverse effects

- A rare idiosyncratic aplastic anaemia (1/50 000), probably immunological in origin but often fatal
- Reversible bone marrow depression caused by its effect on protein synthesis in humans
- Liver enzyme inhibition.

13.3 Antibiotics for tuberculosis

Tuberculosis (TB) is a major cause of death in many parts of the world. In the developed world, TB is currently undergoing a resurgence, partly because of infection in immunosuppressed patients.

The tubercle bacillus (*Mycobacterium tuberculosis*) is an intracellular organism which may survive for months in dormant forms. Therapy, therefore, needs to be prolonged. Drug-resistant mutants are often present and will proliferate if only single drug therapy is used; hence several drugs are used simultaneously to avoid resistance. Failure of therapy is most often the result of poor compliance with the drugs rather than drug resistance.

Regimens for treating pulmonary TB

These will differ around the world, determined partly by bacterial resistance but mainly by economic factors. Currently recommended treatment in the UK is:

1. rifampicin and isoniazid for 6 months
2. in addition, pyrazinamide and ethambutol for the first 2 months (quadruple therapy).

Some doubt the value of ethambutol and omit it.

Isoniazid

Isoniazid is bactericidal, but the mode of action is unknown. It is the most active of the antiTB drugs. It is well absorbed after oral administration and widely distributed, including into the CNS. It is acetylated by the liver prior to excretion; this shows genetic polymorphism (i.e. variation in metabolism due to genetic differences producing enzymes of different activity) giving rise to fast and slow acetylators, which occur with different frequencies in different populations. For instance, Eskimos are predominantly fast, while Egyptians are predominantly slow, and Europeans are about 50% fast and 50% slow. Acetylation ability may affect efficiency and toxicity in an individual.

Adverse effects

- Peripheral neuropathy (occurs particularly in slow acetylators and is preventable by giving pyridoxine)
- Hepatitis
- Rashes
- Drug-induced lupus syndrome: a syndrome resembling systemic lupus erythematosis.

Drug interactions

Isoniazid is a liver enzyme inhibitor (caution with phenytoin and warfarin).

Rifampicin

Rifampicin inhibits RNA synthesis in bacteria but not in humans and is bactericidal. As well as its use in TB, it is also a valuable broad-spectrum antibiotic but its use is restricted to prophylaxis for the contacts of patients with meningococcal meningitis, and the treatment of *Legionella pneumoniae* and *Staphylococcus aureus*. It is well absorbed after oral administration (best taken on an empty stomach) and is widely distributed. It is metabolised in the liver and excreted in bile.

Adverse effects

- Malaise, headache
- Fever, rashes
- Hepatitis
- Invariably, all body secretions (urine, tears, etc.) become an orange-red colour.

Drug interactions

Rifampicin is a potent liver enzyme inducer and may cause interactions with anticonvulsants, warfarin, oral contraceptives, etc.

Pyrazinamide

Pyrazinamide is bactericidal. It is well absorbed and widely distributed, in particular achieving good penetration of the CNS.

Adverse effects

1. Hepatitis, especially if given at high doses. Liver function tests should be monitored
2. Hyperuricaemia.

Ethambutol

Ethambutol is bacteriostatic but its mode of action is unknown. It is excreted by the kidneys.

Adverse effects

Optic neuritis, which is dose related and rare.

Reserve drugs in TB

Thiacetazone, ethionamide, paraaminosalicylate, capreomycin, streptomycin.

13.4 Antibiotics for leprosy

Leprosy is caused by infection with *Mycobacteria leprae*. A mixture of drugs are used to treat leprosy, depending on the type and severity of the infection and the local resistance patterns. *Rifampicin* is used and *dapsone*, which is related to the sulphonamides and also inhibits folate metabolism. Dapsone is also used to treat dermatitis herpetiformis (see Ch. 16). Its adverse effects include haemolysis, gastrointestinal upsets and rashes.

Self-assessment: questions

Multiple choice questions

1. The following antimicrobials should be avoided in pregnant women:
   a. Gentamicin
   b. Tetracycline
   c. Amoxycillin
   d. Nitrofurantoin
   e. Trimethoprim

2. In treating any infection:
   a. Cultures must always be taken first
   b. The clinical picture is of no help in deciding appropriate antibiotic therapy
   c. Superinfection implies infection with an organism resistant to antibiotics
   d. Antibiotic therapy may be standardised for all patients with each infection
   e. Combinations of antibiotics are sometimes useful

3. Failure to respond to an antibiotic may result from:
   a. Microbial resistance to the antibiotics used
   b. Inappropriate selection of antibiotics
   c. Immunosuppression of the patient
   d. Inappropriate route of administration
   e. good blood supply to the area infected

4. Penicillins:
   a. Are highly lipid soluble
   b. Are excreted by glomerular filtration
   c. May all be destroyed by β-lactamase-producing bacteria
   d. Some may be given orally
   e. Are usually highly effective against streptococcal infection

5. Anaphylaxis:
   a. Should be treated with adrenaline
   b. Is life threatening
   c. May occur within seconds or minutes of administration of a drug
   d. Usually occurs on first exposure to the drug
   e. Is caused by endotoxin release

6. Aminoglycosides:
   a. Cross the blood–brain barrier
   b. Are metabolised by the liver
   c. May cause ototoxicity
   d. Require plasma concentration measurement
   e. Are effective against anaerobic organisms like bacteroides

7. Erythromycin:
   a. May interact with phenytoin
   b. Is well absorbed after oral administration
   c. May cause nausea and vomiting
   d. May be used to treat *Legionella pneumoniae*
   e. Cross-allergy to penicillin may occur

8. Sulphonamides:
   a. May cause drug interactions by displacement from plasma proteins
   b. Inhibit nucleic acid formation in humans
   c. Cotrimoxazole may cause blood dyscrasias
   d. Cotrimoxazole may be used in the treatment of patients with AIDS
   e. Trimethoprim is more likely to cause adverse drug reactions than cotrimoxazole

9. Ciprofloxacin:
   a. Blocks protein synthesis
   b. Is the first choice drug for pneumonia
   c. May cause drug hypersensitivity
   d. Is effective against Gram-negative bacilli
   e. May cause interactions with theophylline

10. Tetracyclines:
    a. Are used to treat acne
    b. Should be taken with meals
    c. Should not be given to young children
    d. Bacterial resistance is rare
    e. Superinfection is common

11. Metronidazole:
    a. Is well absorbed
    b. Is effective in some protozoal infections
    c. Can be used to treat peptic ulcer disease
    d. May cause cerebellar damage
    e. May interact with ethanol

12. The antibiotic:
    a. Vancomycin is an aminoglycoside
    b. Vancomycin may be given orally to treat pseudomembranous colitis
    c. Fucidin and vancomycin are both effective against *Staph. aureus*
    d. Chloramphenicol is widely used for respiratory tract infections
    e. Nitrofurantoin is used for Gram-negative septicaemia

13. In treating TB:
    a. Multiple drug therapy is usual
    b. Treatment for 1 month is considered adequate
    c. Isoniazid is metabolised at different rates in different races
    d. Isoniazid may cause hepatic failure
    e. Isoniazid may cause liver enzyme induction

14. In treating TB:
    a. Rifampicin is only used against TB
    b. Rifampicin inhibits the metabolism of warfarin
    c. Rifampicin may cause the urine to change colour
    d. Pyrazinamide may cause hepatitis
    e. Patients about to start taking ethambutol should have their eyes checked first

Case histories

History 1

> A 23-year-old woman presents with a urinary tract infection causing cystitis.

1. What general advice should be given to her?
2. What antibiotics should be considered?
3. If the woman were pregnant, how would this alter your choice of antibiotic?

History 2

> A 54-year-old alcoholic man with no fixed address is found to have tuberculosis with acid- and alcohol-fast bacilli seen in the sputum.

1. Is he infectious?
2. What drugs should be administered and in what regimen?
3. Do his social circumstances pose any problems?

History 3

> A 65-year-old man with a long history of chronic obstructive airway disease develops acute bronchitis: his doctor decides to prescribe an antibiotic.

1. What antibiotics would be appropriate first choices?
2. A week later, the patient returns to the doctor complaining of severe diarrhoea: what diagnosis should be considered?
3. If this diagnosis is confirmed, how should it be treated?

Essay question

List some strategies that can be adopted to reduce the risks of bacterial resistance to antibiotics developing.

Self-assessment: answers

Multiple choice answers

1. a. **True.** Aminoglycosides and vancomycin may cause 8th nerve damage in the fetus.
   b. **True.** Teeth, bone deformities may occur in the fetus.
   c. **False.** Widely used.
   d. **False.** May be used but should be avoided in late pregnancy or breast-feeding.
   e. **True.** Folate antagonist and possibly teratogenic.

2. a. **False.** This is an ideal but not always possible, e.g. in severely ill patients.
   b. **False.** The clinical picture often gives clues, e.g. a lobar pneumonia is most often caused by *Streptococcus pneumoniae* and benzylpenicillin is appropriate.
   c. **True.** At least to the antibiotic which has led to the superinfection.
   d. **False.** Although broad guidelines may be given, each case must be judged on its own merits (as occurs elsewhere in medicine).
   e. **True.** For example in treating TB.

3. a. **True.** For example, penicillinase-producing *Staph. aureus* will not respond to amoxycillin.
   b. **True.** For example, use of benzylpenicillin to treat a Gram-negative infection would be inappropriate.
   c. **True.** If the patient is known to be immunosuppressed, antibiotic regimens will need to be more sophisticated and aggressive to achieve cure.
   d. **True.** For example, oral antibiotics to treat a septicaemia.
   e. **False.** Poor blood supply to an infected area may prevent antibiotic transport to the site, and importantly will also lead to poor tissue inflammatory responses and healing.

4. a. **False.** They are preferentially water soluble.
   b. **False.** They are excreted actively in the renal tubule.
   c. **False.** For example, flucloxacillin.
   d. **True.** For example, amoxycillin, etc.
   e. **True.** Usually the drugs of first choice for this.

5. a. **True.** This is a physiological antagonist to histamine.
   b. **True.** If not treated promptly.
   c. **True.** Particularly after parenteral administration.
   d. **False.** The patient must have been sensitised to the drug previously, but a history of exposure may be difficult to find; patients have unwittingly been sensitised to penicillin by penicillin in milk.
   e. **False.** Endotoxin release by bacteria is a factor in septicaemic shock.

6. a. **False.** Since they are poorly lipid soluble.
   b. **False.** They are excreted by the kidney: this is a general feature of drugs that are not lipid soluble.
   c. **True.** A major adverse effect.
   d. **True.** To avoid some of the dose-related adverse effects.
   e. **False.** Only effective against aerobic organisms.

7. a. **True.** Erythromycin is a liver enzyme inhibitor.
   b. **False.** Absorption is erratic.
   c. **True.** The most common adverse effect.
   d. **True.**
   e. **False.** Widely used to treat patients thought to be allergic to penicillin.

8. a. **True.** Although enzyme inhibition may also occur.
   b. **False.** Humans cannot manufacture folate and so are not affected.
   c. **True.** Especially in the elderly.
   d. **True.** To treat *Pneumocystis pneumoniae* infection.
   e. **False.** Trimethoprim is part of cotrimoxazole and is far less likely to cause adverse effects than the sulphonamide component.

9. a. **False.** Interferes with nucleic acid coiling.
   b. **False.** Not very effective against *Strep. pneumoniae*.
   c. **True.** Anaphylaxis and other reactions are recorded.
   d. **True.** This is its main use.
   e. **True.** By liver enzyme inhibition.

10. a. **True.** And probably its most common use.
    b. **False.** It will bind to heavy metal ions in the food and not be absorbed.
    c. **True.** Damage to teeth.
    d. **False.** Increasingly common.
    e. **True.**

11. a. **True.** And penetrates most tissues well.
    b. **True.** For example, amoebiasis.
    c. **True.** When peptic ulcer disease is associated with *Helicobacter* infection.
    d. **False.** May cause ataxia, but this is caused by peripheral neuropathy.
    e. **True.** The disulfiram reaction.

12. a. **False.** Although similar in its toxicity.
    b. **True.** Metronidazole is usually first choice on grounds of cost.
    c. **True.** Also flucloxacillin (the most widely used) and rifampicin.

d. **False.** Considered too toxic for anything other than life-threatening indications.
e. **False.** Nitrofurantoin is only effective after concentration in the urine.

13. a. **True.** To reduce resistance.
    b. **False.** Treatment for 6 months is usually the minimum for pulmonary TB.
    c. **True.** Genetic polymorphism.
    d. **True.** Especially in patients who are fast acetylators or who are enzyme induced.
    e. **False.** Liver enzyme inhibitor.

14. a. **False.** Also used for *Staph. aureus* and *Legionella pneumoniae*.
    b. **False.** Rifampicin is a liver enzyme inducer.
    c. **True.** Orange.
    d. **True.** This is rare at currently used doses.
    e. **True.** Since optic neuritis is a major adverse effect.

Case history answers

History 1

1. Copious fluid intake, rest and antipyretics as necessary.
2. Antibiotic choice will ideally be based on urine culture. Amoxycillin, trimethoprim or nitrofurantoin would all be reasonable choices. Ciprofloxacin should be a reserve drug.
3. Treating minor urinary tract infections is more important in pregnant women because of the increased risk of progression to pyelonephritis. Neither trimethoprim nor ciprofloxacin would be appropriate.

History 2

1. Yes: he should be isolated if possible for the first 2 weeks of treatment.
2. Rifampicin and isoniazid for 6 months: pyrazinamide and possibly ethambutol for the first 2 months also.
3. This patient's compliance with long-term medication might be poor. It might be appropriate to admit him to hospital for the duration of his treatment or to otherwise ensure that he takes his medication under observation.

History 3

1. Trimethoprim or amoxycillin or erythromycin would be appropriate.
2. The patient may have pseudomembranous colitis as a result of the use of broad-spectrum antibiotic. A stool sample should be sent for detection of the toxin, and a sigmoidoscopy performed.
3. Metronidazole is first choice with vancomycin for resistant cases.

Essay answer

Make the following points:

1. Restricting drug use to confirmed indications and sensitive bacteria.
2. Using drug combinations if treatment is to be prolonged.
3. Avoid unnecessarily prolonged treatment.
4. Establish a hierarchy or drug usage with more potent drugs reserved for resistant cases.

Chemotherapy for viruses, fungi and protozoa

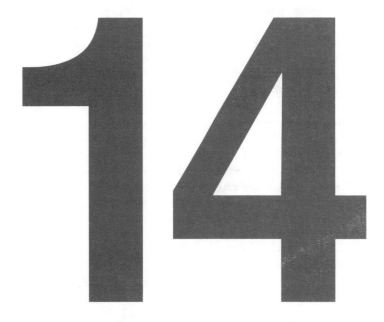

14.1 Antiviral drugs

Antiviral chemotherapy, unlike that for bacteria, is still in its infancy: few of the vast number of viral infections are susceptible to drugs, and many of the available compounds suffer from variable efficacy, unacceptable toxicity or both. Viruses are more difficult 'targets' than bacteria: they are most vulnerable during reproduction, but all use host cell organelles and enzymes to do this, so that antiviral compounds are often as toxic to host cells as to the virus. Viruses have assumed increasing importance in the setting of immunosuppression — both drug induced and AIDS.

Current antiviral drugs are thought to work in one of the following ways:

- inhibition of viral 'uncoating' shortly after penetration into the cell; such drugs are best used prophylactically, or very early in the disease course (e.g. amantadine)
- interference with viral RNA synthesis and function (e.g. ribavirin)
- interference with DNA synthesis by acting as analogues of pyrimidine or purine bases (e.g. idoxuridine, cytarabine and vidarabine)
- inhibition of viral DNA polymerase (e.g. aciclovir and gancyclovir)
- inhibition of reverse transcriptase (relevant only to retroviruses such as HIV; e.g. zidovudine)
- use of complex 'natural' antiviral defences by employing interferon.

Aciclovir

Mode of action

Aciclovir is active against Herpes simplex and Herpes zoster. When taken up into cells infected by virus, acyclovir is phosphorylated by viral thymidine kinase to a monophosphate derivative: host cell thymidine kinase reacts with the drug about 100 times more slowly. Therefore, aciclovir targets virus-infected cells quite specifically, and this explains the drug's relatively low toxicity. The monophosphate is then further phosphorylated to a triphosphate which is a potent inhibitor of DNA polymerase.

Clinical pharmacokinetics

The drug is used topically, orally and i.v. Little drug is absorbed from topical formulations, and the bioavailability of the oral drug is low (about 20%). Acyclovir is widely distributed and crosses the blood–brain barrier. It is mainly excreted in the urine as the unchanged drug. In lactating women it is also excreted in breast milk.

Therapeutic uses

Aciclovir is now the drug of first choice for Herpes simplex and zoster infections, because of greater effi-cacy and lower toxicity than the alternatives. The drug has little activity against cytomegalovirus or Epstein–Barr virus because these lack thymidine kinase.

- Herpes simplex infections of skin, mucous membranes and cornea: these are treated with topical preparations in the immune-competent host
- Life-threatening Herpes simplex infections: encephalitis may complicate immunodeficiency of whatever cause and may also occur in the immune-competent; aciclovir i.v. reduces mortality
- Herpes zoster: this is less sensitive to aciclovir than Herpes simplex, but *early* topical or oral treatment of zoster (preferably at the first sign of erythema) shortens duration and reduces the incidence of post-herpetic neuralgia; aciclovir i.v. is used for life-threatening zoster infection such as pneumonia.

Adverse effects

- Renal impairment: mainly with high i.v. doses in dehydrated patients
- Local inflammation following extravascular administration
- Encephalopathy: mainly at high i.v. doses.

Drug interactions

The renal excretion of aciclovir is impaired by probenecid, and the drug is potentiated.

Zidovudine (AZT)

Mode of action

Human immunodeficiency virus (HIV) is an RNA virus capable of inducing the synthesis of a DNA transcript of its genome, which can then become integrated into the host cell's DNA, thereby allowing viral replication. Synthesis of the initial DNA transcript involves the enzyme reverse transcriptase. Zidovudine, having been taken into the cell, is phosphorylated, and the triphosphate is a potent inhibitor of reverse transcriptase. Because this enzyme is not posessed by the host, zidovudine has relatively specific toxicity for the virus.

Clinical pharmacokinetics

Zidovudine is well absorbed from the gut but subject to first-pass metabolism; bioavailability is about 70%. The drug is widely distributed and crosses the blood–brain barrier. Most of the drug is eliminated by hepatic metabolism (mainly glucuronidation), unchanged zidovudine accounting for about 10% of the dose. In patients with renal or liver impairment, the drug may accumulate, and doses are usually adjusted in these disease states.

Therapeutic uses

This drug is used to prolong life in patients with AIDS and AIDS-related complex (ARC); it probably does not delay the onset of AIDS in HIV-positive patients. The drug usually produces a rise in CD4 cell counts, but eventual deterioration is usual in spite of zidovudine. In patients with late AIDS (often complicated by multiple opportunistic infections) zidovudine is of little use.

Adverse effects

- Bone marrow toxicity: macrocytosis is common, and about one third of patients develop severe anaemia or neutropenia
- Polymyositis: muscle pain and tenderness, accompanied by fever, may respond to NSAIDs
- Headache and insomnia.

Drug interactions

- Paracetamol: the risk of bone marrow suppression may be increased
- Probenecid: zidovudine excretion may be reduced.

Other purine and pyrimidine analogues

Mode of action

These drugs are effective against DNA viruses. The compounds structurally resemble purine and pyrimidine nucleosides; after uptake into the cell they are phosphorylated and incorporated into DNA. The resulting DNA molecule is more easily fragmented, leading to transcription errors. Additionally, these drugs inhibit viral, and to a lesser extent host, DNA polymerase thereby interfering with DNA synthesis.

Examples and clinical pharmacokinetics

Idoxuridine: this drug is not absorbed from the gut, and is used topically.

Vidarabine: cannot be given orally because it is metabolised in the gut; it is usually given i.v., though it may be used topically. The drug is eliminated mainly by metabolism (partly by xanthine oxidase) and has a short half-life.

Therapeutic uses

Idoxuridine: may be used *topically* for Herpes simplex and zoster but is too toxic for systemic use and has largely been supplanted by acyclovir.

Vidarabine: may be used for life-threatening systemic Herpes simplex and zoster infections.

Adverse effects

Idoxuridine: because this drug is only used topically, severe adverse effects are unusual; when given i.v. it causes marked bone marrow depression.

Vidarabine: anorexia, nausea, vomiting, diarrhoea and bone marrow suppression.

Drug interactions

The metabolism of vidarabine is inhibited by the xanthine oxidase inhibitor allopurinol, and toxicity may result.

Ribavirin

Ribavirin is effective against a wide range of DNA and RNA viruses. When taken up by cells it is phosphorylated, and this is the active form. Ribavirin probably works by interference with the 'capping' of viral mRNA.

The drug may be given by aerosol inhalation (the usual route), orally or i.v. Oral bioavailability is about 40%. Ribavirin readily crosses the blood–brain barrier and has a very large volume of distribution, mainly because of cellular uptake. The drug is eliminated by both metabolism and renal excretion, with a terminal half-life of about 2 weeks.

Therapeutic uses

- **Respiratory syncytial virus (RSV) infections:** this virus causes bronchiolitis and pneumonia in young children and may be life threatening
- **Influenza A and B:** in susceptible patients these viruses produce life-threatening disease, and ribavirin aerosol shortens disease duration
- **Lassa fever:** this insect-borne virus is a cause of severe disease in parts of Africa and may be imported into Britain; ribavirin is thought to be beneficial and is usually given i.v.

Adverse effects

- Dose-dependent adverse effects on the marrow are reported when the drug is given systemically, but are not seen with aerosol use
- Gastrointestinal adverse effects are common and include metallic taste, nausea and thirst.

Drugs for cytomegalovirus (CMV) infection

Ganciclovir. This drug inhibits the DNA polymerase of cytomegalovirus (CMV) and, unlike aciclovir, does not require 'activation' by thymidine kinase, an enzyme lacked by CMV. Ganciclovir is used i.v. in the setting of severe CMV infection, most commonly in the immunocompromised host. Ganciclovir causes severe adverse effects including neutropenia, thrombocytopenia and renal impairment.

Foscarnet. This drug has a wide spectrum of antiviral activity, working by inhibition of DNA polymerase. The drug is poorly absorbed from the gut and is usually given i.v. Elimination is mainly as unchanged drug in the urine. Foscarnet is indicated for life-threatening CMV infection, usually in immunocompromised patients. Adverse effects include renal impairment.

Amantadine

The exact mode of action is unknown, but the drug probably works by interfering with the process of uncoating, by which viral nucleic acid is released into the cell. Amantadine is most effective against influenza

A, and has little activity against influenza B. Amantadine is well absorbed from the gut and widely distributed to the tissues, including the mucosa and mucus of the upper airways. Amantadine is mainly eliminated by the kidney as the unchanged drug.

Therapeutic uses

Prophylaxis and treatment of influenza A. Amantadine is useful in the prevention of influenza A in high-risk individuals (e.g. the elderly in residential homes and patients with chronic lung disease) during an epidemic. Prophylactic use of amantadine may halve the risk of acquiring infection. If it is started within 48 hours of symptoms, amantadine reduces the duration and severity of influenza A.

Amantadine is also used in Parkinsonism (Ch. 6).

Adverse effects

Acute CNS reactions are unusual but include seizures and organic psychosis.

Contraindications

- Epilepsy
- Renal failure
- Pregnancy: the drug is teratogenic.

Interferons

This is a group of naturally occurring proteins secreted by virus-infected cells. The therapeutic benefits of the interferons are still being assessed, and their mode of action is incompletely understood. Interferons seem to impair viral mRNA, by altering its translation at the ribosome and by activation of RNAases, which degrade viral RNA. Their use remains experimental but has been tried with some success against chronic active hepatitis secondary to infections with hepatitis B and C viruses. Adverse effects include fever, alopecia, anaemia and gastrointestinal upset.

14.2 Antifungal drugs

Fungal infections are usually confined to the skin, mucous membranes and nails, and systemic disease is unusual in the immunocompetent. Systemic fungal infections are more frequent in tropical countries and in the growing number of patients with AIDS. Fungi synthesise a unique sterol, *ergosterol*, which is incorporated into their plasma membranes, and binding to ergosterol is involved in the mode of action of nystatin, the imidazoles and amphoteracin B. The mode of action of griseofulvin is unknown, but it may involve binding to cellular microtubules.

Drugs for cutaneous and mucous membrane infections

Nystatin. This drug is too toxic for systemic use and is not absorbed from the gut. Nystatin is used *topically* for cutaneous, oral, oesophageal and vaginal infections with *Candida albicans* and various dermatophytes. Nystatin is not beneficial against fungal nail infections.

Griseofulvin. This is used *systemically*, particularly for fungal nail infections; treatment must last for several months. Absorption of griseofulvin is very variable and is increased by fatty foods. Griseofulvin is relatively non-toxic but can produce allergic reactions; it is an inducer of hepatic drug-metabolising enzymes and can affect warfarin therapy.

Imidazoles. Miconazole and clotrimazole are usually employed topically, when drug absorption is negligible.

Drugs for systemic infections

Imidazoles. Ketoconazole and fluconazole, though structurally similar to clotrimazole and miconazole, are less toxic. They may be given orally for systemic infection. Both are well absorbed and widely distributed, but ketoconazole undergoes extensive first-pass metabolism and does not readily cross the blood–brain barrier, and fluconazole is preferred for fungal CNS infection such as cryptococcal meningitis. Ketoconazole and fluconazole are both hepatotoxic, and ketoconazole can cause gynaecomastia. Neither of these drugs should be used for trivial infections. Both are enzyme inhibitors and interact with warfarin.

Amphoteracin B. Amphoteracin is not absorbed from the gut; its oral formulations are, therefore, for topical use only and are relatively free from adverse effects. The drug is given intravenously for life-threatening systemic fungal infections and then has frequent and severe toxicity. Rigors, fever and malaise are usual (they may be reduced by corticosteroids); renal failure, hepatic dysfunction and anaemia are common.

14.3 Antiprotozoal drugs

There is a wide range of antiprotozoal drugs, the most important of which are summarised below.

Quinine. The mode of action of quinine is unknown. It may be given orally (for mild malaria) but is mostly used parenterally for severe malaria. At high dose adverse effects are common but rarely serious if standard regimens are used: deafness, vertigo and nausea are common, and ECG abnormalities may occur. In overdose quinine is very dangerous, causing blindness, shock and severe arrhythmias.

Chloroquine. Chloroquine works by inhibiting haemoglobin digestion by malaria parasites. It may be given orally or parenterally for the prevention and treatment of malaria. Because of its very long half-life, chloroquine is given once weekly for malaria prevention; treatment courses are given over a period of 3 days. Resistance to chloroquine is now widespread. Severe adverse effects are unusual with standard doses, but high doses given for many years can cause retinopathy. In overdose, chloroquine causes severe shock and arrhythmias.

Pyrimethamine. This is an antifolate drug similar to trimethoprim in some respects. It is usually combined with a sulphonamide for the treatment of uncomplicated malaria or for toxoplasmic encephalitis in AIDS patients. The doses used for malaria are usually without severe toxicity (though patients may develop allergy to the concomitant sulphonamide), but the high doses used for toxoplasmosis cause bone marrow suppression. This can be reversed using folinic acid.

Pentamidine. This drug has many effects on *Pneumocystis carinii* and is mainly used as an aerosol in the treatment of *P. carinii* pneumonia. The main adverse effect is hypoglycaemia which is common at high dose (unusual with aerosols).

Self-assessment: questions

Multiple choice questions

1. The following drugs reach high CNS concentrations when they are given by mouth:
   a. Nystatin
   b. Amphoteracin B
   c. Ketoconazole
   d. Aciclovir
   e. Fluconazole

2. Aciclovir:
   a. Is as effective for Herpes zoster as it is for Herpes simplex infections
   b. Is effective for all Herpes virus infections
   c. Must be metabolised before it becomes active
   d. Interacts with allopurinol
   e. Interacts with probenecid

Case histories

History 1

> A 40-year-old with a renal transplant takes cyclo-sporin A as an immunosuppressant. He develops a painful rash on his trunk and thinks it might be shingles (Herpes zoster). His doctor agrees and starts oral aciclovir. A week later the patient is very unwell with fever and breathlessness: he is admitted to hospital as an emergency.

What may have happened?

History 2

> A 30-year-old man is diagnosed HIV positive and found to have oral candidiasis, retinal features of cytomegalovirus infection and a low CD4 count.

What drugs are indicated?

Self-assessment: answers

Multiple choice answers

1. a. **False.** Nystatin is not absorbed from the gut.
   b. **False.** Amphoteracin B is not absorbed from the gut.
   c. **False.** Ketoconazole undergoes extensive first-pass metabolism and does not readily cross the blood–brain barrier.
   d. **False.** Aciclovir is poorly absorbed.
   e. **True.**

2. a. **False.**
   b. **False.** Aciclovir is very effective against Herpes simplex, less so against Herpes zoster and ineffective against Epstein–Barr virus and cytomegalovirus.
   c. **True.** Must be metabolised by thymidine kinase.
   d. **False.** Allopurinol (Ch. 9) inhibits xanthine oxidase and potentiates 6-mercaptopurine, an anticancer drug.
   e. **True.** Probenecid inhibits the renal tubular transport of some drugs including penicillin and aciclovir.

Case history answers

History 1

Immunosuppressed patients are at risk of disseminated herpes, which can cause pneumonia and other systemic illnesses. Aciclovir is the drug of first choice, but its bioavailability is very low. The drug may be given i.v. (which would require hospital admission) to particularly high-risk patients.

History 2

Zidovudine might increase his CD4 count and improve his immune function. The oral candidiasis will often not respond to topical drugs, like nystatin, in AIDS patients: fluconazole is probably the first-choice drug. CMV retinitis is very serious and threatens sight. Gancyclovir is the drug of first choice, but it must be given into a central vein as it causes phlebitis when given peripherally.

Anticancer chemotherapy

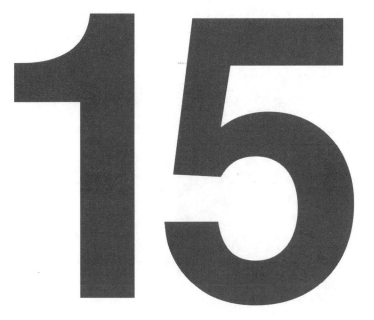

15.1 Cancer

Malignant neoplasms account for a high proportion of deaths in industrial countries. Their prevention continues to elude us because, despite strong epidemiological data linking certain high-risk activities (such as smoking) to cancer, changing the habits of a population is extremely difficult. Treatment options comprise surgery, radiotherapy and chemotherapy; the first two are outside the scope of this book.

Cancers may kill through the local effects of the primary lesion, such as compression of vital stuctures or invasion of major blood vessels, but more usually do so through organ 'failure' (e.g. liver, marrow, lung and brain) caused by metastases. The treatment of a patient with cancer may aim to:

1. give palliation, for example prompt relief of unpleasant symptoms such as superior vena cava obstruction from a mediastinal tumour
2. induce 'remission' so that all macroscopic and microscopic features of the cancer disappear, though disease is known to persist
3. cure, for which all the cells of the clone must be destroyed.

The above options are ranked in increasing order of difficulty, and cure is often impossible with current drugs.

Unfortunately healthy cells, particularly those undergoing replication, for example those in the marrow, mucosa, skin and gonads are also very susceptible to chemotherapeutic drugs, but *less* so than the malignant clone. A basic principle of anticancer therapy is that chemotherapy is given in *courses*, interspersed with 'gaps' of varying duration to allow recovery of normal cells (Fig. 49).

Another principle of chemotherapy is the use of *drug combinations*: though different drugs have additive (sometimes synergistic) therapeutic effects, aspects of their toxicity need not be additive. This approach has the further benefit of reducing the risk of tumour cell

resistance to a particular drug: rather like tuberculosis (Ch. 13), malignant clones contain cells with inherent drug resistance, and use of one drug may allow this population to flourish.

There is a wide range of drugs available, and the more common examples are considered below. All are used, almost exclusively, for haematological and solid malignancies; consideration of regimens for specific diseases is beyond the scope of this book.

15.2 Supportive care during chemotherapy

Synergistic drug combinations and gaps between courses of drugs minimises drug toxicity, but even so cancer chemotherapy cannot be used without extensive supportive care, which is as important to the patient's survival as the chemotherapy itself.

Infection. Predictable periods of agranulocytosis from marrow failure may cause life-threatening infection. Patients are routinely placed in reversed barrier nursing conditions and are given broad-spectrum antibiotic combinations at the first sign of infection. Granulocyte infusions are of limited use.

Thrombocytopenia. Marrow failure predictably causes thrombocytopenia and a risk of severe bleeding. *Intramuscular injections are absolutely contraindicated.* Platelet infusions may be valuable.

Anaemia. Anaemia is often less of a problem because of the long half-life of red cells compared with platelets or white cells. However, transfusions are often needed. In the case of irreversible marrow failure induced by drugs and radiotherapy (e.g. in an attempt to cure certain leukaemias) bone marrow *transplantation* is often needed (usually from a related donor).

Nausea. This is often the worst symptom and requires aggressive management. Antiemetics are discussed in Chapter 11. Prophylaxis against peptic ulcer is commonly given (Ch. 11).

Hair loss. Though seemingly 'trivial' this may have a profound effect on morale. Patients must be warned if depilation is anticipated, and wigs should be made available.

Terminal care. This subject is beyond the scope of this book. Terminal care requires great medical and nursing skill, together with the appropriate use of drugs including analgesics (Ch. 7), antiemetics (Ch. 11) and laxatives (Ch. 11).

15.3 Anticancer drugs

Methotrexate

Methotrexate binds strongly to the enzymes dihydrofolate reductase and thymidylate synthetase (Fig. 50),

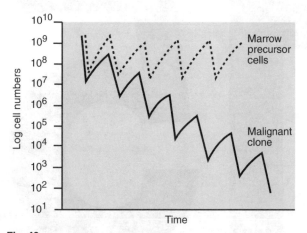

Fig. 49
Giving chemotherapy in courses allows recovery of normal cells.

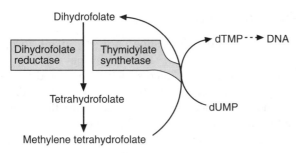

Fig. 50
The folate pathway. dUMP, uridylate; dTMP, thymidlate.

interfering with pyrimidine and, therefore, also DNA synthesis. Methotrexate may be given orally (it is well absorbed by an active uptake mechanism), i.v. or intrathecally. Much of an oral dose may be retained in the liver. The drug is cleared unchanged, by renal excretion. Caution is needed in patients with renal impairment.

Adverse effects

- Marrow suppression, which manifests as agranulocytosis, thrombocytopenia and (to a lesser extent) anaemia; this may be overcome using folinic acid
- Mucositis, comprising ulceration and impaired function of the oral and intestinal mucosa; symptoms include stomatitis, nausea, diarrhoea and weight loss
- Hepatitis, which varies between mild and life threatening
- Neurotoxicity, particularly with the high local concentrations achieved with repeated intrathecal administration.

Drug interactions

Methotrexate increases the toxicity of fluorouracil, cytarabine, 6-mercaptopurine and 6-thioguanine.

The marrow toxicity of methotrexate is reduced by folinic acid.

6-Mercaptopurine

This purine analogue, which is itself a metabolite of azathioprine (Ch. 9), is metabolised to a nucleotide, which is the active form. The nucleotide is probably incorporated into DNA, thereby interfering with transcription, and probably also obstructs the interconversion of purines. 6-Mercaptopurine may be given orally or i.v. The drug is subject to extensive first-pass metabolism; it is metabolised by xanthine oxidase. Excretion of parent drug and metabolites is mainly via the kidney, and care is needed in renal failure.

Adverse effects

- Bone marrow suppression
- Mucositis
- Hepatitis, often idiosyncratic and not dose related
- Pneumonitis.

Drug interactions

Allopurinol inhibits xanthine oxidase and potentiates the toxicity of 6-mercaptopurine.

Daunorubicin, doxorubicin and bleomycin

These are antibiotics isolated from a fungus. They are thought to work by:

- binding to DNA, causing interference with transcription and mitosis, and causing chromosomal breaks
- generation of free radicals, which damage organelles.

Daunorubicin and doxorubicin are not absorbed from the gut and must be given i.v. They do not cross the blood–brain barrier but are otherwise widely distributed. Both are extensively metabolised (some metabolites retain activity) and are predominantly excreted in the bile. Enterohepatic circulation occurs (see Ch. 1). These drugs must be used with caution in patients with liver function impairment.

Bleomycin may be given i.v., i.m. or may be instilled into cavities (such as pleura or peritoneum). Bleomycin does not cross the blood–brain barrier but is otherwise widely distributed. It is mainly excreted unchanged, and renal impairment prolongs the half-life.

Adverse effects
Daunorubicin and doxorubicin:

- Marrow suppression, usually of short duration
- Severe or total hair loss
- Cumulative cardiac toxicity; this manifests as congestive cardiac failure and is usually avoided by careful recording of the cumulative dose given.

Bleomycin:

- Pulmonary fibrosis, which may affect 10% of patients; this is dose related and is more common in older patients
- Anaphylactoid reactions
- Mucositis, which may be severe
- Marrow suppression: unlike most other anticancer drugs, bleomycin causes little myelosuppression, though it may be seen in patients with renal failure and drug accumulation.

Cyclophosphamide and chlorambucil

These agents are structurally dissimilar but act in much the same way by donating alkyl groups, principally to DNA. This causes transcription errors, cross linkages within the DNA coil and DNA fracture.

Cyclophosphamide is a prodrug and may be given orally or i.v. Cyclophosphamide is well absorbed from the gut and widely distributed; it crosses the blood–brain barrier well. It is metabolised in the liver to its active forms, which include the metabolite responsible for bladder toxicity. Most of a dose of cyclophospha-mide is excreted as metabolites in the urine.

Chlorambucil is given orally and is well absorbed. Chlorambucil has a short half-life and is almost entirely metabolised to inactive derivatives.

Adverse effects
Both drugs:

- Marrow suppression is severe, dose related and often of long duration
- Gonadal failure
- Pulmonary fibrosis
- Carcinogenesis
- Gastrointestinal upset is common and nausea may be severe.

Cyclophosphamide:

- Cystitis is a common problem caused by drug metabolites; this is usually avoided by co-administration of mesna, whch protects the bladder epithelium
- Cardiac toxicity, manifesting as arrhythmias and/or heart failure, may be seen at high doses.

Vinca alkaloids

Vincristine and vinblastine are of plant origin (Periwinkle) and work, like colchicine (Ch. 9), by effects on the cellular microskeleton: they bind to and disrupt tubulin polymers. Both drugs must be given i.v. and cause necrosis if they leak into the tissues. Vinblastine does not cross the blood–brain barrier; vincristine does, and this may contribute to its greater frequency of neurotoxicity. Both drugs are cleared by hepatic metabolism: the half-life of vincristine is much longer than that of vinblastine.

Adverse effects

- Neurotoxicity: this is more severe and frequent with vincristine than vinblastine; the effects may comprise peripheral neuropathy, cranial nerve lesions, autonomic dysfunction and seizures
- Marrow suppression is not usually marked
- Gastrointestinal problems are common but usually mild; however, paralytic ileus may occur.

Self-assessment: questions

Multiple choice questions

1. Methotrexate:
   a. Is antagonised by folic acid
   b. Is antagonised by folinic acid
   c. Enters cells by an active uptake mechanism
   d. Is potentiated by intracellular metabolism
   e. Is potentiated by hepatic disease

2. At standard dosage, the following drugs commonly cause the adverse effects to which they are linked in the question:
   a. Bleomycin and bone marrow suppression
   b. Cyclophosphamide and bladder carcinoma
   c. Daunorubicin and cardiac failure
   d. Methotrexate and macrocytosis
   e. Vincristine and peripheral neuropathy

Essay question

Describe giving examples, the mechanisms by which drugs used for cancer chemotherapy work. What adverse effects as the named drugs cause?

Self-assessment: answers

Multiple choice answers

1. a. **False.**
   b. **True.** Methotrexate is a competitive inhibitor of dihydrofolate reductase (Fig. 50) the enzyme which reduces dihydrofolate back to tetrahydrofolate. The latter is a cofactor in the conversion of uridylate (dUMP) to thymidylate (dTMP). Folic acid therefore 'precedes' the inhibited step. Folinic acid can 'bypass' this by conversion to methylene tetrahydrofolate (Fig. 50).
   c. **True.** Methotrexate is taken up by the same system which imports preformed folate into the cell; the lack of this system in microorganisms explains the lack of antimicrobial effect of the drug.
   d. **True.** Within the cell methotrexate becomes attached to glutamic acid residues: the polyglutamated form of the drug has activity against thymidylate synthetase (Fig. 50).
   e. **False.** Methotrexate is cleared unchanged: it is potentiated by renal disease.

2. a. **False.**
   b. **True.** Transitional cell carcinoma, resulting from chronic inflammation of the mucosa, is a problem unless mesna is used.
   c. **True.** This is an avoidable cumulative effect.
   d. **True.** Inhibition of DNA synthesis in red cell precursors results in fewer divisions and larger circulating cells.
   e. **True.**

Essay answer

Outline the modes of action of different drugs and deal with adverse effects.

Modes of action. Alkylating agents (e.g. cyclophosphamide and chlorambucil) transfer alkyl groups to nucleotide components of the DNA molecule. This results in mis-reading of the code, fragmentation of DNA and crosslinkage of DNA. Because alkylating agents interfere with transcription, their effects are not confined to rapidly dividing cells: any cell group may be affected.

Antimetabolites (e.g. methotrexate, 6-mercaptopurine) competes with the substrate for the enzyme and inhibits enzyme function. Methotrexate resembles dihydrofolate, the substrate for the enzyme dihydrofolate reductase. Methotrexate also binds to, and inhibits, thymidylate synthetase, another enzyme important in the synthesis of pyrimidine nucleotides. The net effect is inhibition of DNA synthesis. 6-Mercaptopurine is an analogue of the purine bases adenine and guanine; it inhibits the enzymes responsible for interconversion of purines and is probably also incorporated into DNA. Antimetabolite drugs are mainly effective against rapidly dividing cells.

Vinca alkaloids (e.g. vincrystine and vinblastine) bind to, and disrupt, the cytoskeleton (tubulin molecules). They produce arrest of mitosis and are effective mainly against rapidly dividing cells.

Antibiotics (e.g. daunorubicin) have been isolated from microbes (often fungi). They bind to DNA and block transcription and new DNA synthesis. They, therefore, have their effects on any cell, not just those which divide frequently.

Adverse effects. Suppression of bone marrow and mention the clinical consequences of this. All the above drugs, except the vinca alkaloids, produce marked marrow suppression.

Mucositis is produced by all the drugs to some extent, except the vinca drugs.

All the drugs produce nausea (the vinca drugs to a lesser degree); mention its management briefly.

Alopecia occurs particularly with the antibiotics.

Specific organ toxicity can occur:

- Pneumonitis: 6-mercaptopurine, bleomycin, methotrexate, antibiotics
- Heart muscle damage: daunorubicin
- Cystitis: cyclophosphamide (mention mesna)
- Neurotoxicity: vinca drugs in particular
- Hepatitis: any of these drugs, but particularly methotrexate and 6-mercaptopurine.

Drugs and the skin

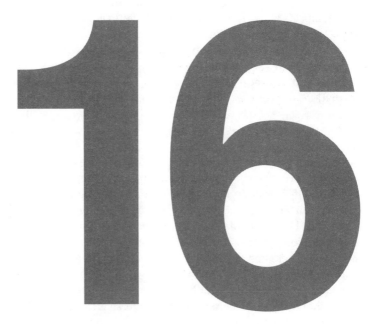

16.1 Skin

The skin normally forms a water-resistant barrier and prevents loss of fluid. It also generally prevents entry of drugs, although certain drugs are now specifically formulated to enter through the skin; this avoids first-pass metabolism and achieves direct entry into the systemic circulation. Sustained release preparations are usually used with the drug contained in a reservoir held in place by an adhesive. Examples include glyceryl trinitrate, oestradiol and progesterone (Chs 3, 12).

Primary skin diseases

The skin may suffer from a variety of conditions, usually not life threatening but perhaps disfiguring. The skin may also be secondarily involved as part of a systemic illness. In the treatment of skin diseases, it is important to remember that the vehicle for the drug (i.e. the ointment, cream or lotion in which the drug is delivered) may itself be very important, affecting the hydration of the skin and aiding the penetration of the active drug.

Emollients

Emollients are bland substances which smooth and hydrate the skin and reduce irritation; they are useful in conditions where the skin is dry and scaly. Examples include aqueous cream or emulsifying ointment. These may be used as vehicles for drugs.

16.2 Skin disorders

Eczema

This is an inflammatory response of the skin to either external or internal factors, acting either singly or in combination. These factors may be simple irritants, or there may be immunological mechanisms involved (there is an association of some forms of eczema with atopy). It may vary greatly in severity from dryness, scaling and itching, to severe itching with redness, formation of vesicles and perhaps exudation with crusting.

Treatment
An attempt should be made to identify and remove any causative irritants; dietary modification may occasionally help. If simple dryness of the skin and itching are present, an emollient to preserve the moisture of the skin may be adequate. In more severe cases, topical glucocorticoid creams and ointments are used; a variety of such creams are available, of varying potency and strength. (See Ch. 12 for their mode of action.) The weakest preparation compatible with successful treatment should be used because of the adverse effects of topical glucocorticoids, including cutaneous atrophy and striae (it is particularly important to use topical glucocorticoids sparingly on the face). When they are withdrawn, a rebound exacerbation of the condition may occur. Rarely, systemic absorption of high-dose topical glucocorticoids leads to systemic adverse effects and hypothalamic–pituitary–adrenal axis suppression.

Examples: hydrocortisone and betamethasone are both available as creams or ointments. In acute severe eczema, with extensive exudate, potassium permanganate soaks are used initially. Oral antihistamines are sometimes useful to reduce the itching.

Psoriasis

Psoriasis is a chronic inflammatory reaction of the skin of unknown aetiology, although there is often a family history. A form of psoriasis can arise after a streptococcal infection. The affected skin appears as thickened scaling plaques, often on the elbows, knees and scalp, although any area may be involved.

Treatment
Topical keratolytic preparations containing coal tar or salicylic acid are effective but not pleasant to use. They act by softening and removing hardened skin and also have an antiinflammatory effect. Dithranol acts in a similar manner and can be used for more severe disease; it is, however, irritant and can stain normal skin, so care must be taken to apply it only to the affected plaque. It is covered with a dressing for an hour and then washed off.

It was observed coincidentally that psoriasis improved in patients taking vitamin D. Calcipotriol, a vitamin D derivative, was developed for topical use in psoriasis. It has no effect on systemic Ca^{2+} balance but should nevertheless be avoided in patients with disordered Ca^{2+} metabolism. It is irritant, and local or generalised skin reactions can occur.

Specialist treatment: ultraviolet light can improve psoriasis, and patients having this treatment may take a psoralen (a drug which increases the sensitivity of the skin) beforehand. This treatment needs careful supervision and is available in specialist centres only. Topical glucocorticoids are also used, but rebound of disease is a problem and they should be used only by specialists. In severe cases, systemic immune suppression may be necessary: methotrexate (Ch. 15) is used. This is clearly associated with increased risks, but in some patients there may be no alternative.

Acne

Acne is a chronic inflammatory condition that particularly affects the face and back, characterised by the presence of comedones (blackheads), papules, pustules and cysts, which in severe cases may resolve leaving permanent scarring. It arises with the activation of the sebaceous glands at puberty, causing increased greasiness of the skin, and tends to clear with age. There may also be colonisation of the skin and sebaceous glands by *Propionibacterium acnes*, a bacterium which breaks down fats in the sebum to form irritant fatty acids.

Treatment

Benzoyl peroxide kills the bacteria and peels the skin, unplugging the follicles: it can be irritant to the skin and a weak solution is applied to the face for a short period and then washed off; gradually, the duration of exposure and the strength of the preparation is increased. In moderate cases, long-term systemic or topical antibiotic treatment, usually with tetracycline or one of its derivatives or erythromycin, is effective.

In very severe cases, vitamin A derivatives such as isotretinoin can be used, given orally. Its adverse effects include hepatitis and altered serum lipids; most importantly, it is teratogenic and is usually given only to males or to females who are using careful contraception (for at least a month before treatment and for at least 2 years afterwards, because isotretinoin concentrates in body fat and is only slowly cleared). Because of these hazards, isotretinoin can only be prescribed by

hospital specialists. Tretinoin is a vitamin A derivative available for topical use, and the systemic adverse effects are avoided.

16.3 Skin and adverse drug reactions

The skin is also a common site for manifestation of drug adverse effects, often allergic in nature. Rashes or itching can occur shortly after the drug is first taken, but sometimes not until 2–3 weeks later. Almost any type of reaction may occur, and these can mimic many skin conditions, including rashes, itching, photosensitivity, hair loss, purpura, blistering and pigmentation. A fixed drug eruption is a drug reaction which occurs in the same place on each exposure. Some reactions are particularly associated with certain drugs:

- morbelliform (measles-like): ampicillin, amoxycillin
- lichen planus-like: gold, antimalarials
- exfoliative dermatitis: penicillin, gold.

Self-assessment: questions

Multiple choice questions

1. The following statements are correct:
   a. The skin prevents the entry of all drugs
   b. Topical corticosteroids may cause systemic adverse effects
   c. Psoriasis is treated with keratolytic agents or vitamin D derivatives
   d. Acne is treated with topical corticosteroids
   e. Vitamin A derivatives are teratogenic

2. The following statements are correct:
   a. Isotretinoin is used to treat herpes simplex
   b. Adverse drug reactions often affect the skin
   c. Methotrexate is used topically in severe psoriasis
   d. Eczema of the face is treated with high-potency fluorinated glucocorticoids
   e. Topical treatment is adequate for all skin conditions

3. The following drugs may be applied directly to the skin for systematic therapeutic effect (i.e. can affect the whole body)
   a. Hydrocortisone
   b. Oestrodiol
   c. Aspirin
   d. Glyceryl trinitrate
   e. Fucidin

Self-assessment: answers

Multiple choice answers

1. a. **False.** Many preparations take advantage of this.
   b. **True.** If used in very high dose.
   c. **True.** Keratolytics to reduce the scaling; calcipotriol's mode of action is unknown.
   d. **False.** Peeling agents and some antibiotics are used: corticosteroids would make things worse.
   e. **True.** So only given to women of child-bearing potential if they are using effective contraception.

2. a. **False.** Isotretinoin is used to treat acne and other skin disorders.
   b. **True.** A very common site of manifestation of adverse drug reactions.
   c. **False.** Used systemically.
   d. **False.** This would cause striae, etc. on the face. Less potent steroids may be used with great care.
   e. **False.** For example, methotrexate, dapsone, etc.

3. a. **False.** Commonly used in dermatology for local effect, but will not have a systematic effect. More potent corticosteroids may if applied in sufficient quantity have a systematic effect, as proven by adrenocortical suppression.
   b. **True.** Used in oestrogen patches for systematic effect in the treatment of postmenopausal problems.
   c. **False.** Too irritant to use topically at all, although some salicylates are used in traditional rubefacients for relief of musculoskeletal pain. These do not have a systematic effect.
   d. **True.** Used in patches to treat angina.
   e. **False.** Although used topically to treat local infections, for instance in the eye.

Drug overdose and poisoning

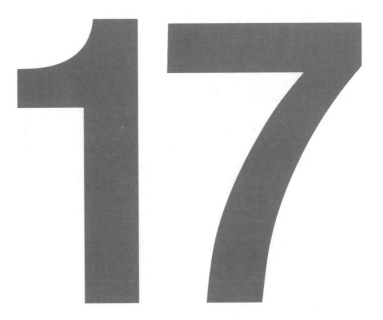

17.1 General measures

Drug overdose is one of the most common medical emergencies. In the majority of cases, it is deliberate, the result of social pressures or psychiatric illness, but accidental overdose by children remains common, despite 'child-proof' medicine containers. In an industrial setting, inadvertent acute poisoning can occur from a variety of non-therapeutic compounds, including heavy metals, insecticides and gases such as cyanide and carbon monoxide. Initial resuscitation (if needed) and assessment of level of consciousness and vital signs should be followed by an attempt to discover what drug(s) or toxin(s) (remember that several different drugs may be taken together), what dose(s), have been taken (empty bottles can be very useful) and roughly when (though the patient's assessment of time lapse can often be unreliable). Management comprises initial decontamination, supportive care and specific measures to reduce toxicity through the use of 'antidotes' or to enhance elimination.

Stopping absorption

Most drug overdoses are taken orally, and if the patient is seen within 6–12 hours of ingestion there may still be drug in the stomach. *Syrup of ipecac* (ipecachuana) is a useful emetic for both children and adults. In adults, a better result is often obtained with *gastric lavage* using a wide bore tube. However, in both cases it is essential that the airway be protected, and if the patient is unconscious this involves use of a cuffed endotracheal tube. *If the patient has ingested corrosive substances, emetics and gastric lavage are contraindicated because of the risk of exacerbating oesophageal damage.* Activated charcoal binds many drugs and toxins, it is either swallowed or introduced via the stomach tube after lavage.

Supportive care

Detailed consideration of supportive care is beyond the scope of this book, but the student should be aware of the principal ways in which poisoning can cause death and the measures by which death can be averted.

Coma. Many drugs cause CNS depression in overdose or in combination (e.g. sedative-hypnotics, opiates, alcohol, tricyclics and anticonvulsants). Death may result from obstruction of the airway by soft tissues, by aspiration of vomit or by depression of the 'respiratory centre'. Protection of the airway, by lying the patient on his/her side with the head down and/or by the use of a rigid airway or endotracheal tube will often suffice. However, ventilatory failure necessitates temporary mechanical ventilation.

Seizures. CNS excitation, resulting in seizures, can co-exist with profound coma. Overdose with tricyclics and theophyllines are particularly associated with seizures. Death may result from compromise of the airway and/or ventilatory failure. Antiepileptic drugs, such as diazepam or phenytoin, may be needed, and resistant cases may need to be ventilated.

Cardiovascular toxicity. Many toxins cause death through circulatory collapse caused by arrhythmias (fast or slow), reduced stroke volume, vasodilatation or a combination of these. Examples include tricyclics, chloroquine, quinine, quinidine, other antiarrhythmic drugs, digoxin and opioids. Temporary pacing, positively inotropic drugs and carefully selected antiarrhythmic drugs may all be needed in supportive care.

Methods of enhancing elimination

Manipulation of urinary pH. Some drugs become unionised at urinary pH and may be reabsorbed in the distal tubule. Relatively small changes in urinary pH produce relatively large changes in the fraction of drug unionised (see Ch. 1 for the Henderson–Hasselbach equation which describes this relationship) and alter renal clearance. This is of practical value with overdoses of the acidic salicylates and phenobarbitone, where alkalinisation of the urine by giving i.v. sodium bicarbonate increases the ionised fraction and enhances elimination. Such *alkaline diuresis* is often 'forced' by administration of i.v. fluid together with loop diuretics, though this confers little additional benefit.

Haemodialysis and haemoperfusion. Drugs with relatively small apparent volumes of distribution (VD) are largely restricted to the plasma, whereas those with large VD are extensively distributed to the tissues (see Ch. 1). Drugs of small VD may be removable by haemodialysis (the extracorporeal pumping of blood across a large surface area of semi-permeable membrane) or haemoperfusion (the pumping of blood through a column of adsorbent material, such as charcoal). Factors influencing the utility of these measures for a particular drug include molecular weight, water solubility and protein binding. Haemoperfusion has fewer indications than haemodialysis.

17.2 Specific drugs

Paracetamol

In therapeutic doses, paracetamol is principally metabolised to non-toxic, water-soluble conjugates. However, in overdose, conjugation becomes saturated and 'excess' drug is oxidised to a toxic metabolite. The toxin forms covalent bonds with proteins, both structural and enzymic, thereby denaturing them. Cells employ glutathione as a defence against such toxins: it forms non-toxic conjugates with the toxin. However, intracellular glutathione 'stores' are soon exhausted after significant paracetamol overdose, resulting in cell death, mainly in the liver.

Patients are relatively asymptomatic between ingestion of the drug and development of liver impairment between 2 and 3 days thereafter: the insidious nature of this problem probably contributes to its mortality since patients can present too late for help. Prolonged prothrombin time and elevated transaminase levels are the first indication of impending illness; thereafter clinical features of acute liver damage develop.

Management

Hepatotoxicity can be averted in the majority of cases by using the specific antidote, N-acetyl cysteine. This compound is a precursor of glutathione (which cannot be used itself because of its inability to enter cells) allowing replacement of glutathione 'stores'. Though very safe, N-acetyl cysteine is not without risk (allergy) and should not be used indiscriminately. Risk of liver damage correlates well with plasma paracetamol concentration, and this measure is used to guide therapy. Because drug absorption may not be complete within the first 4 hours after ingestion, measurement of plasma paracetamol should not be done within this period. Thereafter, patients with a plasma paracetamol above the 'treatment line' (on a graph of drug concentration versus time — these graphs are available in every Casualty Department) should be given N-acetyl cysteine (as an i.v. loading dose, followed by i.v. infusion). Beyond 14 hours after paracetamol overdose, the benefits of N-acetyl cysteine are less clear, though many units would still try using it even in late presenters. Established acute liver failure needs to be treated in specialist centres and carries a high mortality rate; transplantation may be required.

Salicylate

In overdose, the pharmacokinetics of aspirin become *zero order* (Ch. 1) so that with increasing doses, half-life lengthens. Furthermore, while most aspirin is protein bound at therapeutic doses, in overdose this is saturated and the unbound fraction (which is the toxic fraction) rises. Aspirin has several metabolic effects: it stimulates the respiratory centre, interferes with carbohydrate and lipid metabolism and is itself a relatively strong acid. Stimulation of the respiratory centre, which causes hyperventilation, results in early *respiratory alkalosis*. To compensate for this, there is renal loss of bicarbonate ions, which reduces buffering capacity, and higher salicylate concentrations then induce *metabolic acidosis* readily (both directly and by changes in carbohydrate and lipid metabolism).

Salicylate poisoning gives symptoms soon after drug ingestion: abdominal pain, nausea, tinnitus, deafness, vertigo and hyperpnoea. If the overdose was large, fever, dehydration, metabolic acidosis, renal impairment and cardiovascular collapse may follow.

Management

Severity of poisoning can be assessed by measuring plasma salicylate levels: plasma salicylate over 750 mg/l, 6 hours after drug ingestion, confirms severe poisoning (though better guidance is given by serial measurements to establish whether levels are rising). Rehydration is an important part of general care. Drug elimination can be enhanced by alkalinisation of the urine or, in severe cases, by haemodialysis.

Opioids

Sedation, cough suppression and respiratory depression occur as a direct consequence of stimulation of μ-opioid receptors. This results in deep coma with pinpoint pupils and (less frequently) hypotension and hypothermia.

Management

Patients with ventilatory failure should receive the specific antidote *naloxone* as an i.v. injection. This is an opioid receptor antagonist and will cause prompt improvement in the level of consciousness (unless other sedative drugs have been taken); however, its duration of action is very short, and it may need to be given frequently. *Buprenorphine*, a synthetic opioid, may not be reversed by naloxone (Ch. 7).

Benzodiazepines

The GABA-agonist action of the benzodiazepines causes CNS depression. However, benzodiazepines have a relatively flat dose–response curve and do not induce surgical levels of anaesthesia even after overdose. They are consequently safer than the barbiturates in this setting. However, patients may still vomit and aspirate, and those with chronic pulmonary disease are still at risk of ventilatory failure. *Flumazenil* (a specific benzodiazepine antagonist) is very expensive and can precipitate seizures in patients addicted to benzodiazepines; its use is therefore restricted to:

- making a diagnosis: sometimes the nature of the overdose is not clear and a single dose of flumazenil may help clarify the situation. Prompt improvement in level of consciousness can be expected unless other sedative drugs have been taken
- patients in unrousable coma, particularly where arterial gases show evidence of ventilatory failure; flumazenil has a short duration of action and may need to be repeated frequently.

Tricyclics

Tricyclics have complex pharmacological effects (Ch. 6) including inhibition of reuptake of noradrenaline into neurones, anticholineric actions and quinidine-like antiarrhythmic effects. Combined effects on the CNS cause agitation at lower concentration but result in profound CNS depression and seizures at higher levels. Anticholinergic effects cause tachycardia, while the quinidine-like action results in QT prolongation and ST changes in the ECG and reduced stroke volume.

Early features may include blurred vision, retention of urine, dry mouth and agitation. Features of severe poisoning include coma, seizures, arrhythmias and shock.

Management

Because anticholinergic effects delay gastric emptying, gastric lavage (or emesis) is indicated even beyond 12 hours after ingestion. There are no accepted means of enhancing elimination, and no specific antidote is available; management is supportive.

Heavy metals

Lead. Lead poisoning can present with encephalopathy and peripheral neuropathy. *Chelators* include EDTA, penicillamine and calcium edetate.

Mercury. Mercury poisoning can present with tremor, encephalopathy and renal impairment. *Chelators* include dimercaprol and penicillamine.

Iron. Iron is a common overdose in children who mistake the tablets for sweets. Clinical features include gastrointestinal ulceration and liver damage. *Desferrioxamine* chelates iron: it is not absorbed from the gut but is given both orally (to chelate unabsorbed iron) and parenterally.

Self-assessment: questions

Multiple choice questions

1. Poisoning with benzodiazepines:
   a. Causes seizures
   b. Causes respiratory depression
   c. Should be reversed with flumazenil in all cases
   d. Is more severe in the presence of respiratory disease
   e. Can be reversed by haemodialysis

2. In the case of iron poisoning:
   a. Gastric lavage is hazardous
   b. Oral desferrioxamine is adequate to chelate the fraction of the dose which has been absorbed
   c. Oral desferrioxamine is useless
   d. Patients may be discharged within 24 hours of poisoning
   e. Serum iron concentrations give a good idea of prognosis

3. Following paracetamol poisoning:
   a. Symptoms and signs develop quickly
   b. Serum paracetamol levels should be estimated as soon as possible after poisoning
   c. Estimation of the International Normalised Ratio is the most useful guide to severity of poisoning in patients who present late
   d. *N*-Acetyl cysteine works by chelating paracetamol
   e. *N*-Acetyl cysteine should be given to all patients irrespective of their drug levels

Case histories

History 1

> A man takes a deliberate overdose of amitriptylline, but 1 hour later regrets this and presents to hospital.

1. How essential is it to measure drug levels?
2. Should he be given any prophylactic drugs?

> Gastric lavage is done, and he is sent to the ward. His plasma potassium is 2.9 mmol/l (reference range 3.5–5.0 mmol/l). His heart rate is 140 per minute, regular, and his blood pressure is 110/60 mmHg.

3. Should anything be done at this stage?

> Later, he becomes unconscious, has a series of generalised fits and his pulse rate rises to 180 per minute with a BP of 100/60. The doctor gives him physostigmine for the coma and convulsions.

4. Why physostigmine?
5. Was this the drug of first choice for convulsion in a tricyclic overdose?
6. Should an antiarrhythmic drug be given?

History 2

> A 50-year-old woman is admitted comatose after a probable overdose. She is given naloxone i.v. and her level of consciousness improves. Gastric lavage is performed and she is admitted and sent to the ward.

What else must be done?

Short question

Consider the following model illustrating volume of distribution (VD): 1 g each of two compounds A and B are added simultaneously to a small glass beaker, of unknown volume. The beaker is filled with water and has some black powder (looks like charcoal) in the bottom. We lack the means to measure the volume of the beaker directly but can measure the concentrations of A and B: that of A is about 1 g/l, that of B is about 0.001 g/l.

1. What are the VD values of A and B?
2. What is the probable explanation for the difference?
3. What does the charcoal represent in this model?
4. If the relative VDs of A and B are the same in vivo, which is more amenable to removal by dialysis in the event of overdose?

Essay question

What are the main effects of an overdose of aspirin? Discuss the management of severe aspirin poisoning.

Self-assessment: answers

Multiple choice answers

1. a. **False.** Benzodiazepines cause sedation, and seizures are very uncommon.
   b. **True.** Respiratory depression is rarely severe enough to threaten life.
   c. **False.** Flumazenil should be given where there is diagnostic difficulty and where there is respiratory failure (arterial partial pressure of O_2 less than 8.0 kPa).
   d. **True.** Precipitation of respiratory failure is more likely in patients whose blood gases are usually poor.
   e. **False.** Benzodiazepines have very large volumes of distribution.

2. a. **False.** Gastric lavage is contraindicated for corrosive substances (such as bleach) but not iron.
   b. **False.** Desferrioxamine is not absorbed; it must be given parenterally to chelate absorbed iron.
   c. **False.** When desferrioxamine is given into the stomach, it chelates unabsorbed iron.
   d. **False.** The symptoms of serious iron poisoning evolve over several days.
   phase 1 is characterised by gastrointestinal features and may involve severe ulceration; it evolves over about 6 hours.
   phase 2, between 6 and 24 hours, comprises resolution of symptoms — most patients have no further problems
   phase 3, 12 to 48 hours after serious poisoning: a minority of patients develop shock, acidosis and renal/hepatic failure
   phase 4 comprises late complications (2 to 6 weeks after poisoning) from high intestinal or pyloric strictures.
   e. **True.** Serum iron >90 µmol/l indicates the need for parenteral desferrioxamine. Though desferrioxamine is safe, adverse reactions to it include anaphylaxis, hypotension and visual/hearing impairment.

3. a. **False.** Most patients remain asymptomatic until they develop hepatic necrosis (takes about 24 hours to become apparent).
   b. **False.** Estimates made in the first 4 hours after ingestion are not reliable because drug absorption is still in progress.
   c. **True.** Clotting abnormality is a sensitive indicator of developing liver damage.
   d. **False.** N-Acetyl cysteine is a glutathione precursor which forms adducts with reactive paracetamol metabolites.
   e. **False.** N-Acetyl cysteine does causes anaphylaxis occasionally and should be reserved for those

patients with drug concentration above the 'treatment line' on the standard graph.

Case history answers

History 1

1. There is no antidote for tricyclics, and no means of increasing their clearance, so knowing drug levels will probably not alter management. All cases of tricyclic poisoning should be admitted, and most physicians would want to observe for 48 hours because of the tendency for late complications.
2. No. Vital signs should be observed, and electrolyte concentrations should be measured.
3. He is hypokalaemic: this predisposes to tachy-arrhythmias and should be corrected using an i.v. infusion of KCl diluted in 0.9% saline or 5% glucose. His tachycardia is currently insignificant, and his BP is well maintained — antiarrhythmic drugs are not indicated. A cardiac monitor should be used, and the patient should be nursed in a high-dependency area (such as a coronary care unit).
4. Tricyclics have marked antimuscarinic properties which may cause coma and fits. Physostigmine is an anticholinesterase (Ch. 8) which potentiates acetyl choline; furthermore, it crosses the blood–brain barrier.
5. However, the effects of physostigmine are short lived, and it is not considered first-line therapy: i.v. diazepam is probably preferable to terminate fits, and if coma becomes a problem (through respiratory failure) ventilation is indicated.
6. His BP is still well maintained, so the arrhythmia is unlikely to be life threatening at the moment. However, an ECG should be done and the arrhythmia should be identified. If it is anticipated that the present arrhythmia is likely to deteriorate to a more serious type (e.g. ventricular tachycardia may deteriorate to ventricular fibrillation), then induction of alkalosis (using dilute i.v. sodium bicarbonate) may be helpful (this increases the degree of plasma protein binding, see Ch. 1). Antiarrhythmic drugs should be reserved for life-threatening arrhythmias; their early use will often make the situation worse.

History 2

Naloxone has a very short duration of action, and repeat doses may be needed: ward doctors should be warned of this, and close observations made of level of consciousness. Opioids like dihydrocodeine and dextropropoxyphene are formulated in compound tablets with paracetamol, and patients often take more than one type of pill: unless paracetamol levels are measured this poisoning may go un-noticed until liver failure ensues. Salicylate levels should also be measured, given the ready availability of this drug, to judge whether alkaline diuresis is required.

Short answers

1. For compound A, VD = 1 g ÷ 1 g/l = 1
   For compound B, VD = 1 g ÷ 0.001 g/l = 1000 l.
2. The likeliest reason for the difference is that compound B binds avidly to the charcoal.
3. In this model, charcoal represents the tissues.
4. A will be more readily removed from the body.

Essay answer

Discuss pertinent pharmacokinetics: that aspirin has a small volume of distribution, that much of the drug is eliminated unchanged, that aspirin is an acid and that tubular reabsorption of aspirin can be reduced if the urine is made alkaline. Mention also that salicylate pharmacokinetics become zero order at high concentration and that the protein binding of the drug can be saturated at high plasma concentration (so that the unbound drug fraction rises, explain the importance of this).

State that management is heavily influenced by plasma salicylate concentrations. Mention that salicylate concentrations often need to be measured more than once (in case absorption is slow).

Decontamination of the gut (lavage or emesis) is indicated up up 12 hours after ingestion. Supportive care is important and comprises: rehydration and correction of hypokalaemia, hyperglycaemia and severe acidosis. Drug clearance is increased by alkalinisation of the urine if plasma salicylate exceeds 750 mg/l: 1.4% sodium bicarbonate is infused i.v., giving 225 μmol over 3 hours to achieve a urine pH between 7.5 and 8.5; loop diuretics are often needed if urine output does not match the infusion rate of bicarbonate. Input by i.v urine output and central venous pressure should be measured. In severe poisoning (plasma salicylate >1000 mg/l), or poisoning complicated by renal failure, haemodialysis may be required.

Drug dependency and abuse

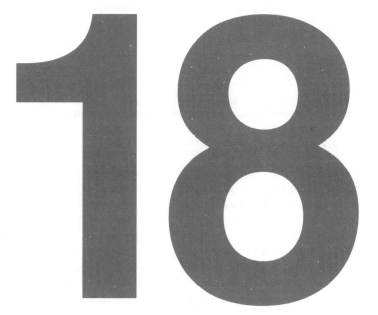

18.1 Drug use

A wide variety of legal and illegal drugs and substances can be used to create a sense of well being or to escape from an unpleasant situation. Most societies have legal restrictions on the use of such drugs. There are a number of risks associated with drug use:

- overdose
- direct physical or mental damage from a drug, e.g. cirrhosis with alcohol abuse
- inappropriate behaviour and legal difficulties, e.g. driving while drunk
- distortion of perception and response to environment: self-neglect, drift into criminal subculture (perhaps to finance illegal drug use)
- users of illicit drugs may not know what they are using: adulteration is common
- spread of disease, e.g. hepatitis B or HIV disease by sharing needles between injecting drug abusers
- drug dependency.

Definitions

Drug dependency (addiction) is a compulsion to continue taking a drug, either because of its pleasant effects or, more commonly, because of fear of drug withdrawal. Dependency is sometimes described as physical where there is a clear physical withdrawal syndrome, or psychological where the drug is used for pleasure or as support and there is no clear withdrawal syndrome. Drug dependency may be stable if the patient has an easily obtainable supply but may have severe detrimental effects on the individual and society if the supply is difficult, when the patient may resort to criminal behaviour to obtain the drug.

Tolerance. The body may adapt to the continual presence of a drug so that greater doses are required to achieve the same effect. This occurs with many drugs of abuse and may occur because of increased metabolism of the drug (alcohol, barbiturates) or because of altered receptor sensitivity (opioids).

18.2 Drugs abused

Alcohol (ethanol)

Alcoholic drinks contain from 4% (weak beer) to 45% (whisky, brandy) ethanol in water. It is the most widely abused drug and a major cause of drug dependency (alcoholism).

Clinical pharmacokinetics

Alcohol is rapidly absorbed after ingestion, although this may be slowed by food. It is metabolised in the liver by two pathways: a specific alcohol dehydro-

genase and the less specific microsomal enzymes. These microsomal enzymes are inhibited by acute alcohol intake but induced by chronic intake; this is a possible source of drug interactions. Small amounts are excreted unchanged in urine and in the breath. The metabolism is saturable, i.e. at high doses, alcohol exhibits zero-order metabolism and the clearance of alcohol is not exponential but is at a steady rate (see Ch. 1). Women are in general less tolerant of the acute and long-term effects of alcohol than men.

Psychological effects. Alcohol is a depressant and causes disinhibition and relaxation, with slowing of mental function. Aggression and confusion may occur. Tolerance and drug dependency may develop with prolonged use.

Physical effects:

- *short term — in overdose:*
  — incoordination
  — injury because of intoxication
  — unconsciousness
  — death
- *long term — in high doses:*
  — hypertension
  — peripheral neuropathy
  — damage to the cerebrum, partly caused by vitamin deficiencies
  — cirrhosis
  — nutritional deficiencies (especially vitamins)
  — cardiomyopathy.

Withdrawal. On withdrawal, delirium tremens (DTs) may occur; the patient becomes tremulous, confused and may suffer convulsion, coma and death.

Treatment

Disulfiram inhibits alcohol dehydrogenase, so that ethanol is broken down to acetaldehyde and other toxic derivatives. It is used to dissuade alcoholics from taking alcohol, as if they drink while taking it, they will experience unpleasant adverse effects, with nausea and vomiting and flushing; severe cases may be fatal. It is useful in a small number of alcoholics who are determined to stop drinking.

Sedatives/hypnotics

Benzodiazepines

The potential for benzodiazepines (see Ch. 6) to cause tolerance and dependence was not recognised by doctors for many years. As a result, doctors unwittingly caused many cases of dependence by over-prescribing of these drugs. They are widely available legally. These drugs are also abused illegally, either alone or in combination with other drugs. They may be taken orally, or the tablets may be crushed and dissolved in water or other solvents and then injected. Temazepam is a widely used hypnotic which is particularly favoured by injecting drug abusers.

The psychological effects are similar to those of alcohol. The physical dangers are less, although injury may occur. Overdose, accidental or deliberate, is rarely fatal unless there is underlying cardiac or respiratory disease or other drugs are abused simultaneously. The withdrawal syndrome consists of increased anxiety, insomnia and sometimes convulsions.

Barbiturates

Barbiturates (Ch. 6) were widely used as hypnotics and sedatives before the benzodiazepines were available. They are now rarely used for medical purposes and hence are not readily available as drugs of abuse. Their effects are similar to those of alcohol. Barbiturates are metabolised by the liver, and are liver enzyme inducers. Tolerance therefore occurred in regular use. Barbiturates are particularly dangerous in overdose, when coma and cardiovascular collapse may occur. Withdrawal often caused severe confusion, agitation and convulsions.

Cannabis

Cannabis is widely used as a relaxant and mild intoxicant. The dried leaves of the cannabis plant may be smoked or eaten (marihuana). A more concentrated form is the resin from the plant, compressed into blocks (hashish). There are several active compounds in cannabis; Δ-9-tetrahydrocannabinol is the most important.

Psychological effects. Relaxation, talkativeness and increased awareness of sensation occur. Concentration and coordination are impaired. Occasionally, a user will experience anxiety and paranoia, and even a toxic psychosis. The long-term effects of the drug are debated; many claim it has none, others point to evidence of brain damage in some users. Users of cannabis are more likely to use other drugs. A mild withdrawal syndrome is described in heavy users.

Amphetamines

Amphetamines are stimulants and indirect sympathomimetics, i.e. they stimulate the release of endogenous catecholamines and so activate the sympathetic nervous system. Initially, they were used for the treatment of depression and as appetite suppressants; now they are used very rarely in medicine, to treat narcolepsy. Amphetamines are widely abused; most amphetamines are now made in illegal laboratories. They may be taken orally, sniffed or injected.

Effects. The physiological and psychological effects are similar to those of adrenaline: hypertension, tachycardia (sometimes reflex bradycardia), mydriasis; in large doses, cardiac arrhythmias, angina or sudden death may occur. The user may become exhilarated, energetic, loses his appetite and feels that his physical and mental abilities have been expanded; with long-

term use, anxiety and irritability may occur. In high doses, confusion and psychosis may be seen. The amphetamines postpone fatigue rather that prevent it and, after use, many users feel exhausted. On withdrawal, depression is common, and amphetamines are said to be psychologically but not physically addictive. Tolerance occurs with chronic use.

Methylenediaminemethamphetamine (MDMA, Ecstasy) is an amphetamine derivative which has, in addition to the effects of amphetamines, hallucinogenic properties (see below). It has become particularly widely used in recent years and has caused a number of deaths as a result of cardiac arrhythmias or as a result of myolysis and subsequent renal failure.

Cocaine

Cocaine is derived from the coca leaf. It is an indirect sympathomimetic and a membrane stabiliser and is still used by ear, nose and throat surgeons as a local anaesthetic (see Ch. 8). Cocaine hydrochloride is a white powder that can be injected but more commonly is sniffed and absorbed through the nasal mucosa. In this form, cocaine has been an expensive drug popular with wealthy users. Cocaine freebase is powder treated with alkali to form nuggets ('crack') which can be smoked. It is said to give very rapid effects and has been sold relatively cheaply.

Effects. The effects are similar to amphetamines: exhilaration, loss of appetite and fatigue, occasionally anxiety, panic or psychosis. After inhalation, the effects last for about 15–30 minutes and repeated doses are usually used. After effects include fatigue and depression. Physical effects include tachycardia and hypertension, and possibly angina, acute myocardial infarction, cardiac arrhythmia and sudden death. Cocaine sniffing will cause intense vasoconstriction of the nasal mucosa and may cause necrosis of the nasal septum. Cocaine is said to be psychologically rather than physically addictive.

Opioids

Opioids (see Ch. 7) can all be abused; the partial agonist drugs *(pentazocine, buprenorpine)* were developed in an unsuccessful attempt to produce an analgesic with no abuse potential. Raw opium was widely smoked in the Far East. The refined alkaloids, morphine and codeine, are taken orally, injected or smoked. *Diamorphine (heroin)* is a potent morphine derivative which is particularly widely available and abused.

Effects. When injected, the user experiences a 'rush' or sensation of intense pleasure, the chronic user in contrast mainly uses it to avoid the unpleasant effects of withdrawal. In large doses, sedation is more prominent. Overdose can occur with respiratory depression and death. Tolerance occurs quickly. Physical dependence also occurs within a few weeks of regular use and a severe withdrawn syndrome occurs within a few hours of the last dose; muscle aches, sneezing and rhinorrhea, and yawning, progress on to chills and piloerection ('going cold turkey'). There is also psychological dependence. Abuse by injection is associated with the infectious hazard outlined above. Sniffing or inhaling the fumes of heroin ('chasing the dragon') is increasingly common. Chronic users of opioids often abuse them with other drugs in an attempt to regain the 'rush'.

Methadone is an opioid with a long half-life, active after oral administration. It is used to avoid the withdrawal symptoms in opioid users, its advantages being that it can be given once per day under supervision. The dose can be gradually reduced over a period of a few weeks or months until total withdrawal is achieved.

Hallucinogens

LSD (lysergic acid diethylamide) is a synthetic ergot derivative and a hallucinogen that is widely used. It acts largely by blocking 5-HT receptors. Users report intensification of all the senses and synaesthesia (merging of the senses, e.g. seeing music or feeling colours). Distortions of the senses occur and the user may see pseudohallucinations (which he knows to be false) or true hallucinations. Some users describe mystical experiences, others severe anxiety, disorientation or acute psychosis. Rarely LSD users may harm themselves or others during the 'trip'. Many users experience 'flashbacks' where they may reexperience the effects of LSD without having taken any. Occasionally long-term psychotic reactions may occur in LSD users. Physical effects do not occur, nor does physical dependence.

Other hallucinogens. Many other naturally occurring alkaloids can act as hallucinogens, including atropine, muscarine and psilocybin from fungi or mescaline (from a cactus).

Solvents

Many organic solvents can be inhaled to produce effects similar to those of alcohol: disinhibition, euphoria, disorientation and dizziness leading to stupor. These can be found in glues, dry cleaning fluids, paints, nail varnish remover and many other household substances. They are commonly put into a plastic bag from which the user inhales. Because organic solvents are lipid soluble, the acute effects clear quickly when the use is stopped. Solvents are particularly abused by children. The adverse effects in short-term use are injury and occasionally sudden death caused by sensitisation of the myocardium to catecholamines by the solvent. In the long term, the adverse effects include poor concentration, liver and kidney damage and possibly permanent brain damage.

Self-assessment: questions

Multiple choice questions

1. The following statements are correct:
   a. Drug dependency describes a compulsion to continue taking a drug
   b. Tolerance means that an increased dose of the drug has no effect
   c. Alcohol is associated with a physical withdrawal syndrome
   d. Alcohol is mostly excreted unchanged in the urine
   e. Disulfiram is used to treat alcohol dependency

2. The following statements are correct:
   a. Benzodiazepine abuse is common
   b. Tolerance occurs to benzodiazepines
   c. Benzodiazepines may cause liver enzyme induction
   d. Barbiturates are safe in overdose
   e. Physical withdrawal syndromes are seen with benzodiazepines

3. Amphetamines:
   a. Cause catecholamine release from nerve endings
   b. May cause angina
   c. May cause weight gain
   d. Withdrawal may cause rebound depression
   e. Are usually diverted from legal medical use

4. The following statements are correct:
   a. Cocaine is a local anaesthetic
   b. Sniffing cocaine may destroy the nasal septum
   c. Dependency only occurs after intravenous use
   d. Withdrawal syndrome includes constipation, drowsiness and miosis
   e. Methadone is a long-acting opioid used to treat dependency

Case histories

History 1

A 24-year-old man is found unconscious in a public toilet and is brought to a casualty department. There are no signs of injury and blood sugar is normal. He has needle track marks on his arms and is noted to have small pupils and slow, shallow respiration.

1. What is the likely diagnosis?
2. What treatment should be given immediately?
3. The patient recovers consciousness initially but an hour later becomes unconscious again. What has happened?
4. What are the effects of sudden withdrawal of the drugs to which this patient is addicted?
5. What other drugs are commonly abused intravenously?

History 2

A 60-year-old man is found to have hepatomegaly. He admits to drinking a bottle of whisky a day.

1. What is the likely cause of the hepatomegaly?
2. What is considered a 'safe' maximum weekly intake of alcohol?
3. Will the patient's capacity to metabolise drugs be increased or decreased?
4. What drugs are synergistic with alcohol in affecting the CNS?
5. What antibiotic should be avoided in such a patient?

Matching item question

Theme: Drug abuse

Options

A. Cirrhosis	J. Tolerance
B. Heroin	K. Hepatitis B
C. Cocaine	L. Dependency
D. Hepatitis A	M. Ecstasy
E. Disulfiram	N. Benzodiazepines
F. HIV	O. Thiamine
G. Pethidine	P. Methadone
H. 'Cold turkey'	Q. Delirium tremens
I. Barbiturates	R. Naloxone

Problem 1
A 40-year-old man comes to his GP complaining of unsteadiness when he walks, and is noted to have an enlarged liver. On questioning, he admits to drinking about half a bottle of whisky per day as well as wine and beer.

i. Choose one liver complication caused by alcohol abuse.
ii. What vitamin deficiency is likely in heavy drinkers?
iii. What may happen to a heavy drinker who suddenly stops drinking?
iv. What drug might be used to diminish the severity of the withdrawal syndrome?

Problem 2
A 24-year-old man comes to the dentist requesting treatment. He is generally dishevelled, and the dentist notes marks on the patient's left forearm which the patient says were due to a cat scratch. The patient also has small pupils. On examining the oral cavity, the dentist finds dental caries and candidiasis.

i. Choose one drug which this patient could be abusing.
ii. Choose one infectious complication of drug abuse which the dentist should consider in this patient.
iii. Patients on such drugs often require escalating doses to achieve the desired effect. What is this phenomenon called?
iv. What drug is used to try to avoid a withdrawal syndrome and maintain such addicts?

Self-assessment: answers

Multiple choice answers

1. a. **True.** A distinction is sometimes made between dependency and addiction but we consider this spurious.
   b. **False.** Tolerance means that an increased dose is needed to achieve the same effect.
   c. **True.** This may be very severe.
   d. **False.** Mostly metabolised.
   e. **True.** By inhibiting alcohol dehydrogenase, toxic metabolites of alcohol are formed.

2. a. **True.** Often iatrogenic.
   b. **True.** Tendency to increase the dose occurs, even in therapeutic use.
   c. **False.** No effect.
   d. **False.** On the contrary, one of the most dangerous of overdoses.
   e. **True.** Including insomnia, anxiety, etc.

3. a. **True.** The definition of an indirect sympathomimetic.
   b. **True.** May cause tachycardia and hypertension.
   c. **False.** May cause loss of appetite and weight loss.
   d. **True.** Hence a psychological compulsion to continue taking the drug.
   e. **False.** Amphetamines have few medical uses today.

4. a. **True.** Still used by ENT surgeons.
   b. **True.** Because of intense vasoconstriction.
   c. **False.** Although obvious, this is a common misunderstanding by opioid users.
   d. **False.** These are all opioid effects: the withdrawal syndrome is, therefore, the opposite of these.
   e. **True.** It has relatively little potential for abuse itself and avoids the withdrawal syndrome in well-motivated users.

Case history answers

History 1

1. Opiate (probably heroin) toxicity.
2. Intravenous naloxone.
3. Naloxone has s short half-life, unlike many commonly abused opiates: the naloxone has probably been cleared allowing the opiate effects to reappear.
4. Muscle aches, sneezing and rhinorrhea, yawning, mydriasis, progressing on to chills and piloerection ('cold turkey').
5. Drug abusers may abuse many drugs intravenously and often use mixtures of drugs. Commonly used are a variety of opioids, benzodiazepines, amphetamines and cocaine.

History 2

1. Alcoholic hepatitis, fatty infiltration of the liver or cirrhosis (with regeneration). Patients with cirrhosis are at risk of hepatomas also.
2. Roughly 21 units per week for men and 14 for women (a unit is half a pint of beer, a short of spirits or a glass of wine — about 15 g of alcohol).
3. Alcohol acutely inhibits liver enzyme drug metabolism, but in the long term is a liver enzyme inducer; this is the likely condition in this patient when he is not acutely drinking.
4. Any CNS depressant, especially benzodiazepines.
5. Metronidazole; disulfiram-like effect.

Matching item answers

Problem 1
  i. A
     Cirrhosis is common. Alcoholic hepatitis may occur, but not hepatitis A or B which are infections.
 ii. O
     Thiamine deficiency is common, and may cause serious neurological and cardiac problems
iii. Q
     This is confusion, agitation, and fitting in some cases. In severe cases, it may be fatal.
 iv. N
     Diazepam or other benzodiazepines are used to diminish the risks of sudden withdrawal.

Problem 2
  i. B or G
     This patient is using an injected opioid - probably heroin (diamorphine), but pethidine is also possible
 ii F and/or K
     Hepatitis B and HIV are often spread between drug abusers who share needles and other injecting equipment. Medical and paramedical staff may be at risk because of their contact with blood and other body fluids. The presence of oral candidiasis is strongly suspicious of HIV disease in this patient.
iii. L
     Users need to increase the dose to achieve the same effect as the number and sensitivity of opioid receptors is decreased (down regulation).
 iv. P
     Methadone has a long half life and can be given orally once per day under supervision. It is useful to avoid withdrawal symptoms in patients who are opioid dependent. Some argue against its use since some addicts will use methadone and other illicit opioids, or may become addicted to the methadone.

Drugs in pregnancy, breast-feeding, children and the elderly

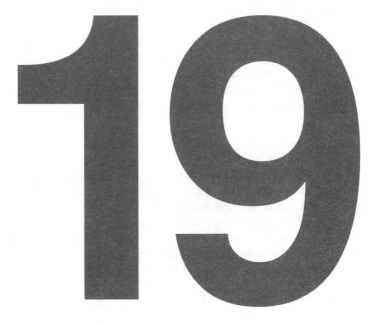

19.1 Pregnancy

Drug use in pregnancy is now limited by doctors' and patients' awareness of the possible harm which may be done to the fetus. This was brought home by the thalidomide disaster of the 1960s, when thalidomide used as a sedative by pregnant women caused deformities of the limbs in the fetus. Despite the risks, some medical conditions require drug treatment during pregnancy and the benefits and risks of this need to be carefully weighed.

Drugs and the fetus

Drugs may adversely affect development of the fetus and cause deformities (teratogenic), particularly during the first trimester of pregnancy when the major organs and limbs are being formed. The list of teratogenic drugs is long: some such as cytotoxics might be anticipated; others may be unexpected and found during animal testing (although this is not completely reliable — thalidomide had not been identified as a teratogen in animal studies, partly because it had been tried only in rodents) or found tragically by chance. It must be remembered that 1–2% of all births are of a child with a malformation of some kind, and it is important not to over- or underestimate the potential of a drug to cause deformity. Not all exposures to a teratogenic drug will cause a malformation, e.g. warfarin causes deformities in only about 5% of cases. A teratogenic drug may be taken by a woman before she realises that she is pregnant; in some cases, the risks of using a teratogenic drug may be outweighed by the benefits, e.g. warfarin in a patient with a prosthetic heart valve.

Some teratogenic drugs:

- phenytoin: craniofacial and limb abnormalities
- carbamazepine: craniofacial and limb abnormalities
- sodium valproate: neural tube abnormalities, spina bifida
- ACE inhibitors: abnormalities of the skull
- alcohol: growth retardation and cranial abnormalities
- stilboestrol: adenocarcinoma of the vagina in the daughters of women exposed during pregnancy.

After the first trimester

The second and third trimesters are mainly stages of growth and development, and drugs taken by the mother may still affect the fetus. Antithyroid drugs may lead to goitre or hypothyroidism in the fetus. Tetracyclines may interfere with bone and teeth formation. There are many other drugs that may have adverse effects on the fetus; a full list should be consulted before prescribing for a pregnant woman. The possibility of pregnancy or of becoming pregnant should also be considered when prescribing for any woman of child-bearing age.

Drugs in the pregnant mother

The pharmacokinetics of drugs may be altered in pregnant women.

Absorption. Gastrointestinal motility is slowed, which increases absorption of poorly soluble drugs such as digoxin.

Distribution. Plasma volume and extracellular fluid increase up to 50% and this will reduce the plasma concentration of drugs with a small volume of distribution for a given dose. Changes in albumin also occur: these fall by around 20% while α_1-acid glycoprotein, to which basic drugs bind, increases by about 40%. This will mean increased free drug for a given concentration for acidic drugs (phenytoin, valproate), while for basic drugs (propranolol, chlorpromazine), the free fraction will fall for a given plasma concentration. This may be of importance if therapeutic drug monitoring is undertaken.

Elimination. Renal plasma flow increases but this is important only for few drugs, such as ampicillin, where larger doses may be needed. For most drugs, renal elimination is relatively unaltered. Liver metabolism is induced by progesterone in pregnancy and so the clearance of drugs metabolised by the liver may be enhanced.

Some common chronic conditions in pregnancy

Epilepsy

There is an increased incidence of congenital deformities in the children of pregnant epileptic women, probably largely because of the use of anticonvulsant drugs. Although most anticonvulsants are teratogenic, the risks to the mother and to the fetus of uncontrolled epilepsy outweigh any risks of teratogenesis, and so pregnant epileptic women are advised to continue their medication. Carbamazepine is probably the least likely to cause deformities, although little comparative evidence is available.

Altered pharmacokinetics may make drug treatment for epilepsy difficult in pregnancy; total anticonvulsant concentrations tend to fall because of increased volume of distribution and enhanced metabolism, although this may be slightly countered by decreased protein binding. Plasma concentration measuring at frequent intervals is advised during pregnancy, with dosage adjustment as necessary. It is not usually possible to measure free drug, and so to compensate for this, it is common practice to keep the plasma concentration at the lower end of the therapeutic range; however, as in all therapeutic drug monitoring, the well-being of the patient and not the plasma concentration is the major measure.

Infections

Urinary tract infections in particular are common in pregnancy, and appropriate drug treatment must be determined by sensitivity testing. Suitable drugs include penicillins, cephalosporins and nitrofurantoin.

Antimicrobials to avoid in pregnant women:

- tetracyclines: teeth, bone deformities; hepatitis more common in pregnant women
- metronidazole: possibly teratogenic
- trimethoprim: folate antagonism, possibly teratogenic
- quinolones: may damage growing cartilage
- isoniazid, rifampicin: use with great care because of risk of hepatitis
- aminoglycosides: 8th nerve damage in the fetus.

Diabetes mellitus

DM may become unstable in pregnant women and some pregnant women may develop gestational diabetes for the first time. All such women need careful specialist monitoring and very tight control of the DM. Some diabetic women may be adequately controlled on diet, but many will require insulin. Oral hypoglycaemic drugs should not be used.

Hypertension

Pregnant women may develop hypertension with proteinuria as part of toxaemia of pregnancy, in which case fetal loss is high. Alternatively, they may have hypertension as an incidental problem. Few antihypertensive drugs have been evaluated in pregnancy. *Methyldopa* has been established by long usage to be safe, as has *labetalol* and *hydralazine*. Diuretics, ACE inhibitors and calcium-channel blockers are not suitable. The role of other beta-blockers has been questioned as, although effective in treating hypertension, they do not seem to improve the fetal prognosis. Bed rest is also important in the management of hypertension in pregnancy. Occasionally, hypertension is sufficiently severe to require early delivery of the fetus.

Hyperthyroidism

Carbimazole can cross the placenta and cause hypothyroidism and goitre in the fetus. The lowest possible dose of carbimazole should, therefore, be used, along with beta-blockers to control symptoms.

19.2 Breast-feeding

Although many drugs taken by the mother may be detectable in breast milk, in many cases the concentrations are low and the dose to the child clinically unimportant.

Drugs that can be given safely to mothers who are breast-feeding:

- penicillins, cephalosporins

- theophylline or β-agonists
- glucocorticoids (although high doses may affect the fetus and cause adrenal suppression)
- anticonvulsants
- tricyclic antidepressants
- neuroleptics such as chlorpromazine
- antihypertensives such as methyldopa, hydralazine
- warfarin or heparin.

Drugs to be avoided in mothers who are breast-feeding:

- aspirin
- ergotamine
- sulphonamides, ciprofloxacin, tetracyclines, chloramphenicol
- benzodiazepines
- lithium
- antithyroid drugs or iodine
- sulphonylureas
- antineoplastic drugs.

Drugs which inhibit lactation:

- bromocriptine
- oestrogens and progestogens (high doses)
- thiazides.

19.3 Children

Half of all children visiting GPs' surgeries will be issued with a prescription, usually for short-term medication, especially antibiotics. Using drugs properly in children requires an understanding of the alterations in pharmacokinetics and pharmacodynamics that occur, especially in neonates (age up to one month) and infants (age up to 4).

Pharmacokinetics

Distribution. Children and neonates have a higher body water/fat ratio than adults, which will result in relatively higher concentrations of water-soluble drugs. Lipid membranes may be more permeable in neonates: in particular, the blood–brain barrier will not be effective. Protein binding will be reduced in neonates.

Metabolism. In neonates, this will be reduced: in older children, it may be relatively greater than in adults. For instance, children may need relatively higher doses of theophylline or phenytoin than adults (based on dose/kg body weight) to attain therapeutic levels.

Excretion. Neonates have diminished glomerular filtration rate and tubular excretion compared with adults: this decreases the clearance of such drugs as penicillin. Older children have renal function similar to that of adults.

Pharmacodynamics

Some drugs will demonstrate a reduced effect in neonates compared with adults or older children (e.g.

digoxin), while some have an increased effect (e.g. CNS depressants). This is sometimes the result of altered pharmacokinetics (for instance, the volume of distribution of lipid-soluble CNS depressants); in other cases, there are alterations in tissue sensitivity.

Adverse effects

These may differ slightly from those seen in adults; for instance, long-term glucocorticoid use may lead to impaired growth, while theophylline may lead to over-activity and learning difficulties. Aspirin may cause Reye's syndrome (hepatic failure).

Doses in neonates and children

Altered pharmacokinetics and pharmacodynamics make determination of doses difficult in children. Doses are sometimes calculated on the basis of mg/kg body weight; the use of mg/square metre of body surface area is better, usually derived from nomograms of height and weight. However, effective doses with minimal adverse effects are often determined only by experience. It is vitally important to consult an appropriate source of doses related to age, etc., before prescribing for young children.

19.4 **The elderly**

Drugs are widely used in the elderly: the elderly (greater than 65 years) account for about 15% of the general population but about 40–45% of prescriptions. The elderly are prone to many chronic degenerative diseases, which promotes prescribing, and may have several medical problems that may lead to multiple drug therapy (polypharmacy) (Fig. 51).

Often there are difficulties of diagnosis in the elderly, and doctors may be excessively enthusiastic in their desire to treat symptoms. Some complaints may be inappropriately treated with drugs, e.g. dizziness caused by age-related loss of postural stability might be treated with prochlorperazine, which may lead to Parkinsonism and further treatment. Many problems of the elderly are psychosocial and cannot be expected to respond to drugs. Often, drugs are started in the elderly and not discontinued although the original indication for the drug has long since resolved.

Adverse drug reactions

These are more common in the elderly and may result in one in ten admissions of elderly patients to hospital. The adverse drug reactions are largely related to increased drug action (type A, see Ch. 21), rather than the idiosyncratic adverse effect (type B). There are several reasons:

- *Increased use* of drugs makes adverse reactions more likely, and *polypharmacy* increases the risks of drug interactions

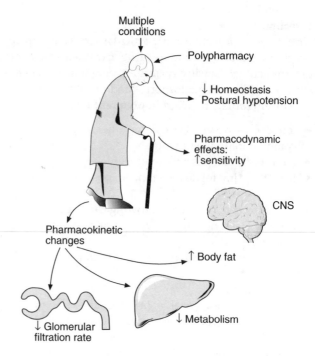

Fig. 51
Drugs in the elderly.

- *Altered pharmacokinetics:* many drugs have not been adequately studied in the elderly
  — absorption may be slower in the elderly
  — distribution may be altered because of decreased serum albumin concentrations and a relative increase in body fat and decrease in body water. Lipid-soluble drugs may have an increased volume of distribution which, coupled with reduced elimination, may prolong the duration of their effects
  — elimination of many drugs in the elderly is reduced; glomerular filtration rate and tubular secretion will be reduced: this may increase adverse reactions from drugs such as cimetidine or digoxin. Liver size and hepatic blood flow and hence enzyme metabolism will also be reduced in the elderly; this is particularly important for drugs which undergo first-pass metabolism, which will have greater bioavailability in the elderly, e.g. propranolol or verapamil
- *Altered pharmacodynamics*, with increased organ or receptor sensitivity: this applies to many CNS depressants, such as benzodiazepines, for reasons that are not entirely clear, and to other drugs such as antihypertensives.
- *Diminished homeostatic reserve*, so that many drugs that affect homeostasis in vital organs have a disproportionate effect in elderly patients, e.g. antihypertensives may lead to postural hypotension because of reduction of the normal reflex responses.
- *The disease state* may influence the response to drugs; for instance, patients with rheumatoid arthritis may be more prone to suffer gastrointestinal bleed after NSAIDs.

Compliance

Compliance with prescribed drugs may be poor or sporadic in the elderly, especially where several drugs are prescribed together. This may be the result of poor understanding by the patient and poor explanation by the doctor of the purpose of the prescription.

Recommendations for prescribing in the elderly

1. Assess the clinical situation carefully, considering other drugs, previous history and the need to prescribe at all.
2. Keep the drug regimen as simple as possible and treat only major problems.
3. Start with the lowest effective dose (often 50% of the usual adult dose) and build up the dose gradually as necessary. Consider carefully the choice of drug in the elderly and work from a limited range of drugs with which the prescriber is very familiar.
4. Explain carefully to the patient the proposed therapy, its purposes, administration and its adverse effects. Verbal explanation may need to be supplemented with written material. Issue a clear prescription for the pharmacist.
5. Avoid inappropriate and overenergetic treatment: consider the patient as a whole and not as a collection of symptoms or diseases.
6. Review medication and compliance frequently and be alert for adverse drug reactions which may mimic other disease or present in a non-specific manner in the elderly.

Self-assessment: questions

Multiple choice questions

1. The following drugs may be safely given to a pregnant woman in the first trimester:
   a. Carbamazepine
   b. Prednisolone
   c. Ciprofloxacin
   d. Cotrimoxazole
   e. Etretinate

2. In pregnant women:
   a. The plasma volume decreases
   b. The free portion of acid drugs rises
   c. Plasma drug concentrations monitoring is accurate
   d. Carbimazole may cause fetal goitre
   e. Sulphonylureas may be used to manage gestational diabetes mellitus

3. In prescribing for children:
   a. Children are basically small adults
   b. Doses for children are best calculated on a simple body weight basis
   c. Adverse drug reactions may occur of a type which are not seen in adults
   d. In a child aged 5 years, the liver metabolism of drugs is proportionately less than that of an adult
   e. Children have relatively high water to fat ratios

4. In prescribing for the elderly:
   a. Pharmacokinetic alterations may occur compared with younger patients
   b. Increased sensitivity to doses of benzodiazepines is an example of pharmacodynamic changes
   c. Polypharmacy is common
   d. Homeostatic mechanisms are well maintained
   e. Compliance with prescribed drugs is variable

Case histories

History 1

> An epileptic woman becomes pregnant, while taking phenytoin.

1. Is she at an increased risk of having a child with a congenital defect?
2. Concerned about the safety of her child, she wishes to discontinue her antiepileptic medication; what do you advise her?
3. If her dose remains unchanged, how will the pregnancy affect the total and free plasma phenytoin concentration?
4. Is this of clinical significance?
5. Can she breast-feed without risk to the child?

History 2

> A 75-year-old man is diagnosed as hypertensive and the doctor wishes to institute drug treatment with a water-soluble beta-blocker.

1. Is this patient in general more likely to suffer adverse drug reactions than a younger patient?
2. Will the clearance of the drug prescribed be affected by the patient's age?
3. The patient subsequently complains of falling episodes and is found to have postural hypotension. What should the doctor do?
4. The patient later develops Parkinson's and is given L-dopa and selegeline, and later still digoxin because of atrial fibrillation. What problems might the use of so many drugs pose?

Self-assessment: answers

Multiple choice answers

1. a. **False.** It may cause fetal abnormalities but nevertheless it is the anticonvulsant of choice in pregnancy, as it seems to be the safest of the antiepileptic drugs.
   b. **True.** As generally used. Very high doses for long periods might be harmful.
   c. **False.** There is a theoretical risk of damage to fetal cartilage.
   d. **False.** Risk of teratogenesis as trimethiprim is a folate antagonist.
   e. **False.** A vitamin A derivative and highly teratogenic.

2. a. **False.** Substantially increased.
   b. **True.** As albumin binding is proportionately decreased.
   c. **False.** Although free drug levels remain much the same, total drug (which is what is measured in therapeutic drug monitoring) is altered because of changes in protein binding.
   d. **True.** Also neonatal hypothyroidism.
   e. **False.** Insulin therapy must be instituted.

3. a. **False.** This is a common but potentially dangerous mistake. Children should be considered quite separately from adults.
   b. **False.** The best way is probably on a dose per body surface area basis.
   c. **True.** For example, Reye's syndrome on aspirin, or stunted growth on glucocorticoids.
   d. **False.** Children have relatively well-developed liver drug-metabolising enzyme systems.
   e. **True.** Hence they may need lower doses than predicted of many water-soluble drugs.

4. a. **True.** For example reduced clearance, etc. If this were an essay question could you discuss it with examples?
   b. **True.** Again, a slight change to this question would make it suitable for an essay or short answer.
   c. **True.** Because of increased illness and perhaps poor prescribing. Around 75% of elderly patients have taken a therapeutic drug within the preceding 2 weeks compared to 33% of younger patients.
   d. **False.** These become increasingly impaired with time.

   e. **True.** Often poor, especially if the patient is required to take a complex drug regimen: occasionally too good, with the patient taking excessive drug.

Case history answers

History 1

1. Yes, probably from both the epilepsy and the drugs. Harelip deformities are associated with phenytoin.
2. It would have been desirable to have this patient on carbamazepine before she became pregnant. Now, however, the risks to her and to her child of stopping therapy outweigh those of continuing.
3. The total plasma phenytoin will fall because of the increased volume of distribution, and because of the reduction in serum albumin. However, the free phenytoin will remain roughly the same.
4. The free drug is active, and since this remains largely unchanged, the change in total drug is of little clinical consequence. However if a doctor measures total plasma concentrations and finds them low, he may mistakenly increase the dose of the drug.
5. Yes.

History 2

1. In general yes, for many reasons: the most important of which is increased drug use in this age group.
2. Yes: water-soluble beta-blockers are cleared by the kidney through glomerular filtration and this will fall with advancing age. The dose of beta-blocker used should be low initially and titrated for effect. The use of a low starting dose is advisable for other reasons also, such as increased sensitivity to the effects of drugs.
3. There are many factors that need to be considered in causing postural hypotension in the elderly, but a reasonable first step would be to stop the beta-blocker. It might be worth trying another antihypertensive (e.g. a thiazide). However, if the patient shows a poor tolerance for such drugs, even if he is hypertensive off treatment, it may be best to leave the hypertension untreated.
4. There may be an increased risk of drug interactions and of poor drug compliance.

Effects of disease state on drug response

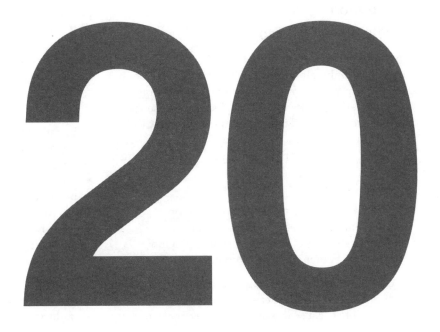

For the majority of drugs, clinically serious inter-individual variation in response is not a frequent problem — most have fairly reproducible effects. However, certain diseases alter drug response predictably, necessitating dose alteration to avoid either toxicity or therapeutic failure. Disease may affect either pharmacokinetic factors (absorption, distribution, metabolism or excretion) or pharmacodynamic factors (concentration-response relationships).

20.1 Pharmacokinetic factors

Disease state can affect:

- absorption
- distribution
- metabolism
- excretion.

Absorption

Blood flow. Most drugs are taken orally, and though acute reduction in gut blood flow can occur, it only rarely compromises drug absorption. However, during emergency surgery, reduction in pulmonary blood flow caused by shock predictably impairs the absorption of inhaled, highly soluble general anaesthetics (e.g. halothane, see Ch. 8), causing slower achievement of effective drug levels. Similarly, the i.m. route of administration is prone to slow absorption if muscle blood flow is reduced, as it can be in shock.

Altered transit time. Acute gastrointestinal infections, both viral and bacterial, may increase motility, reducing transit and hence drug absorption. The severe chronic diarrhoea often seen in AIDS patients may reduce the absorption of anti-TB drugs.

Distribution

Plasma protein binding

Drugs are transported in the plasma bound to plasma proteins, mainly albumin and α_1-acid glycoprotein. Diseases which change plasma protein concentrations alter drug effect by increasing or decreasing the drug concentration unbound in the plasma water (see Ch. 1).

Albumin concentrations may be markedly reduced by disease (e.g. chronic liver disease and nephrotic syndrome).

Clinical example:

- phenytoin (Ch. 6) has serious concentration-dependent adverse effects, including ataxia and sedation, which are dependent on its unbound fraction and potentiated by hypoalbuminaemia.

Concentrations of α_1-acid glycoprotein are low in health but rise in some diseases, for example, myocardial infarction, because it is an acute-phase reactant.

Clinical example:

- propranolol is extensively bound to α_1-acid glycoprotein and its unbound fraction may fall after myocardial infarction, reducing the drug effect.

Tissue distribution

Most drugs have their effects in specific tissues, diffusing out of the plasma to reach effective local concentrations. Inflammation of membrane barriers and changes in local pH may affect this process.

Clinical examples:

- the penicillins are polar compounds which do not readily cross the blood–brain barrier. However, in meningitis, this barrier becomes inflamed, allowing greater partition of the antibiotic into the CNS. The danger comes as meningitis resolves, because care must be taken that CNS drug concentrations are maintained to achieve full resolution
- changes in tissue pH are particularly relevant to the use of local anaesthetic drugs (LAs). To have an effect, LAs must diffuse across neuronal membranes but can only do this in the unionised form. Local infection causes tissue pH to fall, thus favouring ionisation of LA molecules and failure of anaesthesia.

Drug metabolism

Of the effects of disease on pharmacokinetic processes, serious alteration in drug metabolism is among the most commonly encountered in clinical practice. Predictably, the drugs concerned (a) are extensively metabolised to inactive derivatives, (b) have serious concentration-dependent toxicity and (c) have narrow therapeutic indices.

Most drugs are metabolised in the *liver*. This organ has tremendous reserve, and changes in drug effects may not be seen until there is loss of much of the parenchyma. Even so, caution is recommended in both acute and chronic liver disease. Both first-pass metabolism and systemic metabolism may be reduced. The following examples deserve specific mention:

- **opioids:** are absolutely contraindicated in patients with significant parenchymal liver disease. Even 'weak' analgesics such as codeine may precipitate hepatic coma (this is partly due to a failure to clear opiates and also to increased sensitivity to their effects)
- **neuroleptics:** may also precipitate coma
- **benzodiazepines:** must be used with caution and at reduced dose
- **theophyllines:** must be used at low dose; cardiac and CNS toxicity may otherwise be seen
- **metformin:** should be avoided because of the risk of drug accumulation and resulting lactic acidosis.

Metabolism in the liver can also be decreased by renal failure.

Other organs, such as the kidney, can also metabolise some drugs; for instance, metabolism of vitamin D or insulin may be reduced in renal disease.

Drug excretion

Again, the main drug examples have serious concentration-dependent toxicity and narrow therapeutic indices, but they are usually drugs that are excreted unchanged.

Both acute and chronic renal failure reduce drug excretion rate in proportion to the reduction in glomerular filtration rate. Some major examples are:

- aminoglycosides
- digoxin
- sulphonylureas
- captopril.

The liver also has an excretory role for larger molecules which are conjugated, e.g. oestrogens. Effects on conjugation of these drugs are probably more important than effects on their excretion in liver disease. Enterohepatic circulation may also be affected.

20.2 Pharmacodynamic factors

Reduction in drug effect

Less responsive target

Disease may compromise the function of target organs or alter their receptor status.

Clinical examples:

- the loss of function caused by chronic renal failure reduces the response to diuretics, necessitating very high doses to achieve an effect
- gross obesity is thought to reduce insulin receptor numbers, causing insulin resistance.

Endogenous drug 'antagonists'

If the disease allows the accumulation or increased synthesis of endogenous compounds with the opposite effect to that of the drug, it will be rendered less efficacious.

Clinical example:

- the gastric hormone **gastrin** is normally metabolised in the kidneys and accumulates in patients with chronic renal failure, opposing the effects of H_2 blockers such as ranitidine.

Enhanced drug effect

More responsive target

Disease may already 'mimic' the desired drug effect, so that addition of the drug causes unexpectedly marked response.

Clinical examples:

- most clotting factors are synthesised in the liver, and parenchymal disease often prolongs tests of intrinsic and extrinsic clotting cascades. Use of warfarin or heparin in patients with unrecognised liver disease may cause uncoagulable blood: *tests of coagulability should always be done before starting treatment*
- clotting factors II, VII, IX and X are dependent upon vitamin K, a lipid-soluble vitamin, for their synthesis. Patients with vitamin K deficiency (e.g. those with long-standing bile duct obstruction) will be more sensitive to the effects of warfarin than most patients
- aspirin and other NSAIDs may exacerbate the bleeding diathesis of liver disease by their effects on platelet function and gastrointestinal mucosa.

Idiosyncratic responses more likely

The mechanisms underlying so-called idiosyncratic adverse drug reactions are often poorly understood. Certain diseases seem to render patients more likely to such reactions.

Clinical example:

- AIDS seems to predispose towards frequent reactions to sulphonamides and chemically related compounds. The mechanism is unclear, but impaired cell detoxification of chemically reactive drug derivatives has been suggested as the cause.

Self-assessment: questions

Multiple choice questions

1. Response to the following drugs is affected adversely by the disease state:
   a. Morphine and hepatic failure
   b. Propranolol and phaeochromocytoma
   c. Chlorpropamide and renal failure
   d. Sulfinpyrazone and renal failure
   e. Aminophylline and cirrhosis

2. The following statements are correct:
   a. The only determinant of the effect of liver disease on response to a drug is the degree to which it is cleared by hepatic metabolism
   b. The only determinant of the effect of renal disease on response to a drug is the degree to which it is cleared, unchanged, by the kidney
   c. Heart failure has little impact on drug response
   d. Aminoglycosides should be avoided in myasthenia gravis
   e. Digoxin should be avoided in pre-excitation syndromes (such as Wolff–Parkinson–White syndrome)

Case histories

History 1

> A middle-aged man with alcoholic chronic liver disease is given phenytoin for generalised tonic/clonic seizures. His liver-function tests are as follows:
>
> Albumin 37 g/l (32–42), bilirubin 14 mmol/l (2–17), gamma-glutamyl transferase 230 µg/l (<50), prothrombin time 32 seconds (control 27 seconds).
>
> The plasma phenytoin level is closely watched for 3 years thereafter: the level remains within the therapeutic range and seizure frequency declines. He becomes lost to follow-up. The patient is admitted to hospital 5 years later with severe ataxia. His plasma phenytoin concentration is well above the therapeutic range and his liver function tests are as follows:
>
> Albumin 17 g/l, bilirubin 50 mmol/l, gamma-glutamyl transferase 350 µg/l, prothrombin time 125 seconds (control 22 seconds).

Comment on the case: what are the likely mechanisms of the adverse reactions, and in what ways might they have been avoided?

History 2

> An elderly woman develops atrial fibrillation, and is given digoxin to control her ventricular rate. Relevant blood results at the time are:
>
> Na^+ 140 mmol/l (135–145), K^+ 3.9 mmol/l (3.5–5.4), urea 14 mmol/l (2.5–7.0), creatinine 140 µmol/l (50–130).
>
> Two years later she develops peripheral oedema and nocturnal breathlessness. Her doctor diagnoses congestive heart failure, starts a thiazide diuretic and later adds an angiotensin-converting enzyme inhibitor. Her symptoms improve. Two years later, she is admitted to hospital in complete heart block with the following blood results:
>
> Na^+ 138 mmol/l, K^+ 1.4 mmol/l, urea 45 mmol/l, creatinine 360 µmol/l.

Comment on the case: what are the likely mechanisms of the adverse reactions and in what ways might they have been avoided?

Self-assessment: answers

Multiple choice answers

1. a. **True.** Morphine may precipitate fatal coma.
   b. **True.** Phaeochromocytoma is a rare cause of hypertension, in which a tumour secretes catecholamines. The main effect is an increase in peripheral vascular resistance caused by noradrenaline. Paradoxically, beta-blockers may worsen blood pressure control by opposing β_2-effects and by preventing the binding of noradrenaline to β_1-receptors, thereby increasing its binding to α-receptors.
   c. **True.** Chlorpropamide is a sulfonylurea hypoglycaemic agent which is mainly excreted unchanged; it produces profound hypoglycaemia in renal failure patients.
   d. **True.** Sulfinpyrazone is a uricosuric used in gout (Ch. 9). For the drug to work, there must be adequate renal function; furthermore, sulfinpyrazone clearance is reduced by renal failure.
   e. **True.** Aminophylline clearance is reduced in chronic liver disease.

2. a. **False.** Hepatocellular disease may cause hypoalbuminaemia: drugs extensively bound to albumin may, therefore, be more potent. Such patients have impaired clotting, increasing the effect of anticoagulants and antiplatelet drugs (such as aspirin).
   b. **False.** The accumulation of metabolic waste in patients with renal failure occupies binding sites on albumin and other plasma proteins: some protein-bound drugs may, therefore, be potentiated.
   c. **False.** Severe heart failure reduces the VD of some drugs (notably lignocaine).
   d. **True.** Aminoglycosides may cause a degree of non-depolarising blockade at the motor end plate. This is usually of no consequence, but in myasthenia gravis aminoglycosides may worsen weakness.

   e. **True.** Digoxin slows the rate of conduction across the AV node and may encourage aberrant conduction in WPW syndrome: this may cause ventricular tachycardia.

Case history answers

History 1

The lack of linearity between the dose of phenytoin and its plasma concentration (i.e. zero-order pharmacokinetics) should be covered. The extensive binding of phenytoin to plasma proteins should be mentioned and the fact that phenytoin is largely cleared by hepatic metabolism. This man had impaired liver function to start with, but during his loss from follow-up the situation worsened: he probably continued to drink. The LFTs give good guidance of this worsening status. Clearance of phenytoin is almost certainly lower and, given the low albumin, its free fraction is probably higher (you should discuss the importance of free drug fractions at this point). This man's problems might have been avoided had regular follow-up been undertaken, but he defaulted. You may want to discuss the problem of giving potentially toxic drugs, like phenytoin or warfarin, to patients who are likely to default.

History 2

It should be stressed at the start that digoxin is cleared almost entirely by renal excretion and that its effects are potentiated by hypokalaemia (the mechanism of this should be presented). This old woman had renal impairment to start with and probably had a low digoxin clearance. Her renal function deteriorated, however (possibly caused by the ACE inhibitor), and this, together with the thiazide-induced hypokalaemia, caused severe toxicity. She should have been followed more closely, with estimations of renal function, K^+ and plasma digoxin concentration.

Adverse drug reactions and drug interactions

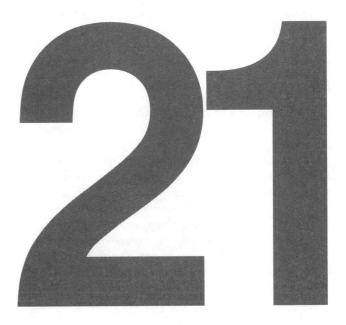

21.1 Adverse drug reactions

Adverse drug reactions (ADRs) can be defined as any unintended harmful effect of a drug. All drugs carry risks and, before prescribing, the potential risks must be weighed against the possible benefits; doctors should only prescribe when the benefits outweigh the risks.

ADRs are very common. It is estimated that ADRs occur in 10–20% of all patients prescribed drugs and are the cause of up to 10% of all GP consultations, 4% of all hospital admissions and about 1 in 1000 deaths. ADRs may mimic natural disease and are generally underdetected by doctors.

Classification

A useful classification of ADRs is as follows:

Type A: the **augmented** or **attenuated** effect, where the ADR is caused by an excessive or inadequate response to the drug and may result from pharmacokinetic or pharmacodynamic problems. In either case, the ADR is predictable from the known effects of the drug and is dose related, e.g. hypotension in patients taking antihypertensives, or excessive sedation in a patient taking carbamazepine. Such effects are very common but are often not severe. Type A ADRs can be managed often by dose modification.

Type B: the **bizarre** effect, which is not predictable from the known effects of the drug and often has an immunological basis: as such, there is often no clear relationship to the dose of drug. Such ADRs are relatively rare but are disproportionately important because the ADR is often very serious, e.g. anaphylaxis with penicillin, or agranulocytosis with carbimazole. Withdrawal of the drug is necessary.

Type C: effects of **chronic** administration of a drug, caused by adaptation, change in receptor sensitivity, etc. For example, rebound angina on withdrawal of beta-blockers, or the on–off phenomenon with L-dopa.

Type D: **delayed** effects, such as carcinogenesis or effects on reproduction, e.g. stilboestrol (Ch. 19).

Drug testing

Premarketing testing of a new drug will involve its administration to an average of about 1500 humans (this number continues to rise as drug testing becomes more rigorous). This will show up many common ADRs, especially type A. However, type B reactions may be relatively rare, perhaps with an incidence of only 1 in 10 000 or less, and so are unlikely to be seen in trials. These may only become apparent after the drug is launched and the numbers of humans treated with it rises. Likewise the late type C and D effects are only likely to be seen after the drug has been available for some years. It may be difficult to connect an adverse event with the drug, especially if the ADR resembles other disease, e.g. liver damage with perhexilene, an antianginal drug now withdrawn, caused histological changes identical to those resulting from alcoholism and was not recognised as an ADR for some years.

It is important, therefore, when new drugs are prescribed that doctors observe closely for any possible adverse effects and report them to the proper authorities. In the UK, the Committee on Safety of Medicines is the statutory body responsible for collecting this data and reports to CSM can be made on special yellow cards, which are widely available. This system has been responsible for identifying many previously undescribed and serious ADRs. In addition, specific postmarketing safety surveillance is often carried out on new drugs by the manufacturer.

Patients particularly at risk of ADRs

- The elderly: little physiological reserve and altered phamacokinetics and pharmacodynamics
- The very young
- Patients with renal disease
- Patients with liver disease
- Genetically predisposed patients, e.g. with glucose 6-phosphate dehydrogenase deficiency who may get haemolysis when treated with many drugs such as sulphonamides or antimalarials such as primaquine, or patients with acute intermittent porphyria who may get exacerbations if given many drugs that are metabolised by the liver and interfere with haem breakdown, such as oestrogens.

21.2 Drug interactions

Drug interactions may be harmful or beneficial. Not all interactions are of clinical importance, and, like ADRs, they may not occur in every patient. Constant vigilance is, therefore, required to avoid drug interactions and to spot them when they do occur. Many lists of possible drug interactions are available. Rather than learn lists off, it is better for the most part to consider which patients are at risk, which drugs are most likely to be involved and what the possible mechanisms are. Some common or dangerous interactions are mentioned but the list is not complete: check carefully if there is any doubt before prescribing. Many general practitioners now prescribe using computers and many pharmacies also use computers in their dispensing: suitable software is available to aid the detection of potential interactions.

Patients who are at risk of interactions

- The elderly (see Ch. 19); polypharmacy, poor homeostatic mechanisms, etc.
- Severely ill patients: for similar reasons and also because a drug interaction may be difficult to

distinguish from the natural history of the disease, e.g. heart failure treated with diuretics may be exacerbated by NSAIDs, which cause fluid retention

- Patients who depend on prophylactic therapy for disease suppression, e.g. epileptics, patients on immunosuppressants or oral contraceptives
- Patients with liver or renal disease
- Patients with more than one doctor, when confusion may arise over what drugs the patient is taking
- Patients who take non-prescribed drugs, e.g. those bought 'over the counter' such as theophylline, pseudoephidrine in decongestants and, of course, ethanol.

Drugs at risk

Some drugs are particularly likely to be involved in serious interactions.

- Drugs with a narrow therapeutic index (Ch. 1), e.g. warfarin, digoxin, cytotoxics, lithium, aminoglycosides, theophylline
- Drugs with a steep dose–response curve (Ch. 1), where a minor change in plasma concentration may make a major change in effect, e.g. oral hypoglycaemics, warfarin
- Drugs with a major effect on a vital process such as clotting (warfarin)
- Drugs where a loss of effect may lead to disease breakthrough, e.g. antiepileptics
- Drugs which may induce or inhibit mixed function oxidase enzymes and so may decrease metabolism of other drugs, and drugs which depend on these enzymes for their metabolism (e.g. theophylline, warfarin, phenytoin, oral contraceptives, cyclosporin and many others).

Mechanisms

Drug interactions may be pharmacodynamic or pharmacokinetic.

Pharmacokinetic mechanisms

Where the interaction causes a change in the plasma concentration of one or other drug leading to a greater or lesser effect.

Absorption. Drugs such as cholestyramine may bind to other drugs (e.g. digoxin, thiazides) in the gastrointestinal tract and prevent their absorption.

Some drugs (e.g. opiates) may slow transit time and so may slow absorption, but the total amount absorbed may be unchanged. Some drugs depend on enterohepatic circulation, e.g. they are excreted in a conjugated form in bile, the conjugation is broken down by bacteria in the gastrointestinal tract and the free drug is reabsorbed, enhancing drug effect, e.g. oral contraceptive oestrogens. If this is prevented, for example by amoxycillin altering gut flora, the drug may lose its effect.

Metabolism. Enzyme inducers (e.g. phenytoin, carbamazepine, rifampicin) will decrease the effects of many drugs; since enzyme induction requires synthesis of new protein, it may take 2–3 weeks to reach its maximum effect. Enzyme inhibitors (erythromycin, ciprofloxacin, isoniazid, cimetidine, sodium valproate, metronidazole, allopurinol, dextropropoxyphene, sulphonamides and many others), however, are effective very rapidly. Problems may arise, therefore, when a patient stable on a drug is prescribed either an enzyme inducer or inhibitor. Problems may also arise if a patient is stabilised on a drug while receiving an enzyme inducer or inhibitor, which is then withdrawn.

Distribution. Only free drug is pharmacologically active, but many drugs are heavily protein bound, e.g. warfarin to albumin. If another drug with a high affinity for protein is prescribed, the result may be a displacement of warfarin from the protein-binding sites, increasing the free drug and its effects (but this is transient, see Ch. 1). This may cause confusion if therapeutic drug monitoring is used, because this usually measures total rather than free drug.

Excretion. Drugs can interfere with excretion, for example thiazides and NSAIDs interfere with the excretion of lithium. This effect can be beneficial, e.g. reducing the clearance of penicillin by giving probenecid.

Pharmacodynamic mechanisms

These are in general more common but are predictable from the known effects of the drug, e.g. two antihypertensives may be used to lower the blood pressure more than either alone. Alternatively, the actions of diuretics are opposed by NSAIDs, which may cause fluid retention, or the effects of oral hypoglycaemics may be opposed by thiazides. Other pharmacodynamic interactions can arise from the effects of drugs on electrolyte or fluid balance, e.g. diuretic-induced hypokalaemia enhances digoxin toxicity.

Self-assessment: questions

Multiple choice questions

1. Adverse drug reactions:
   a. Are a common source of morbidity
   b. Type A reactions are rare
   c. Type B reactions are often serious
   d. Type B reactions will generally have been identified before a drug is marketed
   e. Serious adverse reactions to all drugs should be reported to the CSM

2. Drug interactions:
   a. May result from altered metabolism
   b. May be caused by plasma protein displacement
   c. Are always harmful
   d. Are more likely in the elderly
   e. Are more likely in patients with ischaemic heart disease

3. The following drugs may interact:
   a. Glibenclamide and rifampicin
   b. Heparin and phenytoin
   c. Erythromycin and theophylline
   d. Coproxamol and warfarin
   e. Benzodiazepines and ethanol

Case history

> A 68-year-old non-insulin-dependent diabetic woman is treated with glibenclamide. She is found unconscious one evening, and taken to hospital. Her blood sugar is found to be low.

1. How would you classify this adverse reaction?
2. When she has been treated and has recovered, she describes how she was given cotrimoxazole for a urinary tract infection the day before; is this relevant?
3. She is prescribed amoxycillin instead for the infection, but develops bronchospasm for the first time in her life. What class of adverse reaction is this?
4. Will decreasing the dose be adequate to prevent such an adverse effect?

Matching item question

Theme: Adverse drug reactions
Options

A. Glyceryl trinitrate
B. Benzylpenicillin
C. Verapamil
D. Cotrimoxazole
E. Teratogenicity
H. Immune-mediated toxicity
I. Drug accumulation
J. Carcinogenicity
K. Phenoxymethylpenicillin
L. Exaggeration of the therapeutic effect
M. Mutagenicity
N. Atenolol
O. Placental damage

> Problem 1
> A 40-year-old cigarette smoker consults his doctor about episodic chest pain: the doctor finds the patient's feet are a little cold, and that his chest is a little wheezy, but otherwise there are no positive signs. The ECG is abnormal, suggestive of ischaemic heart disease, and the doctor diagnoses the chest pain as angina pectoris: a drug is started. Two weeks later the patient sees the GP again: he is very wheezy, indeed he can hardly talk, and for the past 2 weeks he has been unable to walk because of severe pain in his calves.

i. Which drug did the GP give for the angina?

> Problem 2
> A young woman presents with severe dysuria. Dipstick testing of her urine reveals 'protein +++, blood+++': the doctor diagnoses a urinary tract infection. He prescribes a drug, but 2 days later the woman returns with a florid rash.

i. Which drug?
ii. What is the likely mechanism?

> Problem 3
> A 20-year-old man has a very severe psoriasis and is under the care of a team of dermatologists. They have tried him on a number of regimens without success, and eventually start him on methotrexate. This drug seems to work, and so the man doubles the dose without seeking medical advice; he also defaults from clinic for a month. When he next presents to clinic he is not well: he has a sore throat, conjunctivitis and a temperature of 40° C. His total white cell count is found to be very low at 1.0×10^9/L, and he is anaemic with a haemoglobin of 9.5 g%.

i. The methotrexate has caused this problem, but by what mechanism?

> Problem 4
> A 30-year-old woman is given an antibiotic by intravenous injection for pneumonia. Five minutes later, she is found collapsed with profound hypotension, a generalised rash and is dyspnoeic with wheezing.

i. What antibiotic is she likely to have been given?
ii. What is the mechanism of this reaction?

Self-assessment: answers

Multiple choice answers

1. a. **True.** For instance, in the elderly, adverse reactions may cause between 10–20% of hospital admissions (less commonly a cause in younger patients).
   b. **False.** These are related to the expected pharmacological effects of a drug and are common.
   c. **True.** Often immunological in origin and generally more serious and unpredictable than type A.
   d. **False.** Given their relatively low frequency and the small numbers of patients treated before a drug is marketed, it is less likely that type B reactions will be seen before marketing.
   e. **True.** Also all adverse reactions (serious or not) with new drugs.

2. a. **True.** For example, liver enzyme induction or inhibition.
   b. **True.** These are not usually of major importance, because the body clears free drug and a temporary increase in free drug because of protein displacement will be followed by increased clearance to restore free drug concentrations.
   c. **False.** For example, penicillin and probenecid, ACE inhibitors and diuretics.
   d. **True.** Because of polypharmacy, because of increased susceptibility to the harmful effects of drugs and because of altered pharmacokinetics and dynamics.
   e. **False.** More likely in patients with congestive cardiac failure, liver or renal disease.

3. a. **True.** The metabolism of glibenclamide and other sulphonylureas is increased because of enzyme induction by the rifampicin and the result may be hyperglycaemia.
   b. **False.** But phenytoin does interact with warfarin.
   c. **True.** Concentrations of theophylline may rise and cause serious adverse effects.
   d. **True.** Coproxamol is a combination of paracetamol and dextropropxyphene (a drug-metabolising enzyme inhibitor) and so may increase warfarin concentrations and cause bleeding.
   e. **True.** A pharmacodynamic interaction leading to increased drowsiness.

Case history answers

1. At first glance, this seems to be type A (augmented effect) adverse drug reaction. Given its severity, the doctor should report it to the CSM.

2. Now it seems more likely to be a drug interaction, caused by protein displacement and liver enzyme inhibition by the cotrimoxazole.
3. This is a type B (bizarre, not predictable from the pharmacological action of a drug) adverse drug reaction.
4. No; the offending drug must be withdrawn.

Matching item answers

Problem 1
 i. N
 These are classical adverse reactions to betablockers (even relatively cardioe\selective ones like atenolol), although rarely seen in such a severe form. This patient was clearly at risk of developing these reactions, and atenolol was a bad choice.

Problem 2
 i. D
 ii. H
 The most likely drug here is cotrimoxazole, and the mechanism is immune-mediated. (The other antibiotics are not commonly used for urinary tract infections, although all might cause a rash.) This is a type B or bizarre reaction, and was not predictable unless the patient had previously had a similar effect.

Problem 3
 i. L
 Methotrexate inhibits the conversion of folic to folinic acid and interferes therefore with purine and ultimately DNA formation. Hence it is used in conditions with a high cell turn over, like some malignant conditions, psoriasis and some inflammatory conditions. What has happened here is predictable from the pharmacology of the drug and is an exaggerated pharmacological effect (type A adverse drug reaction), so that the methotrexate is now affecting the blood precursors

Problem 4
 i. B
 ii. H
 This is classical anaphylaxis. The antibiotics is probably penicillin, and the mechanism is immune-mediated, through IgE. The patient may have had a history of previous penicillin exposure, and possibly previous adverse effects.

Supplementary question: how would you treat this patient? See Chapter 10 for the answers.

New drugs and clinical trials

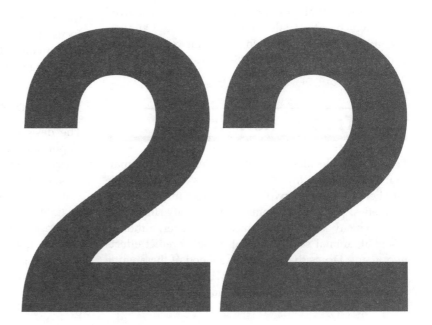

22.1 New drugs

New drugs are developed and marketed, and the drugs learnt by a doctor as a medical student will almost certainly be obsolete within his professional career. The doctor should understand where new drugs come from, how they are developed and licensed and how their value in therapy should be assessed.

How are new drugs found?

In the past, therapeutics was empirical, and drugs were found by chance and experience to be valuable. Most drugs were derivatives of natural substances. With the development of the chemical industry, new synthetic chemicals were produced and screened for activity in various diseases. Existing drugs were purified to extract the active component and ensure more consistent quality. As our understanding of the pathophysiology of diseases grew, drugs were developed to imitate or replace naturally occurring compounds. Later still, the ability to design drugs to attach to a particular receptor developed, and this is the source of most new drugs today.

Increasingly, new drugs are peptides and are often copies of naturally occurring compounds such as hormones and may be produced by recombinant DNA technology. In this, the gene responsible for the production of the substance is identified and inserted into bacteria; when grown in culture media, these bacteria can then produce the drug.

Where do new drugs come from?

Almost all new drugs are the result of research conducted by the pharmaceutical industry. Drug development involves a considerable commercial risk — less than one in a thousand molecules studied reach clinical trials and less than one in a hundred drugs which enter trials are ever marketed. On average, it costs £100–150 million to develop a novel drug, and it can take anything from 8–15 years.

22.2 Testing new drugs

Promising molecules undergo tests initially in animals (but increasingly in *in vitro* systems to reduce the numbers of animals involved) to detect their pharmacokinetics, pharmacodynamics and toxicity, including teratogenicity and carcinogenicity. However, although essential, animal studies do not always predict effects in humans. Drugs that show a likelihood of therapeutic benefit and acceptable toxicity will be subsequently tested in humans. Testing in humans is generally divided into four phases, but the exact duration and

size of these studies will be determined by the nature of the drug and its proposed uses. For instance, an antihypertensive which will be taken for many years needs to be more carefully evaluated in humans and to be less toxic than a cancer chemotherapy drug, which will be used for short periods in patients with a poor prognosis.

Clinical trials are usually considered in four phases:

Phase 1: small studies of the basic clinical pharmacology of a drug involving 50–100 healthy volunteers. These trials will examine pharmacodynamics and pharmacokinetics and will involve the use of various doses.

Phase 2: the early clinical investigations to determine if the drug has the intended therapeutic effect in patients. A group of 50–300 patients will be studied, looking at efficacy and also at pharmacokinetics, pharmacodynamics and adverse effects, using various doses.

Phase 3: if the early trials show promise, advanced clinical investigations will follow. These will involve 300–5000 patients with the relevant condition and will look at efficacy and adverse effects. They may compare the new drug with existing treatments. Study of special patient groups, e.g. elderly, patients with renal disease, etc. will also be undertaken.

If all of these studies show that the drug is effective and relatively safe compared with existing therapies, the company may apply for a licence to market the drug. The evidence will be considered by the licensing authority and if considered satisfactory, a licence will be granted. The drug may then be marketed for specific indications, but testing does not end yet.

Phase 4: The average number of humans studied before a new drug is marketed is about 1500; it is clear that common adverse effects will, therefore, have been identified at this stage, but rarer effects, for instance with an incidence of 1 in 10 000, may not. After marketing, the number of patients who use the drug will rise rapidly and new adverse effects may appear. It is imperative, therefore, that trials continue after marketing: these test the drug as it is used in the real world but focus more on adverse effects and less on efficacy. They may involve 2000–10 000 or more patients. Other trials exploring other uses of the drug will also continue.

Design of clinical trials

The design of clinical trials is complex but of great importance, since poorly designed trials delay progress and waste resources. There are many possible designs depending on the drug and the nature of the condition to be treated. Some of the essential features include:

A clear question to be answered should be established in advance. Investigators must consider the placebo effect whereby patients may seem to improve when given any treatment, effective or not. Trials are often placebo controlled, i.e. patients are divided at random into two groups, half are given a placebo and half the active drug; the difference in response between the two groups gives a measure of the effectiveness of the drug. Often such trials are conducted in a double-blind fashion whereby neither the patients nor the investigator seeing the patients and measuring the effects of the drug know which patients are taking the drug and which the placebo; this avoids possible bias on the part of the investigator.

Comparison with other treatments. Where there is an effective treatment already in existence for the condition in question, it is inadequate simply to compare the new drug with placebo: rather it should be compared with the best current treatment.

The subjects of the trial. These should be appropriate. For example, if the drug for heart failure is to be used mainly in elderly patients, then it should be tested in such patients and not in younger patients.

The duration of the trial. The trial should be of an appropriate duration. For example, for antibiotics a few days may be appropriate, but for an antihypertensive, trials should be measured in months or years.

The trial should be analysed statistically. The statistical analysis of the trial is of vital importance and should be clearly established before the trial is performed. This needs to address questions such as the size of the trial (is it large enough?). How will the results be analysed? In looking at the results of a trial, we need to distinguish statistical significance from clinical significance: a statistically significant result may mean nothing in terms of benefit to patients.

The ethics of the trial should be considered. Trials should be designed so as to minimise any possible harm to the patients who participate. The patients should be made fully aware that they are participating in a trial and consent to this. To protect both patients and themselves, investigators should have the protocol considered by an expert ethical review committee.

Drug licensing

Drugs are licensed for sale according to the evidence presented to the licensing authority. In the UK, the licensing authority is the Secretary of State for Health, guided by the Medicines Control Agency and one of its committees, the Committee on the Safety of Medicines (CSM). Factors considered in the licensing process are the quality of the drug (is it well and safely manufactured?), its efficacy (does it work in the condition for which the licence is sought?) and its relative safety (is it as safe as the existing therapy, or if not, does its greater efficacy justify its greater toxicity? Note that the efficacy of the drug relative to existing drugs is not considered. The CSM is also responsible for monitoring reports of adverse drug reactions and reviewing new knowledge that may allow an extension or a reduction in the terms of the licence of a drug, or even its withdrawal. Many of the current roles of the national licensing authority may in future be taken up by a single agency for the European Community.

22.3 Prescribing new drugs

The true role of any new drug in therapeutics is often unclear at first and may only become apparent with time. Comparative data with existing drugs are often inadequate. Very few new drugs are true innovative advances, and the majority are minor variations on existing drugs ('me-too' drugs). In general, doctors should prescribe new drugs only when they are sure that the new drug is an improvement on existing therapy, in terms of efficacy, safety or cost, and never simply because they are new. New drugs should be prescribed with particular caution and any adverse effect reported to the CSM.

Where do doctors get their information about new drugs?

Many of the most commonly used drugs today were not available at the time that many doctors were medical students. Doctors must, therefore, keep up to date in pharmacology and therapeutics, since existing knowledge may rapidly become obsolete. The most common source of information about new drugs for doctors are the pharmaceutical companies and their representatives; however, doctors must be aware that companies aim to sell their products and that the information they supply may therefore be biased. Doctors should be capable of critically reviewing the evidence presented and should use independent evaluations of new drugs, such as those in the Drugs and Therapeutics Bulletin or in peer-reviewed journals.

Other sources of information about drugs in general and not just new drugs include:

The British National Formulary (BNF), which is updated every 6 months and distributed free to doctors. It lists drugs by their therapeutic uses and provides information on indications for the drugs, formulations and doses, and adverse effects. It also has useful sections on prescribing in general, prescription writing, drugs in the elderly and in children, and in renal and liver disease, as well as drug interactions. It is a most valuable source and prescribing doctors should always carry one and refer to it regularly.

Drug information services are pharmacist operated and sited in regional health authorities. They are available for consultation by letter or telephone (telephone numbers are in the BNF). Many produce local drug information bulletins.

Drug data sheets. A further source is the pharmaceutical industry, which produces drug data sheets and extensive material, some of which is more promotional than informational.

Marketing

Drug companies survive by selling their product, and must make a profit both to fund further research on new products and to remain in business. Companies, therefore, spend large amounts — at least £250 million a year in the UK — promoting their products to doctors, but the enthusiasm of a company for its products sometimes exceeds the critical opinion of an independent reviewer of the value. Doctors should, therefore, exercise particular care in considering promotional material and always seek independent evidence.

Prescribing

Prescribing may be defined as the practical everyday use of drugs. It is, therefore, based on the clinical pharmacology of a drug but also includes factors such as the diagnosis, the patient's previous medical history, as well as other sociological and medical factors. Doctors often prescribe for reasons other than the pharmacological effects of the drug, although this might be deplored: other reasons include the placebo effect, meeting patient demand, maintaining the vital relationship with the patient or even terminating the consultation. Prescribing for these reasons may be wasteful and harmful to the patient.

Good prescribing is:

- appropriate (is a drug needed at all?)
- effective and safe (given the diagnosis and consideration of patient factors, which drug is best?)
- cost effective (takes due account of the costs of drugs: where efficacy and safety are equal then the least expensive drug is the most appropriate; however, more expensive drugs may be justified for a better effect or because they are safer. Doctors should bear in mind that money spent unnecessarily on inappropriate drugs is wasted and deprives other patients of essential care).

Doctors must consider all prescribing as an experiment, in which the outcome may be beneficial or harmful to the patient. In each case, the risks and benefits must be weighed and a drug administered only if the expected benefits outweigh the risks.

How to be a good prescriber

- Stay up to date with information from independent sources
- No one can know all about the 5000 preparations in the BNF. Use a limited range of drugs with which you are familiar. Most doctors do 70–80% of their prescribing from a personal formulary of about 50 drugs. Drugs should be added to or subtracted from this only after careful consideration and review of evidence. Most hospitals have written formularies for their staff to use, and increasingly GPs are developing their own formularies as a useful way to rationalise drug therapy
- Prescriptions should be written with the generic name of the drug and not its proprietary name where possible
- Prescribing should be reviewed regularly, and unnecessary drugs stopped; communication between doctors in hospitals and in general practice is particularly important
- If in any doubt about dose or any other details of a drug, look it up in the BNF or other appropriate resource; be especially careful when prescribing new or unfamiliar drugs
- Individualise prescriptions: consider the patient, the disease, the choice of drug and formulation, the dose, other possible interacting diseases or drugs (including drugs which a patient might buy themselves over the counter without prescription). Consider also patient convenience, keep drug therapy as simple as possible to minimise interactions and adverse effects
- Educate the patient. Drugs may not be the most appropriate way of managing a problem. The patient should know what they have been prescribed and why, how they are to use the medication, and for how long, and what the possible adverse effects are.

In long-term treatment, patients on average take only about 60–70% of prescribed drugs: this is particularly so when patients are unsure of points mentioned above, or when the drug regimen is complex. Both of these may represent failure on the part of the doctor.

Self-assessment: questions

Multiple choice questions

1. The following statements are correct:
   a. Phase I trials involve large numbers of patients
   b. Phase IV trials are completed before a drug is marketed
   c. Drug licensing considers efficacy, safety and cost
   d. New drugs are superior to older drugs and so should be widely prescribed
   e. New drugs may be designed for effect at specific receptors

2. Trials:
   a. That are double blind means that neither the doctor nor the patient know what drug the patient is taking at a particular time
   b. That are placebo controlled are appropriate to show that a new drug is more effective than existing therapy
   c. Should be reviewed by an ethics committee before being undertaken
   d. Results that come from several small but similar trials are inevitably more reliable than the results of a single large trial
   e. Analysed statistically can prove that a new drug is effective

3. The following statements are correct:
   a. The BNF contains up to date information about drugs, doses and formulations
   b. 'Me-too' drugs generally have little advantage over existing drugs
   c. Comparative data on efficiency between new and existing drugs is essential before a new drug gets a licence
   d. All prescribing is an experiment
   e. Drugs should be prescribed by brand name

4. A good prescriber:
   a. Stays up to date
   b. Usually prescribes new drugs
   c. Uses a wide range of drugs to treat all conditions
   d. Never looks anything up
   e. Communicates well with colleagues and patients

Self-assessment: answers

Multiple choice answers

1. a. **False.** Usually involve normal subjects or small numbers of patients if the drug were considered too toxic to give to normal subjects, e.g. anti-cancer agents.
   b. **False.** These are postmarketing surveillance studies.
   c. **False.** Cost may not be considered by law.
   d. **False.** Despite what drug company advertising might have you believe.
   e. **True.** For example, sumatriptan as a serotonin analogue.

2. a. **True.** It is usually possible to break a code to find out what the patient is taking in case of emergency.
   b. **False.** The comparison should be against the best existing therapy (although this is often not the case in advertising).
   c. **True.** To protect both the patient and the investigator.
   d. **False.** Many trials are too small to show a genuine significant clinical effect: a single trial of adequate size is generally superior.
   e. **False.** Statistics can only give a probability, never certainty, especially at commonly used levels of significance such as $P < 0.05$. Statistical significance is also not the same as clinical significance.

3. a. **True.** The best available source and should be carried by all prescribing doctors.
   b. **True.** Again, a drug company may not like to admit this and will go to great lengths to demonstrate a minor or supposed advantage as a selling point.
   c. **False.**
   d. **True.** An important attitude for safe prescribing.
   e. **False.** There are, however, exceptions such as some fixed drug combinations of slow release preparations.

4. a. **True.** Using reliable independent sources.
   b. **False.** A good prescriber will use new drugs where appropriate, i.e. where there is evidence of a clear therapeutic or other advantage.
   c. **False.** In general, good prescribers will work from a formulary of drugs (written or not) of drugs with which he is familiar.
   d. **False.** This attitude smacks of arrogance.
   e. **True.** An essential component.

Index

Penicillins, 133–4, 139Q/141A
  blood–brain barrier in meningitis
    crossed by, 186
Pentamidine, 147
Peptic ulcer, 106–8, 112Q/113A
Pergolide, 64
Pethidine, 74
Petit mal, 58
pH
  tissue, local anaesthetics and, 186
  urinary, manipulation in overdose
    cases, 164
Phaeochromocytoma, 188
Pharmacodynamics, 9–12, 13Q/14A
  altered
    children, 180
    diseases, 187
    elderly, 180
    interactions resulting in, 193
Pharmacokinetics, 4–9, 13Q/14A
  altered
    children, 179
    diseases, 186–7
    elderly, 180
    interactions resulting in, 193
    pregnant women, 178
  parameters, 8–9
Phase 1 drug metabolism, 7
Phase 1 trials, 198
Phase 2 drug metabolism, 7
Phase 2 trials, 198
Phase 3 trials, 198
Phase 4 trials (premarketing), 192, 198
Phenobarbitone, 60
Phenothiazine, 109
Phenoxymethylpenicillin, 133
Phenytoin, 58, 67Q/70A
  disease state affecting response to,
    68Q/71A, 186, 188Q/189A
Phosphodiesterase inhibitors, 98
Physostigmine, 83
Pilocarpine, 19
Pirenzipine, 20
  peptic ulcer disease, 107
Pituitary hormones, 124–5
Pizotifen, 65
Placebos in trials, 198–9
Plasma proteins, *see* Proteins
Plasminogen activator (alteplase), 44
Platelets
  disorders, in anticancer therapy, 152
  inhibitors, 43, 88
Pneumocystis carinii, 147
Poisoning, *see* Toxicity
Postganglionic neurotransmitters in
    autonomic nervous system, 18
Postmenopausal HRT, 121–2, 126Q/129A,
    127Q/130A
Potassium iodide, 123
Potassium-sparing diuretics, cardiac
    failure, 30
Potency, agonist, 11
Prednisolone, 118, 126Q/129A
Preganglionic neurotransmitters in
    autonomic nervous system, 18
Pregnancy, 178–9
  chronic conditions in, 58, 178–9
  drugs in, 178–9, 182Q/183A
    contraindicated, 139, 179
  termination, 122
Premarketing (phase 4) tests, 192, 198
Prescribing, 177–83
  antibiotics, 132
  good, 200, 201Q/202A
  new drugs, 199–200
  pregnancy/children/elderly, 177–83
Probenecid, 91, 93A
Prochlorperazine, 70A
Procyclidine, 64

Progestogen–oestrogen (combined) pill,
    120–1, 125–6Q/128–9A, 126Q/
    129–30A
Progestogen-only pill, 121
Propantheline, 110
Propofol, 82
Propranolol, 27
Prostaglandin analogues, peptic ulcer
    disease, 107–8
Prostaglandin synthase inhibition,
    88
Protamine, 42
Proteins, *see also* Enzymes
  plasma, binding to, 5
    in diseased states, 71A, 186, 188Q/
    189A
  structural, drugs targeting, 11
Proton pump inhibitors, 107
Protozoal infections, 148–9
Pseudocholinesterase, *see* Butyryl
    cholinesterase
Pseudomembranous colitis, 135, 142A
Psoralen and UV, 158
Psoriasis, 158
Psychotropic drugs
  abuse, 172, 173–4
  therapeutic, 56–7, 60–3
Pulmonary disorders, *see* Respiratory tract
    and specific disorders
Purgatives, stimulant, 110
Purine analogues as antivirals, 144, 145
PUVA (psoralen and UV light), 158
Pyrazinamide, 138
Pyrexia, 76
Pyridostigmine, 83
Pyrimethamine, 147
Pyrimidine analogues as antivirals, 144–5

Q
Quinidine, 33
Quinine, 146
Quinolones, 135–6

R
Radioactive iodine, 123
Ranitidine, 107
Reabsorption of drugs, renal tubular, 8
Receptors (for drugs), 10, 13Q/14A, *see
    also specific receptors*
  autonomic nervous system, 18–19
  number, individual variations in, 12
Reflux, gastro-oesophageal, 108, 112Q/
    112–13A, 112Q/113A
Renal system, *see* Kidney
Renin, cardiac failure and, 28
Repolarisation, cardiac cell, 32, 33
  inhibitors, 33
Reproductive system, 120–2, 125–6Q/
    128–9A, 126–7Q/129–30A
Respiratory failure, 99
Respiratory stimulants, 99
Respiratory syncytial virus, 145
Respiratory tract (lower) disorders, 96–9,
    101Q/102A
  infections, 137, 145
Response/effect, drug
  disease state affecting, *see* Disease state
  dose and, relationship between, 11–12
  individual variations in, 4, 12
Retinoids (vitamin A derivatives), 159
Rheumatoid arthritis, 88, 89–90, 92Q/93A
Rhinitis, seasonal, 99, 100–1
Ribavarin, 145
Rifampicin, 138
RSV, 145

S
Salbutamol, 21, 97, 101Q/102A
  as bronchodilators, 97, 101Q/102A

Salicylate, *see* 5-Aminosalicylic acid;
    Aspirin
Salmeterol, 97
Schizophrenia, 62–3, 68Q/70A
Sedation as adverse effects of H₁
    antagonists, 100
Sedatives (anxiolytics; hypnotics; minor
    tranquillisers), 56–7, 67Q/69A,
    67Q/70A, 172–3
  abuse, 172–3
Seizures (in epilepsy), 57–60, 67Q/69A,
    67Q/70A, 68Q/71A, 182Q/182A
  complex partial, 58, 68Q/71A
  drug-induced, 164
  drug therapy, *see* Anti-epileptics
  non-pharmacological techniques, 57
  in pregnancy, 178
  types, 58
Selegiline, 64
Serotonin, *see* 5-Hydroxytryptamine
Sertraline, 61
Serum sickness, 100
Sex hormones, 120–2, 125–6Q/128–9A,
    126–7Q/129–30A
Shingles (zoster), 144, 145, 148Q/149A
Shock, cardiogenic, 21
Short questions, dealing with, 2
Side-effects, *see* Adverse reactions
Simvastatin, 51, 52Q/53A
Skeletal muscle relaxants, 82–3, 84Q/85A,
    85A
Skin, 157–61
  allergies, 99
  fungal infections, 146
Sleep
  drugs adversely affecting, 56–7
  drugs aiding, 56–7
Sodium bicarbonate, 106
Sodium cromoglycate, 97, 101Q/102A
Sodium nitroprusside in hypertensive
    emergencies, 35
Sodium valproate, 58, 59–60, 67Q/69A
Solvent abuse, 174
Somatropin, 124
Spasm, gut, inhibitors, 110
Spironolactone, cardiac failure, 30
Status asthmaticus (acute severe asthma),
    96, 97, 98
Status epilepticus, 68Q/71A
Steroids, *see* Glucocorticoids; Mineralo-
    corticoids; Sex hormones
Stimulant purgatives, 110
Stomach, *see entries under* Gastric
Stones, biliary, 111
Streptokinase, 44
Streptomycin, 134
Stroke risk with oestrogens, 121
Succinylcholine, 83, 84Q/85A
Sulphamethoxazole–trimethoprim, *see*
    Co-trimoxazole
Sulphasalazine
  inflammatory bowel disease, 110
  rheumatoid arthritis, 90
Sulphinpyrazone, 91, 93A, 188Q/189A
Sulphonamides, 135, 139Q/141A
Sulphonylureas, 117
Sumatriptan, 65
Surface area and drug absorption, 4
Suxamethonium (succinylcholine), 83,
    84Q/85A
Sympathetic nervous system, 18
Sympathomimetics (adrenoceptor
    agonists), *see* Adrenoceptor
Systemic lupus erythematosus, 99

T
Tamoxifen, 122
Tardive dyskinesia, 70A
Targets for drugs, 10

Teicoplanin, 137
Temazepam, 56
Temporal lobe epilepsy, 58, 68Q/71A
Teratogens, 178
  anti-epileptics, 59
Terbutaline, 97
Terfenadine, 100
Terminal care in cancer, 152
Testing, *see* Trials
Testosterone, 122
Tetracosactrin, 118–19
Tetracyclines, 136, 139Q/141A
Theophyllines, 98
  cautions in liver disease, 186
Therapeutic window, 12
Thiazides (and related drugs)
  cardiac failure, 29–30
  hypertension, 34
Thiopentone, 82, 85A
Thiouracils, 123
Thrombocytopenia in anticancer therapy,
    152
Thromboembolic disease risk, oestrogens,
    121
Thrombolytics, 43–4, 46Q/47A
Thrombosis, 42–4, 46Q/47A
Thyroid crisis, 123–4
Thyroid disease, 122–4, 125Q/128A,
    126Q/129A
  pregnancy, 179
L-Thyroxine, 124
Time spent at absorption site, 4–5
Tissue, drug distribution in, 5–6
  disease affecting, 186
  volume of, apparent, 6
Tissue plasminogen activator (alteplase),
    44
Tobramycin, 134
Tolbutamide, 117
Tolerance, 172
  definition, 172
  receptor numbers and, 12
  sedatives, 56
Tonic/clonic seizures, 58
Toxaemia of pregnancy, 179

Toxicity/poisoning, 163–9, *see also*
    Adverse reactions
  digoxin, 32
  paracetamol, 78, 164–5, 167Q/168A
  tricyclic antidepressants, 61, 165–6,
    167Q/168A
  other drugs, 164–9
Toxoplasmosis, 147
Tranquillisers
  major (neuroleptics), 62–3, 68Q/70A
  minor, *see* Sedatives
Transformation, *see* Biotransformation
Transmembrane receptors, 10
Transport mechanisms, drugs targeting, 11
Tranylcypromine, 62
Tretinoin, 159
Trials (testing), clinical, 198–200, 201Q/
    202A
  design, 198–9
  phase 1–3, 198
  phase 4 (premarketing), 192, 198
Triamterene, cardiac failure, 30
Tricyclic antidepressants, 60–1, 67Q/69A,
    71A, 165–6
  migraine, 66
  overdose, 61, 165–6, 167Q/168A
Trimethoprim, 135
  sulphamethoxazole and, *see* Co-
    trimoxazole
Trisilicate, magnesium, 106
Tuberculosis, 136–7, 139Q/142A
Tubocurarine, 82
Tubules, renal
  reabsorption of drugs, 8
  secretion of drugs, 8
Tumours, *see* Cancer *and specific tumours*

U

Ulcer, peptic, 106–8, 112Q/113A
Ulcerative colitis, 110
Ultraviolet light and psoralen, 158
Uricosurics, 90–1, 93A
Urinary pH manipulation in overdose
    cases, 164

Urinary tract infection, women, 140Q/
    142A, 179
Uterus
  bleeding (dysfunctional), 122
  general anaesthetic effects, 82
UV light and psoralen, 158

V

Valproate, 58, 59–60, 67Q/69A
Vancomycin, 137
Vasculitis, 100
Vasopressin (ADH), 124
Vecuronium, 83
Venous thromboembolic disease risk,
    oestrogens, 121
Verapamil, 28
Vidarabine, 145
Vigabatrin, 60
Vinca alkaloids, 154, 156A
Viral infections, 144–6
Vitamin A derivatives, 159
Vitamin B_{12} deficiency, 44
Vitamin D, 124, 125Q/128A
  deficiency, 124
Vivas, 2
Volume of distribution, *see* Distribution
Vomiting, 108–9
  ipecac-induced, 164
  levodopa-induced, 63
  prevention, 109

W

Warfarin, 42
  interactions, 43, 89
  in liver disease, cautions, 187
Withdrawal, alcohol, 56, 172

X

Xanthine oxidase inhibitors, 91, 93A

Z

Zidovudine, 144–5
Zopiclone, 57
Zoster, 144, 145, 148Q/149A